THE FIRST RESORT

THE FIRST RESORT

THE HISTORY OF SOCIAL PSYCHIATRY IN THE UNITED STATES

MATTHEW SMITH

Columbia University Press   *New York*

Columbia University Press
Publishers Since 1893
New York   Chichester, West Sussex
cup.columbia.edu

Library of Congress Cataloging-in-Publication Data
Names: Smith, Matthew, 1973– author.
Title: The first resort : the history of social psychiatry in the United States /
Matthew Smith.
Description: New York : Columbia University Press, [2022] | Includes
bibliographical references and index.
Identifiers: LCCN 2022027575 (print) | LCCN 2022027576 (ebook) |
ISBN 9780231203920 (hardcover) | ISBN 9780231203937 (trade paperback) |
ISBN 9780231555289 (ebook)
Subjects: LCSH: Social psychiatry—United States—History—20th century. |
Mental illness—United States—History—20th century. | Mental health
services—United States—History—20th century. | Psychiatric hospital
care—United States—History—20th century.
Classification: LCC RC455 .S594 2022 (print) | LCC RC455 (ebook) |
DDC 362.20973—dc23/eng/20220802
LC record available at https://lccn.loc.gov/2022027575
LC ebook record available at https://lccn.loc.gov/2022027576

Columbia University Press books are printed on permanent
and durable acid-free paper.

Printed and bound by CPI Group (UK) Ltd, Croydon, CR0 4YY

Cover design: Milenda Nan Ok Lee
Cover photo: H. Armstrong Roberts / ClassicStock / Alamy

*To Dashiell and Solveigh and the hope for a kinder world.
And to Gordon Laxer, who taught me that such a
world is possible.*

CONTENTS

CONTENTS

ABBREVIATIONS

AECM	Albert Einstein College of Medicine
AJP	*American Journal of Psychiatry*
AJS	*American Journal of Sociology*
APA	American Psychiatric Association
ASA	American Sociological Association
ASS	American Sociological Society
BMHC	Bristol Mental Health Centre
CMHC	Community Mental Health Center
DSM	*Diagnostic and Statistical Manual of Mental Disorders*
EFO	Ethnic Family Operation
GAP	Group for the Advancement of Psychiatry
IHR	Institute of Human Relations
IJR	Institute for Juvenile Research
ISHL	Illinois Social Hygiene League
JCMHC	Joint Commission on the Mental Health of Children
JCMIH	Joint Commission on Mental Illness and Health
LHMHS	Lincoln Hospital Mental Health Service
MHM	*Mental Health in the Metropolis: The Midtown Manhattan Study*
NCMH	National Committee for Mental Hygiene
NIMH	National Institute of Mental Health

OIA   Office of Indian Affairs
PCMH   President's Commission on Mental Health
SES   Socioeconomic Status
UBI   Universal Basic Income
WHO   World Health Organization
YSMMHH   Yale School of Medicine Mental Hygiene Center

THE FIRST RESORT

INTRODUCTION

The Magic Years

A preventive psychiatry.
—Thomas A. C. Rennie, 1955

I n the archives of the American Psychiatric Association (APA), there exists a dusty old box with a fascinating secret. Inside is an unfinished manuscript called *The Magic Years: The History of Psychiatry, Mental Health, and Mental Retardation, 1945–1970*, written by Daniel Blain (1898–1981), who served as medical director of the APA from 1948 to 1958 and APA president in 1964.[1] Born in China to missionaries, Blain was "rich in family heritage, but poor in finances." He made up for his financial shortcomings by marrying Sarah Logan Wister Starr (1903–1979), a member of a wealthy and longstanding Philadelphia family.[2] Living at the 104-acre Belfield Estate, Blain and Sarah became paragons of Philadelphia society.

The Magic Years cast postwar psychiatry in a warm, rosy glow, describing how, between 1945 and 1970, the field had "moved ahead as never before."[3] Psychiatric knowledge had progressed rapidly, more treatments were available, funding for research had increased enormously, and public and political awareness of mental illness had grown by leaps and bounds. This new psychiatric optimism fomented federal legislation such as the Community Mental Health Act of 1963, which led to the construction of hundreds of community mental health centers (CMHCs) across the United States. Intended to replace the old, crumbling, and often inhumane state hospitals where over half a million Americans were institutionalized, CMHCs were also meant to play a major role in the prevention of mental illness.[4]

These advancements, Blain declared, could stand beside achievements in space travel, organ transplantation, and open-heart surgery. No longer perceiving themselves as the "Cinderellas of medicine and public health," American psychiatrists approached the late 1960s

> with great expectations, increased manpower, strong departments of psychiatry in virtually every medical school, with many of the best senior students going into psychiatry. There is strong financial backing in the Congress . . . increased training in non-professional areas, the relief of pressure on hospitalization, and movement towards less expensive treatment for ambulatory patients . . . a generally encouraging picture over the whole range of psychiatric treatment services.[5]

These developments were possible, Blain explained, because "science and society were undergoing equally dramatic and important changes, perhaps the most concentrated and exciting in the entire history of the world."[6] Psychiatry's insights into the human condition meant that it could help society adapt to these developments. Here, Blain echoed the views of his contemporary, the psychiatrist, administrator, and founder of the Group for the Advancement of Psychiatry (GAP) William Menninger (1899–1966), who argued that psychiatry should be involved in addressing race relations, unemployment, housing shortages, and even foreign policy.[7] For Blain, psychiatry provided "liberal social reformers the weight of medical and scientific opinion to accompany the moral and pragmatic imperatives for progressive change."[8] For psychiatry, these were magic years indeed.

The foundation for Blain's optimism was social psychiatry, an interdisciplinary approach to understanding mental health and illness that combined the insights of the social sciences with those of psychiatry.[9] Emerging partly from the early twentieth century's mental hygiene and child guidance movements[10] and also from the experience of World War II,[11] social psychiatrists studied the epidemiology of mental illness, in particular the socioeconomic factors believed to cause or exacerbate it. After World War II, social psychiatry had significant political influence both within and beyond psychiatry. Most APA presidents during this period were either self-described social psychiatrists or supported social psychiatry. The National Institute of Mental Health (NIMH), founded in 1949, funded a great deal of social psychiatry research during its first two decades. Moreover, social psychiatry convinced many psychiatrists, policy makers, and politicians that it was possible to not only *treat* mental illness in the community but also *prevent* it through progressive social policies. Social psychiatry was a "preventive psychiatry."[12] It gave American psychiatrists—temporarily at least—confidence and a sense of prestige and importance that they had rarely enjoyed.[13] It is social psychiatry and its promise to facilitate the prevention of mental illness in the United States that is the subject of this book.

A VANISHING ACT

Sadly, Blain's magnum opus was never published. Despite being supported by a multiyear National Library of Medicine grant, which paid for—among other things—the assistance of the PhD student Michael Barton (now professor emeritus at Penn State Harrisburg), *The Magic Years* remained incomplete when Blain died in 1981.[14] Notwithstanding Barton's considerable help and support (which included living at Belfield Estate to facilitate Blain's research), Blain had no experience in writing history, and his hope for a rich, contextualized, and comprehensive history proved to be too ambitious.[15] By the time Barton found a tenure-track position, the health of Blain's wife, Sarah, was failing, and, ultimately, the project culminated in a box of incomplete drafts and a five-page article in *Hospital and Community Psychiatry*, a mere fragment of the original project.[16] *The Magic Years* was forgotten, along with social psychiatry.

In contrast to Blain, the history of psychiatry—and its historians—has been unkind to the decades that he regarded so fondly. Far from establishing the foundation for a socially responsible, preventative, and population-based psychiatry, Blain's magic years were swept aside in the wake of another psychiatric revolution, one that had paralleled and even facilitated the changes he lauded: psychopharmacology.[17] Although Blain described the postwar period as being the time when psychoanalysis finally came of age in the United States, by the 1970s it was already being replaced by biological explanations for mental illness and pharmaceutical treatments. In 1973, for example, when Blain was still toiling away on *The Magic Years*, the APA decided to replace the psychoanalytically based second edition of the *Diagnostic and Statistical Manual of Mental Disorders* (*DSM-II*), published in 1968, with a radically different third edition. *DSM-III* (1980) was grounded in biological psychiatry and succeeded in rooting out any semblance of psychoanalytic theory.

Concurrently, psychiatry's shift from the asylum to the community was beginning to be questioned as funding for CMHCs dried up and the promise of prevention was overshadowed by the need to treat those already ill. The cumbersome term *deinstitutionalization*, which described how psychiatric care was shifting from residential institutions to the community, was soon joined by the equally clumsy *transinstitutionalization*, denoting the transition of mental patients from the hospital system to the criminal justice system and other institutional settings.[18] Writing amid the rise of the antipsychiatry, radical psychiatry, and psychiatric survivors' movements, Blain also overlooked many arguments articulated during the postwar period that indicated that many people were not satisfied with American psychiatry, not least those with mental health problems.

As psychiatry's path veered away from the trajectory envisioned by Blain, so too have historians diverged from his assessment. No one has gone further in this respect than the psychiatrist and sometime historian E. Fuller Torrey, whose 2013 book *American Psychosis: How the Federal Government Destroyed the Mental Illness Treatment System* depicts the postwar period in almost polar opposite terms. Torrey, whose career in psychiatry, including six years at NIMH during the early 1970s, began essentially when Blain's story finished, describes his account of the period as "a cautionary tale" and frames his interpretation as a story from which lessons can and should be learned. For Torrey, the postwar emphasis on prevention, "the ultimate goal of psychiatry" for early NIMH directors Robert H. Felix (1904–1990), Stanley F. Yolles (1919–2001), and Bertram S. Brown (1931–2020), was chimerical. Focusing resources "on prevention when nobody understood enough about mental illnesses to know how to prevent them," American mental health policy of the postwar period rested on nonexistent foundations and fatally undermined the state hospital system. The false promise of prevention resulted in a federal program that "effectively lobotomized both the existing and the emerging state mental health programs," "failing tragically," and becoming "an ongoing disaster" that precipitated the problems of "the current, chaotic mental health system."[19]

The late Gerald Grob (1931–2015), arguably the most authoritative voice on the history of American psychiatry, also condemned post–World War II mental health policy, contending that the focus on community mental health severed the link between care and treatment, which had been present previously in asylums. CMHCs and the expansion of psychiatric services in general hospitals might have increased the capacity for treating patients in acute need, but "the social and human needs" for chronic patients that asylums had provided "were often ignored or overlooked."[20] Without this basic care being provided by asylums, many people with serious mental health problems became homeless, a problem that continues today.[21] Addressing social psychiatry specifically, Grob concluded in his 1998 presidential address to the American Association for the History of Medicine that its proponents "embodied a touching if naïve faith that the specialty [psychiatry] had an important role in resolving pressing social and economic problems."[22]

Other historians have focused on different problems that emerged in postwar psychiatry, with race looming large. Whereas Dennis Doyle and Gabriel Mendes (both examining Harlem) have described antiracist attempts to provide mental health services to Black Americans, Mical Raz and Jonathan Metzl have argued that racist stereotypes contributed to the pathologization of Black families and the overdiagnosis of Black Americans with schizophrenia.[23] Martin Summers's recent book on St. Elizabeth's Hospital in Washington, DC, is also a vital contribution to the history of race and psychiatry in the United States, demonstrating that while race imbued all activities at the hospital,

Black patients and their families also exerted agency in their relations with it.[24] None of these studies, however, have focused in particular on social psychiatry.

Outside of the United States, the history of social psychiatry has been discussed occasionally, though the definition of the term has varied across time and place.[25] Focusing on Germany, Heinz-Peter Schmiedebach and Stephan Priebe trace the term "*soziale Psychiatrie*" to a 1903 article by Georg Ilberg, then based at an asylum in Saxony.[26] Ilberg listed a range of factors believed to trigger mental illness, the most important being heredity, syphilis, and alcoholism, and argued that eugenics could be used to prevent such cases. Such ideas would soon be taken up enthusiastically in Germany. Ilberg also claimed, however, that people who were ill suited to their vocation were also susceptible to such problems. While the term was dropped during the first decades following World War II (when it became prominent in the United States), it became popular among reform-minded psychiatrists during the 1960s and 1970s. One example of this was the psychiatrist Karl Peter Kisker, who applied the term to the treatment of psychiatric patients, rather than the prevention of mental illness.[27] Despo Kritsotaki has also explored how the links between welfare reform and social psychiatry influenced mental health approaches in Greece during the 1950s and 1960s.[28] Finally, Harry Wu has examined how some of the epidemiological aspects of social psychiatry shaped the World Health Organization's (WHO) mental health initiatives after World War II.[29]

For the most part, however, social psychiatry, and especially its preventive dimension, has been ignored by many historians and forgotten by many mental health professionals. This is especially the case in the United States, where the most pioneering social psychiatry research was carried out and where it enjoyed the most political influence. One striking example of this can be found in Edward Shorter's *A Historical Dictionary of Psychiatry*, which lacks an entry for "social psychiatry."[30] Although there are a handful of articles and sections of books that have touched on aspects of social psychiatry in the United States, it has lacked a comprehensive history.[31]

SOCIAL PSYCHIATRY: THEN AND NOW

This book addresses this omission. It tells the story of social psychiatry in the United States, charting its rise and fall during the mid-twentieth century and—crucially—analyzing the research that underpinned its preventive approach to mental health. I focus on the four most important social psychiatry research projects, all of which produced novel and continually relevant epidemiological findings. These include Robert E. L. Faris (1907–1998) and H. Warren Dunham's (1906–1985) study of Chicago psychiatric hospital admissions; August B. Hollingshead (1907–1980) and Frederick C. Redlich's (1910–2004) study of class and mental illness in New Haven, Connecticut; the Midtown Manhattan Study, founded by Thomas A. C. Rennie (1904–1956); and Dorothea Leighton (1908–1989) and Alexander Leighton's (1908–2007) Stirling County Study. Using archival material, published documents, and oral histories, I explore how these interdisciplinary studies emerged; what they discovered; how their findings were expressed; how they were received by psychiatrists, social scientists, policy makers, and politicians; and how they were applied to mental health policy and clinical practice.

What this history shows is that while the insights produced by social psychiatry regarding the relationship between mental health and socioeconomic factors were valuable and continue to be relevant, they were only partially applied. Also required in order to prevent mental illness was the reduction or elimination of poverty, inequality, social isolation, and community disintegration in the United States, which was not achieved during the Johnson administration's War on Poverty. Rather than dismissing social psychiatry as flawed, fanciful, or doomed to fail, therefore, we should learn from it and use its story to guide preventive approaches today. This means acknowledging that the prevention of mental illness—while undoubtedly complicated and multifaceted[32]—fundamentally requires progressive political change.

Just as Blain, Torrey, Grob, and others wrote their versions of postwar American psychiatry from a particular perspective, I am writing from mine. In recent years, the WHO has stated that depression, never mind other mental illnesses, is the leading cause of ill health and disability globally, affecting hundreds of millions of people.[33] In the United States, $186 billion was spent on mental health treatment in 2014, according to the Substance Abuse and Mental Health Services Administration.[34] This does not include the cost of lost productivity, estimated at $1 trillion globally.[35] U.S. suicide statistics similarly paint a disturbing picture, with the overall rate increasing in recent years, especially for young people.[36] While these figures have to be taken in the context of concerns about psychiatric overdiagnosis, on balance the evidence points to a deteriorating mental health situation in the United States and elsewhere, which is costing society dearly in financial, social, and emotional terms.[37]

And that was before 2020. The COVID-19 pandemic has increased concerns about mental illness even further. A global pandemic is worrying enough, but its economic and social repercussions have also taken their toll. Lockdown measures, though necessary, have left people isolated and lonely. This has been especially so for those with underlying health conditions who have had to shield themselves for longer than others. The pandemic's economic damage has also made people feel insecure, unsupported, and hopeless, making it likely that, just as during the Great Recession that began in 2007, rates of mental illness will increase.[38] Moreover, the burden of mental illness triggered by COVID-19 will be disproportionately borne by society's poor and disenfranchised, much like the virus's direct impact on physical health. This is because wealthier people have had more ways to escape the isolating effects of lockdown conditions and because they have the financial wherewithal to shield themselves against the economic impact of the pandemic. They also have access to a wider variety of therapies if they do suffer from mental illness.

Similarly, the specter of racial inequality highlighted by the death of George Floyd on May 25, 2020, and the resulting Black Lives Matter protests have also been articulated in terms of mental health. The "I Can't Breathe" slogan signifies not only the asphyxiation of dozens of Black Americans at the hands of police officers but also the relentless weight of racial oppression.[39] As the psychotherapist and author Lola Jaye recently expressed, racism can be experienced as "racial trauma," leading to "depression, hypervigilance, chronic stress and fatigue, bodily inflammation and symptoms similar to post traumatic stress disorder."[40] This is in addition to the fact that racial and ethnic minorities in the United States already "bear a greater burden from unmet mental health needs and thus suffer a greater loss to their overall health and productivity."[41]

In short, 2020 has added even more urgency to the need to prevent mental illness. But it has also presented an opportunity. The pandemic has forced many countries to develop novel economic initiatives to ensure that those made unemployed by COVID-19 continue to receive an income. Government spending for such programs has far exceeded what most economists and political scientists thought possible and has also established a precedent for investing public funds ambitiously in order to prevent even worse calamities from occurring. What if we thought in similar terms about mental health? If anything, the history of social psychiatry demonstrates that the solutions to our current mental health crisis will be anything but "magical." No flick of a wand will prevent mental illness. But innovative, evidence-based investment in addressing the entrenched socioeconomic problems that cause and exacerbate mental illness is a good first step.

OVERVIEW

The First Resort combines an overview of the rise and fall of social psychiatry in the United States in chapters 1 and 6 with case studies in chapters 2–5 of the most notable social psychiatry studies. These address Chicago, New Haven, New York City, and rural Nova Scotia. Other North American psychiatric epidemiology studies were conducted during the mid-twentieth century, but the four I highlight were the most significant in terms of priority, ambition, scope, methodological innovation, and variety of populations investigated. Bringing these four studies together, along with chapters that analyze the rise and fall of social psychiatry, provides a robust—if not completely comprehensive—account of how preventive mental health was envisioned, researched, and carried out in the United States during the middle of the twentieth century.

Before summarizing the book's chapters, however, it might be helpful to frame how I interpret the term *mental illness*. Throughout the book I concentrate on how the historical actors I investigate defined and understood mental illness, rather than impose my own views. Nevertheless, it is worth noting that, as with most historians of mental health and psychiatry during the last half-century, I see mental illness as a highly complex phenomenon that has changed across time and place and will continue to do so. The characteristics that demark an individual as mentally ill in one culture at a particular time in history would not necessarily be deemed pathological in another culture or at a different period in history. I also see mental illness as having a wide range of causes, many of which are poorly understood. Some mental illnesses, such as tertiary syphilis or pellagra-induced psychosis, have clear biological causes. Others are the result of trauma or periods of pronounced stress. Still other mental illnesses, such as ADHD and autism, are socially constructed to varying degrees, the result of changes in how society has defined what are "normal" behaviors or emotional responses. Because of these different causes, which may occur in combination, the degree to which and the ways in which specific mental illnesses can be prevented vary enormously. Putting all these complexities to one side, I have also written this book with the understanding that socioeconomic problems can have a profound effect on the incidence and experience of mental illnesses. In some cases, they may be the precipitating cause, and in others they may exacerbate symptoms, trigger relapses, and undermine recovery. In other words, regardless of how we choose to define mental illness, the social environment in which it is experienced should be central to our understanding of it.

Much like our understanding of mental health, social psychiatry did not emerge in a vacuum. It evolved out of earlier preventive mental health approaches, and its influence was dependent upon significant historical events, most notably the experience of American psychiatry during World War II. Chapter 1 begins by explaining how social psychiatry built on the mental hygiene and child guidance movements of the first half of the twentieth century. These, too, were preventive approaches to mental health that emphasized the role of socioeconomic factors. What differentiated social psychiatry, however, was its focus on interdisciplinary, epidemiological research involving the collaboration of social scientists and academic psychiatrists. The chapter proceeds, therefore, to explore how sociology, anthropology, and other social sciences turned to the investigation of mental health. Chapter 1 concludes by exploring the role of World War II in transforming psychiatry from a marginal medical discipline concerned mainly with running asylums to a major tool in the American war effort. Psychiatrists became convinced during the war that mental illness was far more common in American society than previously thought. They were able to convince politicians of the need to invest more in research into both the extent and the causes of mental illness in the United States, ultimately spurring the foundation of NIMH in 1949. These developments provided the context in which social psychiatry could grow and flourish.

Although World War II acted as a powerful catalyst for the flourishing of social psychiatry, research conducted before the war also helped pave the way for the major epidemiological studies that would follow in the 1950s. Chapter 2 shows how poverty and community disintegration began to be linked with mental health by exploring the first social psychiatry research project, conducted by the University of Chicago sociologists Robert Faris and Warren Dunham during the 1930s. Publishing their results in *Mental Disorders in Urban Areas: An Ecological Study of Schizophrenia and Other Psychoses*, Faris and Dunham helped establish the link between deprivation and mental illness and also convinced psychiatrists that social scientific research was an important tool in psychiatric epidemiology.[42]

Chapter 3 turns to the relationship between class and mental illness through the lens of one of the first social psychiatry projects to emerge after World War II. The Yale-based psychiatrist Frederick Redlich and sociologist August Hollingshead received funding from NIMH in 1950 to research the epidemiology of mental illness in New Haven, Connecticut, resulting in *Social Class and Mental Illness*.[43] The chapter then explores how issues of inequality inflected the development of community mental health during the 1960s and 1970s. It addresses how typically white, middle-class, male psychiatrists attempted to negotiate tensions relating to race, class, and gender in establishing CMHCs. While Hollingshead and Redlich demonstrated that class had a major bearing on both the rate of mental illness and how it was treated, psychiatrists were often unwilling to cede their authority to nonpsychiatrists within CMHCs. Chapter 3 demonstrates that social psychiatric research concerning inequality posed awkward questions for psychiatrists, who were at the top of the mental healthcare hierarchy and among the upper echelons of American society more generally.

Chapter 4 turns to how social psychiatrists investigated the relationship between urban environments and mental health by unpacking the complex story of the Midtown Manhattan Study. While many urban planners argued that inner slums were pathological and had to be replaced with more modern housing stock, some social psychiatrists questioned this. When the study's first volume, *Mental Health in the Metropolis*, was published in 1962, its headline finding, that under 20 percent of New Yorkers had good mental health, seemed to confirm that cities were indeed bad for mental health.[44] But the real message of the study was that mental illness was associated with poverty, social isolation, and inequality, which could be found in both urban and rural environments. Archival records relating to Midtown also reveal the difficulties involved in carrying out large, complex interdisciplinary social psychiatry projects. The large team of researchers often disagreed bitterly about the direction of the study and how to interpret its findings, ultimately undermining its potential impact. Chapter 4 reveals that while social psychiatrists might have been united about the need to prevent mental illness, they also debated vigorously about how to achieve this elusive ambition.

While most social psychiatry research projects studied cities, one of the largest, and certainly the longest, concentrated on the rural environment. This, the Stirling County Study, is the subject of chapter 5. Founded by Dorothea and Alexander Leighton in 1948, it focused on rural Nova Scotia, Canada.[45] In its first phase (roughly 1948–1963) it produced three weighty monographs, which described the nature of mental health in both English- and French-speaking (Acadian) communities and found that mental illness was more common in places that were more socially disintegrated.[46] Chapter 5 proceeds to explore how psychiatry attempted to address social disintegration via the community mental health center movement. CMHCs were not only intended to treat patients outside of the asylum system. They were also designed to be places where preventive mental health occurred. The chapter argues that while CMHCs did admirable work in providing treatment and helping to destigmatize mental illness, their preventive function was never fully realized.

Although the Community Mental Health Act of 1963 symbolizes how influential social psychiatry became during the postwar period, this influence was not to last. Chapter 6 addresses the fall of social psychiatry and its replacement by biological psychiatry. It examines the internal and external factors that contributed to this decline, suggesting that just as social psychiatry benefited from the political context of the 1950s and 1960s, biological psychiatry would benefit from both scientific and political changes in the decades that followed. By the 1990s, social psychiatry—and its focus on prevention—was forgotten.

The epilogue applies the history of social psychiatry to today's fight against mental illness. In recent years, there has been more interest in understanding the social determinants of mental health, with a view toward prevention. I argue that there is little need for more epidemiological research on the relationship between socioeconomic factors and mental health. What is needed, however, is research—and action—on how to translate existing epidemiological evidence into preventive mental health policies. I conclude by suggesting that universal basic income might be just such a policy. UBI is a guaranteed income that is provided by the state to every individual without question or qualification at a level sufficient to take them out of poverty. UBI has risen in popularity during the COVID-19 pandemic, with many governments introducing relief schemes that bear resemblance to it. In addition to transforming how welfare is conceptualized and managed, UBI has the potential to alleviate many of the factors that social psychiatrists blamed for mental illness, including poverty, inequality, and social disintegration. I conclude by demonstrating how UBI, by reducing socioeconomic deprivation and restoring trust in the capacity of individuals to contribute to society, could be the core of a new, preventive public health policy fit for the challenges of the twenty-first century.

1

THE ORIGINS OF
SOCIAL PSYCHIATRY

Causes for Admittance to Oregon State Insane Asylum, 1906
—Oregon State Hospital Museum Display Board

> *Brain Softening*
> *Childbed Fever*
> *Christian Science*
> *Disappointment in Love*
> *General Disability*
> *Idiocy*
> *Lead Poisoning*
> *Masturbation*
> *Menopause*
> *Nervous Prostration*
> *Overstudy*
> *Puerperal Trouble*
> *Removal of Ovaries*
> *Spiritualism*
> *Suppressed Eruption*
> *Tobacco*
> *Worry*

—Willa Schneberg, found poem

I n 1955, Thomas Rennie published "Social Psychiatry—a Definition" in the inaugural issue of the *International Journal of Social Psychiatry*.[1] The term "social psychiatry" had been used in the United States for nearly forty years by the time of Rennie's article, but its meaning had varied. Foreshadowing Rennie, the psychiatrist E. E. Southard (1876–1920) provided the first English-language definition of "social psychiatry" in the first issue of *Mental Hygiene* in 1917. Southard defined it as "a conjugation of social and psychiatric concepts," with the "social" aspects pertaining to "social service investigations and care." He added portentously, but without elaborating, that "it may well be claimed that a good portion of [social psychiatry] is nothing but a pious wish."[2] For Southard and many others before World War II, social psychiatry effectively meant psychiatric social work.[3]

Rennie's definition was more ambitious. At the time, he was directing the Midtown Manhattan Study and had recently been named the first professor of social psychiatry in the United States, a position he held at Cornell University Medical College (see chapter 4). Rennie described how psychiatrists had become "deeply impelled to turn their interest outward from the individual patient to the family, the community, and the whole cultural scene." Despite the fact that he was a psychoanalyst himself, Rennie argued that psychiatrists had been "too one-sidedly preoccupied with the search for dynamics as revealed by the intensive and 'microscopic' study of the intra-psychic dynamics of the person." Although this focus had resulted in "psychiatry taking great strides forward," these advances were "gained at the expense of a relative neglect of . . . family dynamics and of the cultural *milieu* from which the patient came." A shift was required toward examining the relationship between the broader social environment and mental health in order to develop "preventive psychiatry."[4]

The shift Rennie depicted reflected a growing awareness that if psychiatry was "to move into a vigorous period of real preventive work . . . it must begin to look beyond the individual to the forces within the social environment which contribute to the personal dilemma." To do so required the establishment of "a working relationship between the social scientist and the psychiatrist."[5] For Rennie, social psychiatry consisted of this marriage between psychiatry and the social sciences in the quest to understand the complex social environment of the patient and, ultimately, determine how best to prevent mental illness.

Although Rennie asserted *that* a need for social psychiatry had arisen, he spent little time explaining *why* or *how* it had arisen. What had led to this shift in American psychiatry, from a marginalized medical discipline that was either preoccupied with treating individual patients in asylums or in private—typically psychoanalytic—practice to one that was concerned with "the whole social framework of contemporary living"? In this chapter, I address this question, tracing the origins of social psychiatry before 1945. I begin by showing how the preventive focus of social psychiatry was rooted in the mental hygiene and child guidance movements. The prevention of madness had long been a goal of physicians, religious leaders, and Progressive Era campaigners, such as the members of the short-lived National Association for the Protection of the Insane and the Prevention of Insanity.[6] But while nineteenth-century advice on preventing insanity tended to focus on the need to maintain individual moral standards (for instance, by not masturbating or imbibing alcohol to excess), by the twentieth century, attention had begun to pivot slowly toward the social sphere and environmental causes. Prevention was an important goal for mental hygiene and child guidance advocates partly for pragmatic reasons: it was "easier to prevent mental disorders than it was to treat them."[7] One way they attempted to achieve this preventive aim was by establishing multidisciplinary clinics that engaged with families and communities in order to root out problems before they became pathological. To illustrate both the variety of preventive approaches and the difficulties in carrying out such work in practice, I discuss a child guidance case from Chicago and the story of the Yale School of Medicine's Mental Hygiene Center (YSMMHC).

I then turn to social psychiatry's connection to the social sciences. For some, the social origins of mental illness were self-evident. Toward the end of his groundbreaking tome *The Mentally Ill in America* (1937), for example, the journalist and historian Albert Deutsch (1905–1961) speculated on the effect the Great Depression would have upon mental illness. Although he warned that it was too early to assess the full impact of the economic turmoil, he asserted that the "effect of the depression on the mental and emotional life of the unemployed is too obvious to require elaboration."[8] He proceeded to quote Henry C. Schumacher (1893–1971), then director of the Cleveland Child Guidance Clinic, who had written in 1934 that "only the unthinking can question the serious effects of these depression years on the mental health of both adults and children."[9]

For Deutsch, much could already be done to prevent mental illness. He estimated that 40 percent of mental disorders could be prevented "if we utilized to a maximum degree the knowledge of certain disorders already at hand." While much of this knowledge concerned organic causes of mental illness, ranging from syphilis and pellagra to brain injuries caused by accidents, even more could be done by tackling socioeconomic problems. Preventing "the recurrence of cyclic depressions," for instance, could be a powerful preventive measure.[10]

But while Deutsch, Schumacher, and others might have been convinced that it was possible to prevent mental illness based on current knowledge—intuitive or otherwise—about its causes, others were not convinced.[11] Rennie, for instance, contended that "most of what is carried on as preventive psychiatry has been untested by research methods as to its effectiveness. . . . We have practically no studies which convincingly prove, other than by clinical impression, that preventive techniques as currently employed are really effective over a long period of time." Writing in 1955 (eighteen years after Deutsch), Rennie argued that existing studies into the etiology of mental illness were "few and scattered, and the picture they add up to is tentative in the extreme."[12] Social psychiatry was needed to provide a much more robust foundation for preventive psychiatry.

One of the tasks of social psychiatry, therefore, was to provide the scientific evidence that would prove conclusively what people had been suspecting for decades: that socioeconomic problems contributed to mental disorder. To do so, psychiatry turned to the social sciences, which had been exploring the relationship between the environment and mental health since the pioneering work of Émile Durkheim (1858–1917) in *Le suicide* (1897) and Georg Simmel (1858–1918) in "The Metropolis and Mental Life" (1903).[13] Such investigations were soon followed up by U.S. studies, especially those conducted by members of the Chicago School of Sociology.

World War II ensured that the interdisciplinary insights of social psychiatry were heard by the policy makers and politicians who could do something about them. I conclude the chapter by exploring World War II's impact on American psychiatry and on social psychiatry especially. In broad terms, the war provided the opportunity for psychiatry to emerge from the asylum and become a vital part of the American military effort. Psychiatrists helped weed out recruits that were thought to be vulnerable to combat shock and, in turn, rehabilitate soldiers who succumbed nonetheless.

The process of screening recruits and rehabilitating psychiatric casualties also revealed two key insights that were crucial to establishing the political influence of social psychiatry. First, the numbers of psychiatric rejections were far higher than anticipated, suggesting that mental disorder was much more prevalent in American society than previously thought. Second, work by military psychiatrists, such as Roy R. Grinker (1900–1993) and John P. Spiegel's (1911–1991) *Men Under Stress*, highlighted that the psychiatric problems experienced by military personnel were environmental in nature.[14] Although some such factors were specific to combat situations, others had parallels in civilian life. As William Menninger, chief consultant in neuropsychiatry to the Surgeon General of the U.S. Army, explained, "Millions of people became really aware, for the first time, of the effect of environmental stresses on the personality. They learned that such stresses could interfere with or partially wreck an individual's efficiency and satisfaction with life." This realization presented psychiatry with the opportunity "to discover how it can contribute to the problems of the average man and to the large social issues in which he is involved."[15] Overall, the experience of World War II gave rise to the notions that mental illness was a major, yet often overlooked, problem and that social psychiatry had the potential to solve it by identifying its root causes and recommending preventive measures.

MENTAL HYGIENE AND CHILD GUIDANCE

In 1913, Thomas W. Salmon (1876–1927), medical director of the National Committee for Mental Hygiene (NCMH—now Mental Health America), contributed a chapter for a textbook entitled

Preventive Medicine and Hygiene, which was largely written by the influential physician and public health official Milton J. Rosenau (1869–1946). At over one thousand pages, the book was among the first comprehensive treatises on "modern hygiene and sanitation," covering everything from communicable diseases and eugenics to waste disposal and industrial hygiene.[16] Salmon began his chapter, entitled "The Prevention of Mental Diseases," by noting that while many of the root causes of many mental disorders were difficult to determine, some—especially those of an organic nature—were clear. These included general paresis (tertiary syphilis), alcohol psychosis, pellagra (which had by then been linked to corn-based diets but not to niacin deficiency), and insanity caused by infections such as typhoid fever.[17] Next, Salmon mentioned the importance of hereditary causes (including a tentative and qualified discussion of eugenics), followed by some reflections on the role of childhood development within psychoanalytic theory. Following this, he discussed the role of "economic factors," stating:

> Unemployment, overwork, congestion of population, child labor, and the hundred economic factors that increase the stress of living for the poor are often contributing factors in . . . mental disease. . . . everything which makes for the betterment of those upon whom the stress of living falls heaviest will save many from mental disease. For the individual careful training, encouragement, wise counsel, and a little financial assistance in times of especial need are helpful measures.[18]

Taken in its entirety, Salmon's chapter highlights how, during the early years of the twentieth century, mental illness was understood to be rooted in numerous and disparate underlying factors. But while the specific causes differed, underlying them all—and Salmon's hope for prevention—was a desire to "create a better society."[19] Such sentiments were hinted at in Salmon's words about "economic factors," though the specific mechanisms for doing so ("training, encouragement, wise counsel, and a little financial assistance") were rather vague.

As Grob has described, such aspirations were part and parcel of the mental hygiene movement, which flourished between approximately 1909, when NCMH was founded, and the start of World War II. While the term "mental hygiene" can be dated to the mid-nineteenth century, having been discussed by the physician William Sweetser (1797–1875) and the influential psychiatrist Isaac Ray (1807–1881), its meaning had shifted from focusing on individual responsibility to the measures society could adopt in order to promote mental health and prevent mental illness.[20] NCMH itself was largely the brainchild of Clifford Beers (1876–1943), who wrote the revealing autobiography *A Mind That Found Itself* in 1908.[21] Beers had spent time in psychiatric hospitals, and his book recalled the inhumane treatment he had experienced. Its primary purpose was "to expose, reform, and inform" how the mentally ill were treated in the United States.[22] While this was also the initial goal of NCMH, the organization eventually took on a more expansive role: promoting mental health and preventing mental illness.

Placing prevention at the center of mental hygiene, according to Grob, was eminently sensible. Prevention was central to the newly emerging profession of social work. The public was also concerned about the apparent rises in venereal diseases and alcoholism. But prevention chiefly provided opportunities for psychiatry. It allowed psychiatrists to focus on something other than their institutional role, where their ability to treat patients was limited, and associate themselves with public health more generally.[23] As Salmon would state in 1916, "Very few years ago it would have been difficult to justify the inclusion of a chapter on mental hygiene in a general treatise on preventive medicine and hygiene." Now, Salmon continued, it would have been neglectful not to include such a chapter: "The realization that many forms of mental disease depend in a large measure on preventable causes, the rapid growth of psychiatry and its acceptance as a department of scientific medicine, and the newly discovered opportunities for utilizing its resources in practical attempts to deal with social problems have broken down the barriers which so long and so effectually isolated mental medicine."[24] In other words, by focusing on prevention, psychiatry could obtain the scientific legitimacy that it lacked.[25]

But how exactly would such prevention occur? Although mental hygienists, such as Salmon, were fairly certain about what caused mental illness, they were aware that more research was required. As such, NCMH undertook a series of social surveys, beginning in 1915. While many of these investigated the state of the hospitalized mentally ill, others began to explore the nature of mental disorder outside institutions.[26] By revealing the extent of mental health issues outside of hospitals (relating to juvenile delinquency, alcoholism, and prostitution, for example), these latter surveys reinforced the idea that if NCMH was to prevent mental illness, it should develop community-oriented clinics.

One such clinic was the Maryland Mental Hygiene Clinic, which was funded by the Commonwealth Fund in 1927 at the prompting of the pioneering Swiss-American psychiatrist Adolf Meyer (1866–1950) and Edward N. Brush (1853–1933), superintendent emeritus of Shepard and Enoch Pratt Hospital.[27] As with most such clinics, the Maryland Clinic was staffed by a team consisting of a psychiatrist, a psychologist, social workers,

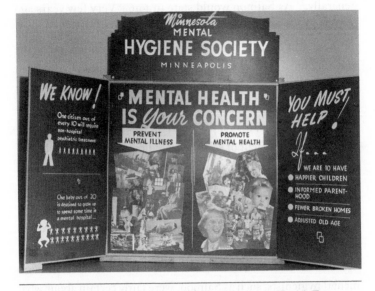

FIGURE 1.1   Poster presentation at the Minnesota Health Fair.
Source: City of Minneapolis Archives. Creative Commons. https://www.flickr
.com/photos/mplsarchives/32243162253.

and clerical support. The breakdown of the clinic's functions indicates how prevention was just one of its many roles:

1. To serve as a center for clinical study and treatment of psychiatric and behavior problems of all ages and color. . . .

2. To serve as the psychiatric out-patient department of the University Hospital and as a teaching center in Clinical Psychiatry for the University of Maryland Medical School.

3. To serve . . . those individuals, who seek the assistance of the clinic directly . . .

4. To assist in a general community mental hygiene program.

5. To cooperate with individual agencies and groups of agencies in . . . relation to mental hygiene educational work.[28]

Mental hygiene could also extend to eugenics, which was also fueled by some of the NCMH surveys—particularly those conducted in the Deep South.[29] Grob describes how there was a "hopeful and benign" side to mental hygiene (generally represented by NCMH) that stressed the role of societal reform and a more pessimistic and "interventionist" side that advised eugenic measures, such as "marriage regulation, immigration restriction . . . involuntary sterilization," and the institutionalization of the so-called biologically unfit.[30] Whereas child guidance and mental hygiene clinics were rooted in the "hopeful" idea that vulnerable individuals could be supported to maintain good mental health, those who believed mental illness to be primarily hereditary in nature looked to eugenics. Ian Dowbiggin has suggested that while the NCMH included some "ardent eugenicists," it could not officially support more radical interventions, such as sterilization, not least because one of its funders, the Rockefeller Foundation, was not supportive.[31] Nevertheless, over 18,000 mentally ill patients in the United States were surgically sterilized between 1907 and 1940. Sterilization laws were instituted at the state level, meaning that while California accounted for over half of such sterilizations, New York's tally was only forty-one (all women), since its law was declared unconstitutional and repealed.[32]

Sterilization laws were still in place in many jurisdictions well after social psychiatry rose to prominence following World War II. But it and other eugenic measures had largely been rejected by social psychiatrists by this time. While people diagnosed with mental disorders continued to be sterilized throughout the 1970s in some states, the concept of eugenics had been indelibly associated with Nazi Germany. Overall, it was the "hopeful and benign" elements of the mental hygiene movement that proved to be more influential in the development of social psychiatry.

These included the parallel and interlinked development of the child guidance movement and the establishment of both mental hygiene and child guidance clinics across the United States.

Children and childhood were of vital concern to mental hygienists. According to Theresa R. Richardson, "the mental hygiene paradigm originated with the premise that society could be perfected through the socialization of children. Happy, healthy children were argued to be society's best assurance of a rational and productive population."[33] The emergence of the child guidance movement highlighted such concerns. As Kathleen W. Jones has described, child guidance was often associated with child guidance *clinics* but also came to represent "a psychodynamic (often psychoanalytic) interpretation of the behavior problems of children; a therapeutic approach to solving the problems; the team of psychiatric, psychological, and social work professionals trained to work together to evaluate and treat problem children; and a critique of parental responsibility for troublesome behavior that was the wellspring of modern 'mother-blaming.'"[34]

In some ways, child guidance and mental hygiene were closely intertwined, both being examples of Progressive Era reforms that came into their own beginning in the 1910s and 1920s. NCMH, for example, was concerned with delinquency and set up child guidance clinics.[35] In turn, children and adolescents were also seen in mental hygiene clinics. Although NCMH was inextricably linked with Clifford Beers, just as the child guidance movement was associated with the psychiatrist William Healy (1869–1963) and Chicago's Juvenile Psychopathic Institute (founded in 1909, the same year as NCMH), others involved in mental health, including Adolf Meyer and William Alanson White (1870–1937), worked with both movements.[36]

But in other ways the two movements diverged. Deviant children, for instance, had been dealt with separately by both institutions (including asylums, workhouses, prisons, and separate
schools) and charities (such as the Society for the Prevention of
Delinquency, founded in 1824) since the nineteenth century.[37]
The work of child guidance also necessitated the involvement and
input of a larger and more disparate group of stakeholders,
including parents, teachers, social workers, and juvenile court
officers. As Jones and others have stressed, child guidance became
influential not least because its proponents were able to convince
these other stakeholders that they alone possessed "the special
knowledge and authority to help caregivers combat troublesome
behavior caused by maladjusted personalities."[38] Although both
child guidance and mental hygiene were interested in preventing problematic behavior, the range of issues child guidance
experts addressed was greater, encompassing everything from
bedwetting and discipline to truancy and adolescent moodi-
ness.[39] In turn, child guidance experts were also consulted on a
variety of matters not related to behavior, such as diet or vaccination. Finally, while psychoanalytic theory was influential in
the mental hygiene movement, the state of U.S. psychiatry more
generally remained "highly eclectic and fragmented."[40] Child
guidance, in contrast, was rooted securely in psychoanalytic theory and its emphasis on early childhood experiences. This was
the case not only for the psychiatrists who worked in child guidance clinics but also for their colleagues in social work. Finally,
child guidance borrowed from the insights emerging at the same
time from child psychology and child development studies.

What child guidance and mental hygiene chiefly had in common, however, was the desire to prevent mental illness and the
willingness to claim the authority over doing so. Just as debates

erupted within the mental hygiene movement between asylum psychiatrists, neurologists, and lay activists, such as Beers, there were limits to the authority of child guidance experts. Within the clinic, disciplinary tensions existed. Although (predominantly male) psychiatrists usually directed such clinics, they had to share their authority with (predominantly female) psychiatric social workers and clinical psychologists (split more evenly between male and female workers).[41] Psychologists focused primarily on testing both intelligence and aptitude, though they would also record their "impressions" of patients.[42] The psychiatrist, in turn, would conduct both physical and psychiatric examinations of patients in order to uncover the factors involved in shaping personality. Last, but certainly not least, the social worker investigated the impact of family background and social setting on patient behavior.[43] This could involve interviewing the patient's parents at the clinic, as well as visiting their home and neighborhood. As Jones beautifully describes, without the scales or test scores of the psychologist to lean on, "social workers relied on the authority of detail to make the case for or against a family and prove their value to the clinic's team."[44]

Ultimately, the insights emanating out of these discrete tasks had to be combined in order to prescribe a program of treatment, education, or rehabilitation for the patient and/or their parents. While the psychiatrist might have been seen as the most authoritative individual within the child guidance triumvirate, Jones asserts that social workers carried considerable influence in many cases. She describes how their status as women and as intermediaries between families (as well as other stakeholders) and the clinic often outweighed the scientific authority of psychiatry and psychology.[45]

Any advice the child guidance team agreed to, however, was worthless unless it was taken up by the families referred to the clinic and seen as authoritative by relevant stakeholders. In effect, child guidance sought to supplant (or perhaps extend) the knowledge about childhood development traditionally held by parents (especially mothers), as well as teachers, religious figures, and the community at large. In some cities, the task of child guiders was made more challenging by the fact that many children came from immigrant backgrounds where there were language difficulties and where different cultural standards could loom large. Most of the delinquent children seen at Boston's Judge Baker Foundation in 1920, for instance, were either immigrants or the children of immigrants, hailing from Italian, Irish, French-Canadian, or Jewish backgrounds.[46] Given the influence of psychoanalytic theory, issues related to sexual behavior, in particular, tended to be raised in most interviews psychiatrists conducted with children. This was the case for both genders but especially so for girls. Using psychoanalytic theory as their guide, child guidance experts often "constructed" links between the "unruly behavior" of children and their "sexual experiences."[47] Such connections could confound both children and their parents.[48]

A CHILD GUIDANCE CASE

Although the links between childhood sexual experiences and behavior problems might have been overemphasized by some child guidance experts, staff at the clinics also engaged with children who had suffered extensive sexual abuse, including incest.[49] An Illinois Social Hygiene League (ISHL) case from 1929, which also involved staff from the Institute of Juvenile Research (IJR), provides an example of the challenges child guidance clinics faced in supporting abused children. It also highlights the aspects of the case, namely, the patient, their family, and their community, on which clinic staff tended to focus, thus providing insights into how child guiders interpreted the varying risks of different childhood experiences.

The case centered on a ten-year-old girl who had been referred to the clinic. She had been diagnosed with gonorrhea after being raped by her brother-in-law.[50] The girl had been attacked when the brother-in-law had called her to his home to do some housecleaning. The girl "was terribly scared and when she got home she was afraid to tell her mother what had happened but because she was crying bitterly her mother threatened to whip her unless she told." The girl's sister (the wife of the rapist), however, did "not apparently feel disturbed" and blamed her sister for it, "intimating that she wanted intercourse and if she had an infection she acquired it from some little boy." She continued to support her husband (who denied any wrongdoing), pushing that he be released early when he was sentenced to one year in prison. The case notes also indicated that the girl's mother initially had doubts about her daughter's account, speculating that she might have acquired the infection from someone else.[51] The clinic staff, however, felt that the girl was genuinely "resentful and very sincere."[52]

On reporting to the clinic, the girl was described as "a nice looking girl with a pleasing personality," as "alert and responsive," and as being "dressed cleanly but cheaply."[53] As with other cases, the staff investigated the girl's family background and living circumstances in considerable detail. The girl's family had immigrated to the United States from Poland twenty-five years earlier, but it had not been an easy transition. The mother still did not speak much English (a translator was required), and the father had struggled to find consistent employment following the failure of a business venture (selling coal) caused by his heavy drinking. The family struggled financially, primarily relying on the income of one of the older daughters, who had a steady job at a factory; their rent and other payments were typically in arrears. Nevertheless, the home visit revealed that their two-bedroom basement flat was kept "spotlessly clean" despite housing between six and eleven individuals, depending on the circumstances.[54] The crowded conditions meant that the girl often had to sleep in the same bed as her twenty-one-year-old brother, who had been in the U.S. Navy but was now home and unemployed.

The school visit indicated that the girl was an average student, attended regularly, and presented few behavior problems. The teacher did note, however, that when the girl started out in her class she was "flirtatious with the boys." Nevertheless, the teacher "was able to settle her down to work and her deportment became average."[55] The teacher added that one of the girl's older sisters (not the wife of her rapist) had been particularly flirtatious and was rumored to have had a baby during a pronounced absence from school.[56] This sister, however, was also "one of the cleverest girls who ever attended" the school, with a particular penchant for drama.

A few months after the initial investigation, a physical examination of the girl was conducted by a psychiatrist based at IJR (the delay's cause was not disclosed). It revealed significant dental decay, head lice, evidence of rickets earlier in life, and an "elongated and ruptured hymen." The case notes also stated that the "psychiatrist finds that at the present time there is no evidence of emotional upset as a result of the rape mentioned in ths [sic] history. The patient has apparently been exposed to a great deal of sexual experiences previous to the sexual attack." No speculation was made as to the nature of these "sexual experiences," though it was recommended that other members of the family be checked for venereal diseases. Indeed, the psychiatrist seemed to be as much concerned with treating the girl's physical health problems (throwing in a ubiquitous tonsillectomy for good measure) as with the potential mental health problems emanating from the rape and subsequent family discord. In contrast to the psychiatrist's assessment, both the girl's mother and another one of her sisters asserted that her behavior had deteriorated following the attack, becoming more "nervous, unstable, and . . . unmanageable."[57]

The IJR psychiatrist advised that the girl be removed from her home, but this went against the judgment of the ISHL social work staff, who stated that the girl's "general home life appeared to be normal" and that she was devoted to at least some members of her family (specifically, her mother, her baby sister, and another sister). While awaiting the psychiatric examination, the girl had been attending the ISHL clinic three times per week for unspecified "treatment." She tended to turn up early and stayed afterward, "playing and helping in the office." After a few months, however, the staff suspected her of stealing money and, after first denying her guilt, the girl fessed up, stating that she gave most of the money to her mother. She was told to show up on time and leave directly after her appointment, which upset the girl because she enjoyed "playing" and "helping" at the clinic. Later, she requested a three-dollar loan on behalf of her mother, which was "of course" refused.[58] There is then a three-month gap in the notes, during which time the girl failed to show up to any of her appointments. Further investigation revealed that the entire family had moved to another state for agricultural employment, and the case was closed.

The final words in this particular case file provide a glimpse of the extent to which child guidance staff attempted to provide support for their clients: "Looked up the town [where the family had reportedly moved] on Atlas, but was unable to locate any such place. The Institute of Juvenile Research will find out whether there are facilities in a nearby town for the family to be under observation."[59] Despite the family leaving for another state, clinic staff still endeavored to help. These final sentences also provide a reminder of how thorough child guidance clinics could be in trying to understand the background of families and in offering support. While this case might have centered on the ten-year-old girl, the clinic also offered support to other family members. The girl's mother, for example, was offered birth control advice and assistance in caring for her sick baby. The girl's brother was offered help in finding employment. Even the girl's sister (the wife of the rapist) was offered support, despite the fact that she was already being helped by other agencies and was generally regarded as a troublemaker who stole from other clients. In determining the family's background, clinic staff not only visited the girl's home and school but also delved deeply into the family's history. They learned that both the father and mother came from peasant stock (perhaps explaining the decision to depart Chicago for farm work) and asked about their remaining family in Poland. Details about every family member were ascertained, including their school and employment history and their standing in the community.

The case also suggests that while mental hygiene and child guidance experts acknowledged that many disparate factors were involved in determining an individual's mental health, the nineteenth-century focus on morality had not been completely abandoned. The themes that loom largest in the case file, for example, focus on the moral failings of the family members, whether the alcoholism of the father, the flirtatiousness of the girl and her sister, or the propensity of the girl (likely prompted by her mother) and other family members to steal. When family members were praised, it tended to be on the basis of their appearance, cordiality, and ability to keep their flat clean; although their crowded living conditions are discussed (mainly with respect to sleeping arrangements), more words were spent describing its tidiness.

In turn, little was said about the structural problems (such as poverty, unemployment, housing, and immigration issues) that either contributed to or caused the family's woes. The petty thefts committed by the girl and various members of her family, for instance, were never blamed on the family's perilous financial situation, despite the fact that they were constantly at risk of being evicted and struggled to pay the costs associated with their unhealthy baby. The family had to borrow money to pay for the baby's milk, they worried about making the payments for her baby carriage, and—as Roman Catholics—they even procrastinated in christening her because of the five-dollar fee. When her condition worsened, the father scrambled to borrow the money for this because the mother "could never forgive herself if the baby should die un-christened."[60] Even the apparently deplorable behavior of the girl's sister in disbelieving her claim about her husband was underpinned by financial insecurity. Her efforts to exonerate her husband were fueled not so much by loyalty to him but because he was that household's sole breadwinner. A few weeks after the rape, it was noted that she intended to leave him, but not before securing an allowance from his wages. Finally, it is notable that the last interaction the family had with the clinic was when the girl requested a loan from a staff member, which was "of course" refused. Of all the many challenges faced by the family, underlying all of them was the lack of a stable and sufficient income. With that in place, the efforts of the clinic in supporting the family might have been more successful. Without it, the attempts of the clinic to "guide" the family were attenuated and fell back on addressing apparent moral failings.

Ironically, the morality of the girl's brother-in-law was barely mentioned at all.[61] As we shall see in subsequent chapters, CMHCs funded during the 1960s were similarly hampered by structural and other factors out of their control, including rapid deinstitutionalization, inconsistent funding, and endemic poverty and racism.

THE YALE SCHOOL OF MEDICINE MENTAL HYGIENE CENTER

While an individual case file can provide an in-depth example of how child guidance and mental hygiene work was carried out in practice, tracing the activities of a clinic over a longer period of time can shed light on other difficulties such clinics faced. In this section, I discuss a very different clinic, the Yale School of Medicine Mental Hygiene Center (YSMMHC) during the late 1920s and early 1930s. Its story helps show how ideas about mental hygiene were applied not only to underprivileged Americans (for example, poor immigrant families living in urban slums) but also to elites: in this case, Yale University students. It also illustrates many of the tensions and challenges that arose in such clinics. These included the difficulty in implementing preventive—as opposed to therapeutic—measures, the unwillingness of some psychiatrists to share authority with psychiatric social workers, and the difficulty in finding appropriate staff to work in such innovative centers. All of these issues would be mirrored in the CMHCs that were established during the 1960s.

During the 1920s, numerous universities began setting up mental hygiene facilities to both prevent and treat the mental health difficulties of their students. At least nine university mental hygiene centers had been established in Minnesota, Michigan, and California by 1925 when plans were afoot to develop one at Yale.[62] In a letter that year to Yale's president, the psychologist James Rowland Angell (1869–1949), NCMH's medical director Frankwood E. Williams (1883–1936) stressed how important mental hygiene was becoming to college administrators. He added that Barry Smith (1877–1952), general director of the Commonwealth Fund (a Yale alumnus), might be interested in funding such an initiative at Yale. Prophetically, however, he concluded by saying that "should work develop in various institutions along hit or miss lines . . . without any well thought out plan, it seems to me that more harm than good would probably be done."[63]

The Commonwealth Fund would fund YSMMHC for a five-year period, providing $50,000 per year primarily for staff costs, including one professor of mental hygiene, one associate professor, two instructors, two psychiatric social workers, one secretary, and two stenographers, along with generous salaries for members of the center's executive committee.[64] The initiative was launched with considerable fanfare, including two articles in the *New York Times*. The first, dated June 23, 1926, quoted Angell as saying that "the inability of our universities to deal promptly with cases of incipient mental or nervous disorders among their students has been most distressing, and they have been constantly seeking some solution."[65] Expectations for the program were high. But YSMMHC would quickly face numerous challenges.

One of the first difficulties involved staff recruitment. Initially, the newly appointed—and Yale's first—professor of psychiatry, Arthur H. Ruggles (1881–1961), was expected to direct the center, but he ultimately declined, as did two other desirable candidates. Ruggles would instead chair YSMMHC's executive committee, earning a generous annual salary of $2,500. With Ruggles taking a back seat, the leadership of the center remained problematic. Equally concerning for the center's Commonwealth Fund backers was the delay in appointing psychiatric social workers. Smith, the fund's general director, had worked for a year at the New York School of Social Work and emphasized the importance of social work in mental hygiene. The Commonwealth Fund's executive assistant, Mildred Scoville (1893–1969), who was responsible for monitoring the progress of YSMMHC's progress, was a psychiatric social worker and was convinced that the center's success was dependent on the effective deployment of such workers.[66] Scoville was one of the founding members of the American Association of Psychiatric Social Workers and a pioneering figure in the child guidance movement. She would go on to serve on the first National Mental Health Council appointed to advise NIMH and was also a member of GAP, ensuring that the interests and views of psychiatric social work were represented.[67] As the archival record shows, she was also highly respected within the Commonwealth Fund and forthright in her opinions.

Despite the influence of Smith and Scoville, however, it was not evident that Yale administrators were convinced that hiring psychiatric social workers was necessary. The fact that most such workers were women was part of the problem. In a 1925 conference to discuss mental hygiene at Yale,

> there was also some discussion as to the possibility of having psychiatric social workers, Dr. Angell feeling pretty strongly that the fathers of Yale students would object to having a woman butting in. He apparently bases this belief on the fact that Yale is so exclusively a man's university. After considerable discussion in which the method of technique of a good psychiatric social worker was explained . . . Dr. Angell seemed to be willing to give the matter a trial.[68]

Although it was agreed to "trial" the use of (female) psychiatric social workers, the appointment of any was delayed, to the chagrin of Smith and Scoville. By the spring of 1927, however, the center had begun to interview candidates. Scoville noted in a memorandum to Smith that the successful candidate should be given "*an adequate salary and with a faculty rating of some sort. I believe that it is very important for the worker to have this rating if she is to receive proper recognition on the campus. Without such a definite standing she may be quite handicapped.*"[69] The search was exhaustive and attracted an impressive array of candidates. Despite being general director of the Commonwealth Fund, Smith was personally involved in the appointment, stating to Ruggles that "the position at Yale is so extremely important . . . as to make it necessary . . . to be certain that we are getting the best person obtainable and one with exactly the proper qualifications." He spoke personally to the shortlisted candidates and shared his views on them. Of one, he stated that although he liked her "very much personally, she does not strike me as quite one hundred percent for that particular job. Perhaps I am unjust and I certainly do not want to put my judgment over everybody else's."[70]

Eventually, Elma Marie Olson, who had previously worked as an educational counselor at a school in La Salle, Illinois, was hired. One of her references was from Frankwood Williams, who described her as "an unusually capable person. She has a good mind and has learned how to use it, is a capable student and with it all has a pleasing and agreeable personality." It soon became clear, however, that Olson was not being asked to do the sort of "social service" work intended for the role, namely, conducting social histories that investigated the social and family backgrounds of students, doing treatment work in the home, and informing the recommendations of the psychiatric staff. Although

Ruggles wrote to Smith in February 1928 to say that Olson was doing well and that "the ice has been successfully broken" regarding psychiatric social work, Scoville was not convinced. Her review of the center in early 1929 (which was damning on many counts) confirmed her concerns. YSMMHC psychiatrists rarely asked Olson to conduct social histories of students, and she ended up spending too much time doing "copying jobs" that should have been done by a clerical assistant. Moreover, Olson "attends staff conferences but does not feel free to suggest that social service be used even when clearly indicated." Overall, she was "aware of the startling defects in the work and has attempted to change some of them but without success." In one case connected to "the lack of followup she established a tickler file that would indicate when the patient should return, and on that date would bring the fact to the attention of the psychiatrist. Within a short time she found her tickler file discarded and stored away unused in the back of a file case."[71]

All of this left Olson "very discouraged" and wanting to leave. Scoville recommended that Olson should—at the very least—receive the support of a secretary and an assistant psychiatric social worker; hiring the second proposed psychiatric social worker was also advised. In addition, Scoville stressed that all cases should be reviewed by Olson for the "study and analysis of social implications." Olson should also participate in a conference with the relevant psychiatrist afterward to "determine the possibility, practicality and desirability of social service for each case." Scoville added that "the psychiatrists' alibi for not using social service more is that the students object to having any one talk with their parents. I believe that this attitude on part of many students could be changed if psychiatrists had the proper professional attitude re: social service. Social work has a real contribution to make in obtaining social histories and doing treatment work in the home and this should be utilized."[72]

Olson, however, would leave at the end of 1930, having become "very unhappy by the whole experience."[73] Scoville was convinced that the YSMMHC psychiatrists did not think that social workers had much to contribute. As Angell's comment about "having a woman butting in" foreshadowed, part of the problem was simply sexism. When E. Van Norman Emery, who had been hired as the chief of staff for Yale's newly founded Division of Mental Hygiene, asked Scoville and Smith if they could recommend a psychiatric social worker, Smith replied revealingly that "possibly some of your difficulties would be overcome if you could secure a man instead of a woman but they are difficult to obtain." Smith added that he and Scoville would hesitate to recommend anyone because, on past evidence, there would not be much for such a worker to do.[74] Overall, according to Smith and Scoville, the problems related to psychiatric social work seriously undermined the successful functioning of YSMMHC because the "social service" work that psychiatric social workers did was the foundation for any attempts to prevent student mental illness. Without psychiatric social work, the center only offered therapeutic services. This was not mental hygiene.

Another problem YSMMHC faced regarded the take-up of their services by students. During its inaugural semester in 1926, the center offered two services to students: (1) a psychiatric consultation service and (2) freshman conferences (or "smokers"), which were to be held "practically every evening." These consisted of a thirty-minute lecture on a topic related to mental hygiene followed by student-led discussion. The intention was that these conferences would lead to individual consultations, but while some of the first sessions were well attended and well received, attendance soon dropped. By mid-November, 530 students had been invited to the conferences, but only 151 had attended (28 percent), and some subsequent sessions attracted no one at all. The quality of participation also deteriorated, from being "snappy, attentive [and] intelligent" to "very disinterested."[75]

Although staff members were not discouraged by the "apparently slow progress in attracting undergraduates," the freshman conferences were nonetheless replaced in early 1927 with one-on-one interviews with freshmen, in addition to physical examinations. Upon interviewing each freshman, the psychiatrist assigned them a score of I, II, or III:

Group I = "clean bill of health during the psychiatric examination"

Group II = "are considered doubtful"

Group III = "those who evidence some manifestations that definitely indicate psychiatric study"[76]

Out of these freshmen, 716 were assigned to group I, 277 to group II, and ninety-five to group III. In her 1929 report, Scoville described how she believed that the students in group II "were extremely important" and required "routine follow-up service" in order to prevent more serious problems from developing. This was because while the students in group III often only had the "rather natural nervousness of a young lad away from home and undergoing all the uncertainty of fitting into a new environment," group II students had "longstanding" and "deep-seated difficulties" that they were able to cover up. And "yet," she exclaimed, "nothing had been done to work out any plan to meet these men!"[77]

Scoville was not impressed with many aspects of the center. In her 1929 report, she criticized the lack of support provided to the center from Yale's deans, who appeared to be ignorant of it and what it offered. This, she determined, was attributable to poor communication from the center's psychiatrists, of whom she had little positive to say. Individually, they provided some effective therapy to students, but they contributed little to mental hygiene. Moreover, the poor administration of the center made it difficult for Scoville to determine exactly *what* the psychiatrists were doing. As she pointedly explained, "All of the men complain about being rushed to death but the output of work does not seem to confirm this."[78] YSMMHC, according to Scoville, lacked both leadership and clear policies to ensure that the psychiatrists achieved their responsibilities.

Despite these difficulties, however, the center continued to receive $50,000 annually from the Commonwealth Fund. Although the lack of "great or entirely satisfactory" progress meant that the fifth and final installment in 1930 was only awarded after some debate, by then Yale's focus had shifted to the foundation of the Institute of Human Relations (IHR), which was funded by a ten-year, million-dollar grant from the Rockefeller Foundation.[79] This new initiative was more focused on research and was framed along the lines of psychology rather than psychiatry.[80] A reconstituted Department of Psychiatry and Mental Hygiene was initially included in the IHR, but it soon separated from the institute, and the importance of mental hygiene at Yale waned.[81] Overall, the story of YSMMHC helps demonstrate that even with significant funding, the involvement of impressive individuals, and media fanfare, mental hygiene was difficult to achieve in practice.

PUTTING THE SOCIAL INTO SOCIAL PSYCHIATRY

Soon after the establishment of YSMMHC, it also became clear that much of its work lacked a foundation in research. In order to remedy this, as the educational philosopher Robert Maynard Hutchins (1899–1977) wrote in 1929, the IHR was established. Included in it were not only academic psychiatrists and psychologists but also social scientists and legal scholars. By bringing these disciplines together, the IHR's founders hoped to overcome "departmental rigidities" and work toward "co-operative research." Hutchins reminded his readers, however, that merely including the social sciences did not necessarily ensure that medicine, which had been distracted from the "human situation . . . through preoccupation in recent years with laboratory experiment," would develop the sort of insights into "human nature" that would result in preventive medicine.[82] The social sciences, he observed, could also be overly remote.

Regardless of Hutchins's concerns, the inclusion of the social sciences in IHR indicates that those involved in preventive mental health, at least within academia, were beginning to acknowledge the role that sociologists, anthropologists, and other social scientists could play. As Rosenau had stated in the preface to *Preventive Medicine and Hygiene* in 1913: "Many of these [medical] problems are complicated with economic and social difficulties, which are given due consideration, for preventive medicine has become a basic factor in sociology."[83] Indeed, by the early twentieth century, European sociologists such as Durkheim and Simmel were beginning to explore the relationship between social factors and mental health. And while similar studies had not yet emerged in the United States, sociologists there were following the work of their European counterparts closely. Durkheim's *Le suicide*, for instance, was featured in an 1898 article on suicide in the newly founded *American Journal of Sociology*.[84] Similarly, Simmel's "The Metropolis and Mental Life" inspired a 1912 *AJS* article that took up the idea that city life was "marked by . . . heightened stimulation."[85] Another telling contribution was from the Belgian sociologist Guillaume de Greef (1842–1924), who included a lengthy analysis of the characteristics and causes of insanity in Belgium and France in his series of eighteen "Introduction to Sociology" articles in 1903.[86] *AJS* also picked up on more obscure European research, such as a fin-de-siècle investigation of the relationship between prisons and asylums in Mecklenburg-Schwerin, Germany, among other studies.[87]

U.S. social scientists were also beginning to publish summaries of articles and reviews of books that dealt with mental health.[88] These included reports on NCMH surveys and brief synopses of articles in the *American Journal of Psychiatry* and other psychiatry journals and articles written by psychiatrists and asylum superintendents.[89] One early and relevant example of the latter was an 1899 article by Jules Morel, superintendent of the State Asylum of the Insane in Mons, Belgium, entitled "Prevention of Mental Diseases."[90] The article highlighted heredity as the most pernicious cause of insanity, but rather than advocating eugenic measures, Morel's advice included "to kindle affection for comrades and animals, and repress egoism by all means," to discourage masturbation, and to encourage a compassionate approach to education.[91] Morel also listed parental alcoholism, religious fervor, career difficulties, and unhappy marriages as potential causes of mental disease.

The development of rigorous U.S.-based sociology exploring the origins of mental health was slower to develop. Early social science literature on mental health tended to take the form of opinion pieces, which were interesting in what they revealed about current thought about various issues but were not examples of sociological research. One early example of a sociologist establishing some of the problems *to* address was Seba Eldridge's (1885–1953) 1915 book *Problems in Community Life: An Outline of Applied Sociology*, which included a section entitled "Care and

Prevention of Insanity and Feeblemindedness." Among the preventive measures Eldridge included were:

Reform of the labor conditions to eliminate excessive and improper work as causes of nervous strain;

Provision of recreational facilities adapted to the needs of various classes;

Improvement of domestic relations through the elevation of housing standards and the readjustment of marriage and correlate economic institutions;

Prevention of procreation by the feebleminded and insane through their retention in institutions;

Sanitary control of syphilis;

Treatment of alcoholism.[92]

While a review of *Problems in Community Life* in *AJS* by the urban sociologist and Chicago School leader Robert E. Park (1864–1944) dismissed it as having "no merits as a work of science" and that it would only be of use "as an aid to the investigations of amateur sociologists," Eldridge's breakdown of preventive measures did succeed in highlighting the range of factors implicated in mental illness at the time.[93]

Psychoanalysis also proved to be of interest to sociologists, with Ernest R. Groves's (1877–1946) 1917 article "Sociology and Psycho-Analytic Psychology" among the first published on the topic.[94] Groves would contribute to an American Sociological Society (now American Sociological Association) roundtable on the sociological implications of psychiatry and then co-chaired another roundtable on sociology and psychoanalysis in 1920; in 1922, a section at the ASS conference called "Psychic Factors in Social Causation" appeared.[95] Although sociologists were not always enamored with Freudian theory, they grew in confidence in terms of discussing and debating psychoanalysis. Upon Sigmund Freud's death in 1939, a special issue of *AJS* discussed the degree to which psychoanalysis had influenced sociology; the issue also identified some of psychoanalysis's shortcomings and how social scientists might address them. This included, as Rennie would later note, going beyond the individual and their immediate family to uncover the role of society more generally.

U.S. anthropologists were also beginning to investigate how mental disease was understood and addressed in different societies. One of the most influential anthropological studies touching on mental health would be Margaret Mead's (1901–1978) *Coming of Age in Samoa* (1928), but there were earlier studies, including those by early European investigators such as Georg A. Schweinfurth (1836–1925), John H. Weeks (1861–1924), and Henri A. Junod (1863–1934), that also reported on mental illness in far-flung parts of the world.[96] One of the early debates, which mirrored disputes about urban mental health, centered on whether primitive tribes were less likely to suffer from mental illness than those in more "civilized" societies.[97] U.S. anthropologists soon began similar investigations, including a 1921 article in *American Anthropologist* by the influential Berkeley anthropologist A. L. Kroeber (1876–1960) that included an analysis of the patients of the Honolulu Hospital for the Insane.[98] The hospital catered to a wide range of ethnicities, which allowed Kroeber, using methods such as participant observation, to speculate on the relationship between ethnicity and insanity. Kroeber observed that certain ethnic groups were disproportionately likely to be admitted. Korean residents of Hawaii, for example, represented only 2 percent of the population but over 10 percent of patients. While they tended to present behavior that was "listlessly apathetic," Portuguese patients (who represented 13.5 percent of patients, while making up 9.5 percent of the population) were "considered the most intractable, insistent, violent, and least likely to recover of all nationalities."[99] Other conditions were diagnosed along ethnic lines, with dementia praecox being common among Chinese patients and manic depression and psychoneuroses likely to be diagnosed in Japanese patients.

After citing the potential role of heredity, syphilis, and cultural factors, Kroeber added: "It . . . would be of exceeding theoretic interest, and no doubt of practical social value also, if the cause of these striking differences could be determined. . . . Considerable painstaking investigation would probably be required to obtain sufficiently accurate data; but once secured, the information might well shed light on the psychiatric problem of the causes of insanity as well as on race problems."[100]

Kroeber's call to investigate the causes of mental illness would be heeded by the 1930s (see chapter 3). Moreover, his interest in how different ethnicities seemingly suffered from different psychiatric afflictions would be reflected in major social psychiatry studies and in the subsequent development of transcultural psychiatry. His emphasis on "painstaking investigation" would also prove prescient, as debates about methodology would come to dominate many social psychiatry projects.

By the 1930s, social scientists were beginning to take ownership over the understanding of various aspects of mental health, including the epidemiology of mental illness.[101] For instance, the term "social psychiatry" was beginning to be employed more regularly by sociologists. In 1932, ASS included a Section on Social Psychiatry at their December annual meeting for the first time.[102] Moreover, the textbook *The Fields and Methods of Sociology* (1934) had a chapter on social psychiatry, which was defined as "a division of sociology."[103] Lawrence K. Frank's (1890–1968) article "Society as Patient," published in *AJS* in 1936, also provides an indication of how sociologists were growing increasingly ambitious in articulating how social problems played a key role in mental illness and in their role in both understanding and addressing them.[104] In part, such interest in mental health was driven by the pronounced focus of mental hygienists and child guidance experts on the social environment. It was also driven by the burgeoning academic, clinical, and cultural importance of psychoanalysis, though the views of social scientists toward psychoanalysis varied considerably.[105]

Developments at the Chicago School of Sociology were also highly influential, especially in terms of articulating how social scientists should tackle the problem of mental illness.[106] Many pioneering Chicago School members either researched mental health directly or discussed it in relation to their own work. These included Robert Park's *The Principles of Human Behavior* (1915), Nels Anderson's (1889–1986) *The Hobo* (1923), Louis Wirth's (1897–1952) *The Ghetto* (1925), Frederick Thrasher's (1892–1962) *The Gang: A Study of 1,313 Gangs in Chicago* (1927), Harvey W. Zorbaugh's (1896–1965) *The Gold Coast and the Slum* (1927), Ruth Shonle Cavan's (1896–1993) *Suicide* (1928), and E. Franklin Frazier's (1894–1962) *The Negro Family in Chicago* (1931).[107] Other leading sociologists, including Ernest W. Burgess (1886–1966) and Ellsworth Faris (1874–1953), wrote regularly about mental health. Among the many studies focusing on mental health to be influenced by the Chicago School was Faris and Dunham's *Mental Disorder in Urban Areas* (1939), which used Burgess's urban concentric zones theory (see chapter 3).[108]

As U.S. sociologists became more interested in mental health during the 1930s, discussions also emerged about the degree to which their work should remain academic or, in contrast, be applied directly to mental health settings. A 1931 article by the Chicago School member Louis Wirth, for example, introduced the term "clinical sociology" and argued that sociologists should play an important role in child guidance centers.[109] But while Wirth's term, along with the older concept of "applied sociology," did attract those eager to follow Durkheim's advice about not watching the "march of events" passively, the role of the social scientists within social psychiatry tended to be more academic than practical.[110]

It was one thing for the social sciences to become interested in mental health; it was another for psychiatrists—who were still mainly working in asylums—to recognize what such studies could offer. According to the sociologist Thomas D. Eliot (1889–1973), before 1940, sociologists were drawn to psychiatry more than psychiatrists were drawn to the social sciences.[111] While the next chapter will discuss how psychiatry took up the insights of social science in the 1930s, there were indications that sociological and anthropological research was being noticed before then. A 1913 article entitled "The Sociology of Insanity," written by J. T. Searcy, the superintendent of the Mount Vernon Insane Hospital in Alabama, for instance, demonstrates that psychiatrists were becoming aware of sociology but had differing views on what it was or could offer. Searcy began by declaring how "sociology may be said to be the study of all those means which render men and women 'more fit' in society." He described how sociologists, as with others, were noticing marked increases in the numbers of people with "psychic defects and deficiencies." Speculating as to why, Searcy pointed to the perils of civilization and, in particular, the role of drugs, including caffeine, nicotine, and alcohol. The other chief cause of insanity, Searcy argued, was "the leading principle in civilization of placing an equal value on all human lives alike." Further, "[it] should be a leading principle of sociology to encourage all measures that lead to the hereditary multiplication of the more capable, and to discourage the multiplication of the less capable, who are increasing."[112] In other words, sociology was a tool in achieving eugenics, which was—according to Searcy—the key to preventive psychiatry. Regardless of their specific views on eugenics, most sociologists would not have seen their role as justifying a particular social policy but trying to understand society itself.

The history of Searcy's asylum (which would be renamed in his honor in 1919) also provides context for his views on eugenics and the role of sociology. The Mount Vernon Insane Hospital was for "colored" patients and would remain segregated until 1969. In 1906, it experienced a pellagra epidemic, the first reported in the United States, which killed fifty-seven patients. Searcy discovered the epidemic himself, noting that the disease affected the "poorer classes" and was related to an insufficient diet (he suspected putrefied corn, along with exposure to the sun and poor hygiene).[113] Although it was not discussed in the article, pellagra would likely have been the root cause of the mental illness experienced by some of the patients, as it was in other parts of the South and in many parts of southern Europe. But despite the prominent role poverty would have played in the lives of many, if not most, of Searcy's patients, he stressed the role of narcotics and degeneration. As Salmon's chapter in *Preventive Medicine and Hygiene* suggested, the preponderance of causes for mental illness meant that psychiatrists—and social scientists— could gravitate toward explanations that suited them. One of the potential roles of the social sciences, therefore, was to subject such ideas to more rigorous investigation and scrutiny.

By the 1920s, some psychiatrists were articulating that their field could benefit from the social sciences. Such interest fitted into the so-called new psychiatry that Adolf Meyer had coined in the 1890s. Meyer's new psychiatry was influenced by both evolutionary biology and the Progressive Era's social ideals.[114] It took root in earnest when psychiatric services began to shift from the large asylums to smaller mental hospitals and clinics. In these more intimate settings, psychiatrists had more opportunity to spend time with patients and understand their family and social background.[115] It took time, however, for psychiatrists to suggest that the social sciences could contribute to psychiatry's understanding of mental illness. One of the earliest to do so was the Berkeley psychiatrist Herman Adler, whose 1927 article "The Relation Between Psychiatry and the Social Sciences" indicated that collaboration between social scientists and psychiatrists could help achieve this end.[116] In that same year, Harry Stack Sullivan (1892–1949) suggested that the ASS form a joint committee with the APA to explore mutual interests. The Committee on the Relations of Sociology and Psychiatry was formed, consisting of Robert Park, W. I. Thomas (1863–1947), and Kimball Young (1893–1972), and it reported at most ASS conferences between 1928 and 1941.[117] In turn, the APA formed the Committee on Relations with the Social Sciences in 1928. The resulting two Colloquia on Personality Investigation were funded by the Laura Spelman Rockefeller Fund.[118] These events, as Naoko Wake has described, did much to encourage collaboration between psychiatrists and social scientists.[119] Psychiatrists, including Sullivan, were also invited to speak at a newly formed (1929) ASS conference section on Sociology and Psychiatry.[120] Along with Sullivan, other prominent psychiatrists, such as William A. White, Trigant Burrow (1875–1950), William Healy, and Adolf Meyer, "were increasingly coming up against problems which were not only sociological in nature, but which demanded the specialized training of a sociologist."[121] Meyer, for instance, spoke of the value of the social sciences in his presidential address to the APA in 1928.[122] As the anthropologist-linguist Edward Sapir (1884–1939) would write in 1937, "psychiatrists are becoming more aware of the social component in conduct while social scientists are becoming more aware of the concerns of psychiatry."[123] Soon they would be working together to address such problems in earnest, becoming, in effect, the first social psychiatrists.[124]

PSYCHIATRY IN A TROUBLED WORLD

A final spur was needed to trigger the truly interdisciplinary research that would flourish as social psychiatry: World War II. During the war, U.S. psychiatry evolved from a medical discipline largely concerned with institutionalized patients into a key player in the drive to improve mental health. The momentum built during World War II was reified in the creation of NIMH, which was made possible through the Mental Health Act of 1946 and formally established in 1949. It also, however, cultivated a strong sense during the postwar period that psychiatry, in conjunction with the social sciences, was fully capable of preventing mental illness.[125]

U.S. military interest in psychiatry was driven by the desire to improve military effectiveness and efficiency, first by screening out mentally unsuitable recruits and second by facilitating the speedy return of psychiatric casualties to combat roles.[126] The U.S. military was motivated to avoid the high rates of shell shock that emerged during World War I.[127] Many shell shock cases were thought to be derived "from so-called weaker personnel who were predisposed to situational stress." In order to prevent such circumstances from reoccurring, "major reliance was placed on psychiatric screening at induction in order to exclude vulnerable individuals." By the end of 1940, Harry Stack Sullivan, a member of the APA's Military Mobilization Committee, had designed the Selective Service System to identify recruits unsuitable for combat.[128]

Despite eventually weeding out a staggering 1.75 million recruits, the effectiveness of the Selective Service's Central Examining Board for Neurology and Psychiatry was—at best—modest. The examinations, for instance, were designed by Sullivan to take fifteen minutes but, in practice, often consisted of "cursory" two-minute interviews by physicians with no psychiatric qualifications.[129] They also screened out recruits on the basis of race, ethnicity, sexuality, and intelligence, as well as predicted propensity for psychosis, psychopathy, mood disorder, or neurosis. Wake has described how homosexual recruits were caught in the net of the screening system, despite Sullivan's liberal approach to homosexuality in his clinical practice.[130] One of the questions asked, for instance, was "Do you like girls?" Ellen Dwyer's research has also revealed that white examiners were quick to reject Black recruits, partly because they often had lower educational scores but also out of racial bias or ignorance. She states that examiners often "resolved uncertainty about Black inductees by rejecting them."[131]

More damning, at least from the U.S. Army's perspective, were the high numbers of psychiatric casualties that occurred despite the screening efforts. Military leaders were irked by the high numbers of rejections, but they also had to face over 1.1 million hospital admissions on psychiatric grounds (though some of these were readmissions). Given that these numbers had major implications for the army's effectiveness, the onus on psychiatry both to treat and attempt to prevent such cases grew considerably. The numbers of psychiatrists supporting the war effort also increased. In December 1941, only thirty-five members of the Army Medical Corps had been assigned to neuropsychiatric roles; by 1944, psychiatry had been given equal status with surgery and medicine within the Office of the Surgeon General, and 2,400 physicians had been assigned to psychiatry.[132] As

William Menninger would declare in his 1949 presidential address to the APA:

> The war experience brought a much wider recognition of the potential contribution of psychiatry and mental health to various services in the federal government. Those of us . . . who so recently served in the armed forces are all too keenly aware of the results of totally ignoring psychiatry in military planning prior to the war and the minimal role it had played in the Veterans Administration. However, psychiatrists now serve in almost every major government department that is concerned with medicine or health.[133]

Menninger and other psychiatrists would capitalize on this newfound influence after 1945.

As World War II wore on, military psychiatrists increasingly employed new preventive and therapeutic measures in trying to reduce the numbers of psychiatric casualties and support the return of those who were hospitalized. Treatment innovations included providing psychiatric "first aid" (which included "mild sedation, a night of sound sleep, and warm food") and dealing with psychiatric casualties closer to the front line rather than sending them to a hospital many miles away.[134] According to the psychiatrist John C. Whitehorn (1894–1974), successful treatment "seemed to depend less upon specific procedures or specific drugs than on general principles—promptness in providing rest and firm emotional support in a setting in which the bonds of comradeship with one's outfit were not wholly disrupted and in which competent psychiatric reassurance was fortified, symbolically and physiologically, by hot food and clean clothes and by evidence of firm military support and command of the situation."[135]

Such measures were mirrored in the steps taken to prevent psychiatric casualties. In order to reduce combat exhaustion, fixed tours of duty were introduced, rather than keeping troops in theater indefinitely, as had previously been the case. Group cohesion, which was observed to be crucial to maintaining morale, was maintained by rotating entire units (rather than individual soldiers). Finally, officers were educated to recognize that all soldiers were vulnerable to psychiatric breakdown and that such episodes were not examples of malingering, cowardice, or weakness, despite the famous scene in *Patton*. By the end of World War II, these preventive and therapeutic measures were reducing the burden of military psychiatric illness.[136]

World War II provided three lessons for U.S. psychiatrists that would influence the development and support of social psychiatry. First, high rejection rates suggested that mental illness was far more common in U.S. society than previously thought. This, combined with the fact that asylums were already struggling from overcrowding and crumbling infrastructure (to be shortly highlighted by Deutsch's *The Shame of the States*), indicated that a new, preventive approach to mental health policy was required.[137] Second—and influencing the approach taken to prevention—was the growing awareness of how environmental factors contributed to mental illness. The stresses of modern war, as Grinker and Spiegel argued, were such that they could trigger mental disorder in any individual.[138] Grinker and Spiegel also hinted, however, that the stresses faced by civilians could be similarly pathological. In order to prevent mental illness, therefore, these environmental factors had to be investigated thoroughly and urgently. Finally, the ascension of psychiatry during the course of World War II from a marginalized medical discipline to one that was central to the war effort—as well as the perception that it had made a substantive difference—gave psychiatrists confidence that they could also succeed in identifying the causes of mental illness and eradicating them. Such faith reflected a broader sense, buoyed by contemporary medical advances such as the development of antibiotics, that medical science was capable of achieving the previously unthinkable. Adding to this optimism was the fact that many physicians exposed to psychiatry during World War II were young and not necessarily shackled to the asylum. Typically rooted in psychoanalytic approaches but also mindful of the role of social factors, these "Young Turks" sought to advance psychiatry—and their own careers—by taking an active part in tackling the problems believed to afflict the United States during the postwar period.

One way these young psychiatrists sought to achieve their ambitions was by forming GAP in 1947, under the leadership of William Menninger, the top military psychiatrist during World War II, and with the financial support of the Commonwealth Fund. As Menninger explained, GAP's founders sought "a way in which American psychiatry could give more forceful leadership, both medically and socially. . . . Those early years of GAP were marked by the feeling on the part of its membership that much needed to be done and quickly."[139] It also sought to "overcome the sluggish and cumbersome machinery of action of the Association [APA]."[140] By 1950, GAP's Committee on Social Issues had produced a report entitled *The Social Responsibility of Psychiatry: A Statement of Orientation*, which stressed the need to redefine "the concept of mental illness, emphasizing those dynamic principles which pertain to an individual's interaction with society"; to examine "the social factors which contribute to the causation of mental illness"; and to develop "criteria for social action, relevant to the promotion of individual and communal mental health." Going further, the committee "had the conviction that social action . . . implies a conscious and deliberate wish to foster those developments which could promote mental health on a community-wide scale."[141]

Another way that the experience of World War II catalyzed the emergence of social psychiatry was through the passage of the Mental Health Act in 1946, which led to the foundation of NIMH in 1949. NIMH had a broad remit, but its founding director, Robert Felix, was particularly eager to fund research into understanding the collective mental health of communities. Among the first projects funded by NIMH included Hollingshead and Redlich's New Haven Study (chapter 3) and the Midtown Manhattan Study (chapter 4). Crucially, NIMH represented a major federal government investment into mental health. Although states would continue to pay for much mental health care in the form of state psychiatric hospitals, NIMH signified that mental health was now also a federal priority. By 1955, Congress had further demonstrated its commitment to mental health by passing another Mental Health Act, which led to the Joint Commission on Mental Illness and Health (JCMIH), which was followed by the Joint Commission on the Mental Health of Children (JCMHC). As Grob explains, Felix's charisma, humor, and bureaucratic skills helped NIMH and its priorities gain influence, especially leading up to the passage of the Community Mental Health Act of 1963, which facilitated the shift from institutional to community mental health care in the United States.[142]

CONCLUSION: FAITH IN PSYCHIATRY

Overall, World War II provided the urgency, enthusiasm, and optimism that would fertilize the flowering of social psychiatry during the next two decades. It helped reconceive the patient as "a social unit" and psychiatrists as capable of providing "leadership and counsel to the family, the community, the state, welfare workers, educators, industrialists, religious leaders and others."[143] It set the scene for the "magic years" that Daniel Blain would describe and provided the confidence required for the momentous changes in mental health policy that would soon come. As a result, the postwar United States "witnessed an extraordinary spike in attention given to the status of Americans' mental well-being."[144] Although some argued that psychiatrists also found themselves "unwillingly and unwittingly in the limelight," it is likely that many relished this opportunity to come out of the shadow of the asylum.[145] In addition to producing psychiatrists keen to make a difference to the nation's mental health, it also played a significant role in shaping the careers of many of the social scientists involved in social psychiatry, as will be discussed in subsequent chapters.

In many ways, however, World War II merely accelerated the desire to prevent mental illness that had existed for half a century. The emergence and influence of social psychiatry during the postwar period was built on longstanding observations about the relationship between socioeconomic factors and mental health and a growing belief that the social sciences were essential to understanding the etiology of mental illness. Some of the challenges that social psychiatry would eventually face in trying to realize preventive psychiatry can also be traced to these origins.

A balance, for example, often had to be struck between the intuitive assumption that socioeconomic problems contributed to mental illness and the need to design robust studies that satisfied both psychiatrists and social scientists. Whereas mental hygiene and child guidance advocates could be accused of supporting policies and clinical practices that were not based on evidence, social psychiatrists were often guilty of the opposite: hesitating to make policy recommendations while waiting for evidence to accrue. Social psychiatry was also borne out of post-war hopes and expectations that it had the insights to prevent mental illness. As William Menninger bullishly exclaimed in 1947: "Of all the potential expansions for psychiatric effort, the field of prevention promises unlimited opportunity. We have every reason to believe that had the manpower and the effort and the time been devoted to the preventive aspects of psychiatry as was given to the preventive efforts in physical medicine, we too could have perhaps demonstrated spectacular achievements comparable to vaccination or DDT."[146]

Such expectations put considerable pressure on social psychiatrists, who were tasked with elucidating the environmental causes of mental illness and—what is more—doing something about them. Given that the findings of social psychiatrists inevitably pointed toward political solutions, it is understandable that such hopes were unfulfilled.

2

FROM HOBOHEMIA TO THE GOLD COAST

*Day after day he roamed about in the arctic cold, his soul filled
full of bitterness and despair. He saw the world of civilization
then more plainly than ever he had seen it before; a world in
which nothing counted but brutal might, an order devised by
those who possessed it for the subjugation of those who did not.*

—Upton Sinclair, *The Jungle*

In late 1935, a thirty-one-year-old man was admitted to
Cook County Hospital in Chicago and diagnosed with
dementia praecox, then a common psychiatric diagnosis
that came with a poor prognosis.[1] Originally from Virginia and
the son of Ukrainian immigrants, he had left home in 1923 after
his parents died and his engagement broke off. He spent two
years in Ohio working as a busboy, and after a failed attempt at
reeducation (he had a sixth-grade education), he left for Chicago
in 1925. There he also found restaurant work and, after initially
living at the YMCA, found suitable accommodation.

The man's life in Chicago began well. Work was steady, and
he saved seven hundred dollars. But within a few years, his life
became unstable. A run on the bank as the Great Depression

loomed left him with only 10 percent of his savings. Following an aborted love affair, he started drinking and gambling. He moved into a rooming house owned by a bootlegger, and soon "every cent I earned went for drink or poker."[2] He eventually left but still struggled to refrain from drinking. One night, while drunk, he was "jack-rolled" (mugged).[3] Upon entering the hospital, his landlady claimed that he owed thirty dollars in unpaid rent. She added that he never had any friends, never brought "girls" back (of which she was glad), and was often drunk: "He was for himself only. He was a queer fellow. . . . He never spoke to anyone here."

The man's case worker attempted to tease out the source of his problems. In an extensive interview over a number of days, he dug for more details, focusing especially on his sexual habits, drinking, and gambling but also on what he read, his dreams, and his religiosity. The case worker repeatedly probed into the events that led to the man's hospitalization but failed to get a concrete answer. The man described how he had been drinking and thinking about his mother's death, but there was no precise trigger. The case worker's questions kept drifting into whether the man masturbated or visited brothels (never; occasionally), as well as his drinking, without determining conclusively what was at the root of his difficulties.

Elsewhere in the file, however, clues could be found. In a section where the man effectively dictated his life story, he described feeling lost and alone in Chicago. Echoing the comments of his landlady, he described how "the trouble with me is that ever since I left home I never had any social environment at all." Without alcohol, he was "bashful" and "sort of slow and hard to get acquainted with . . . when I get drunk I meet many people."[4] He concluded by stating that "since my father died I have had no one in whom to confide." His father had died in 1921, fifteen years before.

These factors would not have been lost on Robert Faris and Warren Dunham. In fact, this man would have been one of the 34,864 individuals admitted to Chicago's psychiatric hospitals between 1922 and 1934 who formed the basis of their landmark study *Mental Disorders in Urban Areas* (1939).[5] The book charted where patients had lived before admission and the socioeconomic conditions found in these communities. In addition to studying the situation in Chicago, the book compared admission statistics in Providence, Rhode Island.[6] When the characteristics of the areas with the highest admissions were analyzed, it became apparent that many patients would have shared the impoverished, chaotic, and socially disorganized lifestyle experienced by the man featured here.

In his foreword, H. Douglas Singer (1875–1940), director of the Illinois State Psychopathic Institute, reflected that while it had been "long recognized" that "the environmental setting is an important factor in the etiology" of mental illness, there had not been any studies conducted that confirmed such assumptions or analyzed them in any detail.[7] Faris and Dunham rectified this issue, Singer explained, by providing "statistical validity" for the connection between socioeconomic factors and mental disorder. Sitting "at the borderland between medicine and sociology," their book demonstrated to both social scientists and psychiatrists that social science methods could help elucidate the epidemiology of mental illness, thus taking the first steps toward preventive psychiatry.[8]

Faris and Dunham's "technique" was rooted in the "ecological" methods that had been developed by members of the Chicago School of Sociology during the previous decades. Under the leadership of Albion Small (1854–1926), who founded both the university's sociology department and the *AJS*, and in the wake of Robert Park and Ernest Burgess's influential textbook *Introduction to the Science of Sociology* (1921), sociology transformed from a largely philosophical enterprise to a social science based on rigorous research.[9] Faris and Dunham were among the first to apply such an approach to studying mental illness. In particular, they followed Burgess's approach to urban sociology, which depicted the various socioeconomic zones of the city as a series of concentric circles.[10] Using this model, Faris and Dunham added nuance to longstanding debates about whether cities were good or bad for mental health (see chapter 4). While some urban zones had particularly high rates of mental disorder, other areas were less afflicted. Identifying why individuals from particular areas were more vulnerable to mental disorder than others, therefore, emerged as the crucial task in understanding urban mental health, rather than damning or praising cities per se.[11] Crucially, they were also able to add weight to the argument of the anthropologist Franz Boas (1858–1942) that social factors were more important than biological or cultural factors in the formation of human behavior.

Nevertheless, Faris and Dunham's work also yielded surprises regarding where certain disorders were to be located in Chicago. Whereas schizophrenia was commonly found in Chicago's deprived regions, manic-depressive psychoses were more evenly distributed. In addition, while racist attitudes within U.S. psychiatry meant that Black Americans in other cities were disproportionately diagnosed with psychoses, Faris and Dunham's findings challenged this assumption, suggesting that other factors, such as social isolation, were more important.[12] Such insights informed the approaches that would be adopted in later studies. In particular, it spurred the incorporation of ever more detailed social sciences methods (including questionnaires and interviews) that could reveal the social factors involved in mental illness.

I begin this chapter by exploring the origins of *Mental Disorders in Urban Areas*, tracing the project's roots in the Chicago

School and how Chicago had been conceptualized in the previous decade of sociological research. I then turn to how Faris and Dunham derived and interpreted their findings, focusing in particular on the project's implications for preventive psychiatry. Finally, I address how the book was received by both social scientists and psychiatrists. Overall, I argue that while the message coming out of *Mental Disorders in Urban Areas* served to support the idea that environmental factors were crucial to the etiology of mental disorder, it also highlighted that uncovering the precise nature of these factors, let alone determining preventive measures, was both complex and divisive. In other words, Burgess was correct in asserting that *Mental Disorders in Urban Areas* was a "pioneer study," but the terrain Faris and Dunham opened up would prove difficult to navigate.

THE CHICAGO OF THE CHICAGO SCHOOL

Mental Disorders in Urban Areas was preceded by many other works produced by the Chicago School that had put the Windy City under the microscope.[13] Subjecting Chicago to sociological scrutiny was a "rich tradition" by the time Faris and Dunham embarked upon their study, and "social disorganization" was a popular topic.[14] The Chicago School approach to social disorganization assumed that "a social problem is a malady of society, but that it is social rather than organismic processes that are deranged and in a pathological state."[15] When the socialization of individuals and the integration of communities were undermined, social problems emerged. The Chicago School sociologists, therefore, often viewed their city through the lenses of homelessness, ghettoization, gangs, juvenile delinquency, suicide, crime, and prostitution in the hope of further understanding the role of social disorganization in cities.[16] Chicago was more than able to provide rich subject material.

Following the Great Fire of 1871, which completely destroyed Chicago's downtown, the city had to be rebuilt. It rapidly transformed from a ramshackle and chaotic sprawl to a carefully designed urban center characterized by a new architectural marvel: the skyscraper. Crucially, Chicago's modern downtown was dedicated almost exclusively to commercial use; former residents moved outside of the central business district to outlying areas. Chicago's position as a railway hub facilitated its rebirth and allowed both American migrants and European immigrants to flock to the city for economic opportunities in lumberyards, meatpacking, manufacturing, and even emergent mail-order companies (for example, Sears and Roebuck, founded in 1893).[17] Following on from Irish and German immigration during the 1840s and 1850s (which could be measured in the tens of thousands of people), immigration to Chicago accelerated rapidly, peaking with 859,000 immigrants coming to Chicago during the 1920s (especially Poles, Italians, and Lithuanians). They were joined by 120,000 Black Americans from the South during the Great Migration, as well as an estimated 300,000 to 500,000 workers who flocked to Chicago annually in search of work.[18]

Although Chicago offered economic opportunities to these migrants, the rapid growth of the city led to social problems. These ranged from desperate living conditions for the city's poorest inhabitants and ethnic and racial tensions (including a major race riot in 1919) to infamous gangland crime and vice. Such problems did not escape attention. As early as 1894, the English editor William T. Stead (1849–1912) had decried Chicago's political corruption, immorality, and crime in *If Christ Came to Chicago!*[19] More significantly, the plight of Lithuanian meatpackers and their families was famously portrayed in Upton

Sinclair's (1878–1968) *The Jungle* (1906). Sinclair's novel might not have achieved the labor reforms he desired (though it did lead to the foundation of the Food and Drug Administration in 1906), but efforts were made by reformers, such as the Nobel laureate Jane Addams (1860–1935), to address the difficulties faced by Chicagoans. Addams and Ellen Gates Starr (1859–1940) founded Hull House in 1889, a "settlement house" that offered immigrants English classes, inexpensive meals, and recreational facilities, including the city's first playground.[20]

By the early 1920s, Chicago had also become the prime subject for Chicago School sociologists. The first monograph to be published in this tradition, Nels Anderson's *The Hobo: The Sociology of the Homeless Man* (1923), might have been written by a sociologist with an unconventional background, but it provided an indication of the sort of topics and approaches that would be adopted later. The son of Swedish immigrants, Anderson had a peripatetic upbringing, living in logging camps, the Nez Perce Indian reservation, Chicago's slums, and finally a farm in Michigan. His early adult years were similarly characterized by wanderlust, and he spent over a decade working in an array of transitory occupations across the American West, often "bumming" as a hobo himself.[21] Convinced to return to education, he studied at Brigham Young University in Utah before journeying to Chicago (his "final effort at riding freight trains") to begin graduate studies.[22] Anderson wrote two of his first essays as a student on the hobo life that he knew so well, and he was encouraged by those interested in Chicago's homelessness problem to take on the topic. With the support of the Chicago Council of Social Agencies and the Laura Spelman Rockefeller Fund (which paid to publish the research of many Chicago School graduates between 1923 and 1930), *The Hobo* was published by University of Chicago Press before he had even graduated with his master's degree.[23]

Anderson's depiction of Chicago's Hobohemia, the section of the city around West Madison Street where the homeless congregated, would influence Faris and Dunham's understanding of what life was like for Chicago's homeless and transient population, as well as the impact of such a lifestyle on the psyche. This was despite the fact that the two projects employed completely different methodologies: while Anderson based his findings on his own experience and participant observation (highly novel at the time), Faris and Dunham's approach was essentially statistical and geographical. A central question, however, bound both studies together: were hobos (for Anderson) and the mentally ill (for Faris and Dunham) born or made?[24] Judging from Park's preface to *The Hobo*, both aspects were involved, but the environment was most important. Comparing the socially derided hobo or "vagrant" to the revered figure of the American pioneer, Park declared how with respect to "biological predisposition, the pioneer and the hobo are perhaps the same temperamental type; from the point of view of their socially acquired traits, they are something quite different."[25] He added that "human nature . . . is very largely a product of the environment, and particularly the human environment in which the individual happens to find himself." Moreover, "every community . . . tends to determine the personal traits as it does determine the language, the vocation, social values, and, eventually, the personal opinions, of the individuals who compose it."[26] Such communities included the 30,000 to 75,000 men living in Hobohemia.[27]

Anderson also raised the issue of mental disorder among the homeless, citing an earlier study of one thousand homeless men in Chicago by the charity worker Alice Solenberger (d. 1910), which determined that, while two-thirds of homeless men had physical and mental ailments, only 5 percent were insane. Solenberger observed that the "life of the true tramp or vagrant, with its excitements, excesses, and irregularities . . . might reasonably be expected to cause insanity in a certain percentage," adding that four out of the fifty-two insane men in her study had become insane during the course of her study.[28] She surmised that the "worry" and—interestingly—"under-nourishment" associated with homelessness were responsible. In sum, however, Solenberger suspected that "insanity acts as a cause of vagrancy more often than vagrancy as a cause of insanity."[29] Anderson acknowledged that some individuals became hobos because of "defects of personality" but added that there were other reasons, including "crises in the life of the person" and the desperate search for seasonal work.[30] Among those with personality defects were the "feebleminded," some of whom found it difficult to cope with the increasingly industrialized workplace, as well as those with dementia praecox, epilepsy, and other disorders. Overall, according to Anderson, it was impossible to single out one explanation or to tease out the precise relationship between homelessness and mental health.

Anderson's Hobohemia resonated strongly in Faris and Dunham's description of the areas of Chicago most likely to house the mentally ill. Other Chicago School projects would also influence *Mental Disorders in Urban Areas*. Harvey W. Zorbaugh's *The Gold Coast and the Slum: A Sociological Study of Chicago's Near North Side* (1929), for example, presented Chicago as a city with clear cultural and socioeconomic divisions, providing important context for Faris and Dunham's analysis.[31] Louis Wirth's doctoral research, culminating in *The Ghetto* (1928), similarly informed how Faris and Dunham understood the features of the city's many segregated ethnic neighborhoods.[32] In many of these immigrant communities "the language, customs, and many institutions of their former culture are at least partly preserved."[33] This cultural continuity helped reduce social disorganization. When these ghettos began to disintegrate—which happened quite rapidly with the arrival of new immigrant groups—social disorganization becomes "severe," with "extreme poverty," "high rates of juvenile delinquency, family disorganization, and alcoholism reflect[ing] the various stresses in the lives of these populations."[34] Wirth's analysis of the ghetto (whether they be "Chinese, Negro, Sicilian, or Jewish") as "not merely a physical fact, but also a state of mind" allowed Faris and Dunham to tease out the specific factors in Chicago's various communities that contributed to mental illness or health.[35] Many of those who attempted to "flee from the ghetto" only to become "disappointed and disillusioned" by the coldness of the outside world would "return to the warmth and the intimacy of the ghetto."[36] Much more pathological than the ghetto was the social isolation prevalent in regions of the city where no such support could be found.[37]

Other Chicago School studies, including E. Franklin Frazier's *The Negro Family in Chicago* (1931) and Clifford Shaw's (1895–1957) *Delinquency Areas* (1929), helped shape Faris and Dunham's understanding of Chicago's neighborhoods and populations.[38] *Delinquency Areas* not only reinforced the view that social problems were attributable to life experiences, rather than constitutional or physiological factors, but its methodological approach also proved to be influential. Funded by multiple agencies, one of Shaw's approaches was to analyze over sixty thousand cases of juvenile delinquency that passed through Chicago's juvenile court.[39] By examining the residences of the juveniles processed, they were able to determine what neighborhoods were most likely to produce delinquency, much like Faris and Dunham would do with respect to psychiatric inpatients. Shaw found that delinquency was most common and most serious in the areas of the city closest to the city's central business district and in areas that were deteriorating physically and undergoing depopulation. As with Faris and Dunham, Shaw's work would also be critiqued by those who suspected "downward drift"; in other words, such areas did not produce delinquency, but rather delinquents (born, not made) gravitated toward them.[40]

The two most influential Chicago School studies for Faris and Dunham in terms of their theoretical perspective and subject matter, however, would prove to be Park and Burgess's *The City* (1925) and Ruth Shonle Cavan's *Suicide* (1928). Burgess's concentric zone theory was central to how Faris and Dunham framed their project (see figures 2.1 and 2.2). Burgess divided the city into a series of circular zones that emanated out from Zone I, the central business district. In Chicago, these zones were bounded by physical barriers, such as the Chicago River, railway lines, and industrial features, such as the expansive Chicago stockyards, as well as by socioeconomic and cultural barriers.[41] Zone I was home to few people apart from "transients inhabiting the large hotels, and the homeless men of the 'hobohemia' section." It did contain, however, offices, light industry, and "places of amusement."[42] Zone II was the "zone in transition," so called because the industrial region of Zone I encroached on its fringes and was expected to soon expand into it. Zone II landlords, therefore, assumed that they would eventually sell the residential dwellings they owned to make way for this industrial expansion and, as a result, did not bother to maintain them. This kept rents low. Zone II was occupied primarily by newly settled immigrants in segregated slums or ghettos, as well as those living in rooming houses. Most occupants consisted of low-skilled laborers and their families. Zone III comprised the homes of skilled laborers and housed a higher percentage of native-born Chicagoans, as well as older immigrant neighborhoods, such as "Deutschland." Finally, Zones IV and V were occupied by upper-middle-class residents and were characterized by much more stable

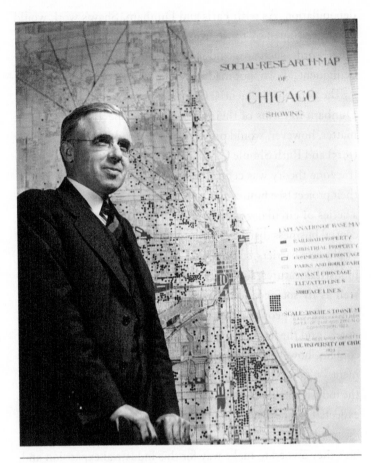

FIGURE 2.1 Burgess and map.

Source: University of Chicago Photographic Archive, apf1-02326, Hanna Holborn
Gray Special Collections Research Center, University of Chicago Library, https://
www.lib.uchicago.edu/about/news/seeing-chicago-sociologists-anew-through-the
-archives/. Permission provided by the Hanna Holborn Gray Special Collections
Research Center, University of Chicago Library.

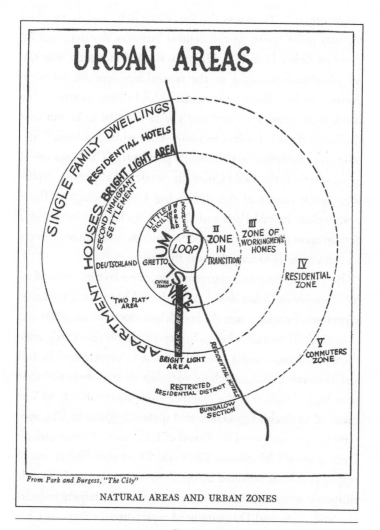

From Park and Burgess, "The City"

NATURAL AREAS AND URBAN ZONES

FIGURE 2.2 Concentric zones.

Source: Robert E. Park and Ernest W. Burgess, *The City* (Chicago: Chicago University Press, 1925).

neighborhoods. There was also the "Black Belt," which stretched for two miles south of the central business district, cutting through Zones II and III. Home to Black Americans, only the neighborhoods adjacent to the central business district were deemed to be subject to "extreme" social disorganization; the Black communities further south were thought to be not dissimilar to those inhabited by native-born white residents.[43] The only other exception to this orderly portrayal of Chicago's social geography was the Gold Coast, the stretch of expensive dwellings in the center of the city facing Lake Michigan. These descriptions helped Faris and Dunham go beyond stating *that* certain areas of Chicago seemed to generate more mental illness and speculate as to *why* this was the case.

Burgess's influence is apparent to anyone who flips open *Mental Disorders in Urban Areas*. As Faris and Dunham's academic supervisor, Burgess wrote the book's introduction, and Faris and Dunham's first chapter began by explaining his concentric zone theory.[44] Burgess had a marked interest in mental health, and unlike some Chicago School sociologists who believed that sociology should retain a distance from their subject, he was involved with child guidance and mental hygiene in Chicago, serving as a member of the Board of Education's Committee on Delinquency.[45] Moreover, Faris and Dunham's liberal use of maps in the book reflected Burgess's concentric zones. But while Burgess's concentric zone map (figure 2.2) was largely impressionistic, Faris and Dunham used representative maps of Chicago to chart rates of mental disorder throughout the city. These nevertheless conveyed Burgess's theory that social disorganization worsened toward the center of the city (figure 2.3). These maps clarified, emphasized, and reified the relationship between mental disorder and the socioeconomic environment, especially for those familiar with the geography of Chicago.

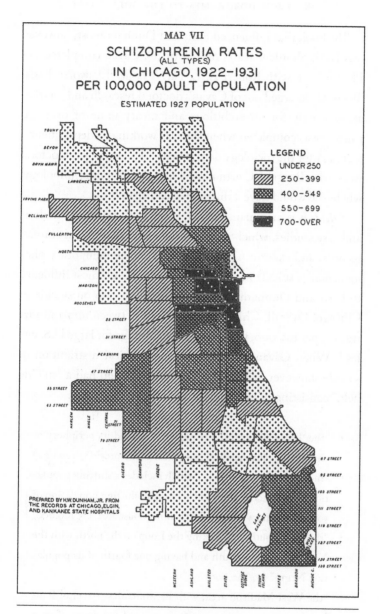

FIGURE 2.3 Chicago map.

Source: Robert E. L. Faris and H. Warren Dunham, *Mental Disorders in Urban Areas* (Chicago: University of Chicago Press, 1939). Permission provided by John Faris.

The book that influenced Faris and Dunham most, however, was Ruth Shonle Cavan's *Suicide* (1928). Cavan completed her PhD in 1926 with Robert E. L. Faris's father Ellsworth Faris. The book emerged out of Cavan's doctoral research and—rather astoundingly for an ambitious and meaty tome of over 350 pages—was completed when she was working as departmental secretary for the sociology department.[46] Following postdoctoral work with Burgess, Cavan moved into the field of criminology, where she would have a distinguished career.[47]

Suicide was an expansive text, using both statistical analysis and case studies, which relied on the use of diaries and coroner records, and examining the historical and contemporary phenomenon of suicide in many global contexts. Of most influence to Faris and Dunham, however, was the section on suicide in Chicago. Overall, Chicago's suicide rate between 1919 and 1921 was 15.3 per 100,000, which was about average for large U.S. cities.[48] When Cavan analyzed the geographical distribution of suicide, however, it became clear that Chicago had a "suicide belt," consisting of four regions with the highest rates:

- "the 'Loop' or central business district and its periphery of cheap hotels for men and sooty flats over stores" (87/100,000)
- "the Lower North Side . . . which includes a shifting population of unattached men and an equally shifting population of young men and women in the rooming house area" (35/100,000)
- "the Near South Side linking the Loop on the north with the Negro area to the south and having one fourth of its population Negro" (59/100,000)
- "the West Madison area, with its womanless street of flophouses, missions, cheap restaurants, and hundreds of men who drift in aimless, bleary-eyed abandon" (40/100,000)[49]

These rates mapped onto the "disorganized" regions of Chicago that Burgess had discussed in *The City*, mirrored Shaw's findings about the geographical distribution of delinquency, and would foreshadow Faris and Dunham's findings regarding mental disorders.[50]

Going beyond the bare statistics, Cavan delved into the characteristics of the regions that made up the "suicide belt." Investigating factors such as race, ethnicity, gender, quality and style of housing, divorce, prostitution, crime, drug and alcohol use, and even the number of pawnshops, she determined that suicide was "co-incident with disorganized communities." As she explained, "the low economic status . . . of the Americans in these areas contribute to their restlessness and mobility, and in the shifting population organized group life has no place." Other communities had more community control over antisocial behavior and "a certain amount of community consciousness and feeling of community ownership and pride." Disorganized communities did not "cause suicide," Cavan added, but were "symptoms of a general condition of personal and social disorganization which in the end may lead to suicide."[51] As with the previous Chicago School work on homelessness, ghettos, and delinquency, Cavan's work in situating suicide in the chaotic, disintegrated regions of the city would have a significant bearing on Faris and Dunham's own interpretations.

MAPPING MENTAL DISORDER

In contrast to the journey Nels Anderson took to get to the Chicago School, the path taken by one half of the duo that wrote *Mental Disorders in Urban Areas* could not have been smoother.

Robert Faris has been described as the "ultimate insider" in sociology.[52] He was the son of Ellsworth Faris, who had taken over from Albion Small in 1925 as chair of the sociology department. Born in Waco, Texas, Robert Faris and his family soon moved to Chicago, where his father, who had previously been a missionary in Africa and a minister, had enrolled in graduate studies, studying under George Herbert Mead (1863–1931). Robert Faris attended the University of Chicago's high school and then proceeded to the university itself in 1924 for his undergraduate, master's, and doctoral studies, which he would complete in 1931. In 1967, perhaps cementing his "insider" status, he wrote *Chicago Sociology 1920–1932*, a history of the Chicago School that overlapped neatly with his time there.[53] According to Faris's son, Jack, the spark that led to *Mental Disorders in Urban Areas* was "virtually accidental"; it also emphasized the debt the book owed to Cavan's *Suicide*.[54] Robert Park asked Faris about his planned dissertation, and Faris replied that he admired Cavan's work on suicide. Park immediately suggested that Faris do the same thing with mental disorder, and the project was born.[55] Jack Faris notes that his father's "apparently capricious" decision in selecting his dissertation topic actually reflected his pragmatic nature. Rather than "fussing about for months (or years, as is sometimes the case), he simply got on with it," completing his PhD a full decade before Dunham did.[56]

H. Warren Dunham may have not had quite the Chicago School upbringing that Faris had, but he still completed all three of his degrees at the University of Chicago, after transferring from the University of Nebraska, his home state, in 1926. Dunham would complete his BA in 1928 but took somewhat longer to complete his graduate studies, finishing his MA in 1935 and PhD in 1941, two years after the publication of *Mental Disorders in Urban Areas*. The delay was in part caused by Dunham's

difficulty in securing funding to complete his graduate studies, which began in 1930. He managed to find a job as a social
worker in 1931, however, and soon began working with homeless
men. Dunham discovered that some of these men attempted to
get committed to state hospitals because the meals and beds
were better than they could find on the street.[57] Burgess then
asked Dunham in late 1931 if he would work as a research assistant at the Elgin State Hospital, which funded the project, col-
lecting case data on first admissions. This would be a welcome
opportunity—he would receive room and board at the hospital
and fifty dollars a month—but meant that he would not begin
his PhD until 1938, by which time *Mental Disorder in Urban
Areas* was virtually finished. Dunham described his "ignorance
of psychiatry" as "colossal" when he started work at Elgin. He
would, however, take a class with the psychoanalyst and psychosomatic pioneer Franz Alexander (1891–1964) and proceeded
to read as many psychiatric textbooks as he could. Burgess then
brought Faris and Dunham together to produce a monograph
based on their research in late 1933. Funding was provided by
both the University of Chicago's Social Science Research Committee and the Illinois State Department of Public Welfare,
though Dunham described it as "infinitesimal." Dunham and
Faris had met previously as undergraduates while painting seats
at Stagg Stadium in Chicago, and they adjusted easily to collaborating.[58] While Dunham would concentrate on the empirical data, Faris contributed the sections on the theory of social
isolation.

Following their work together at the University of Chicago,
the careers of Faris and Dunham diverged. Faris, would spend
most of his career at the University of Washington (after teaching at Brown, Bryn Mawr, McGill, and Syracuse), where he
would serve as department chair for thirteen years. Although he

continued to study social psychology, his interests shifted from mental disorder to the study of ability and the sociology of institutions. He also served as president of the American Sociological Association in 1961—his presidential address made no reference to *Mental Disorders in Urban Areas*—and as part of a policy advisory group for the Johnson administration, where he advised on the environment, foreign policy, and issues related to life expectancy.[59] After the publication of *Mental Disorders in Urban Areas* in 1939, Faris would not do any more significant research on mental illness, though he would review books on the subject.[60]

In contrast, Dunham continued to write about the sociology of mental illness, though he would become hostile to community psychiatry by the 1960s.[61] In a review of his book *Sociological Theory and Mental Disorder* (1959), which brought together Dunham's writing on the subject since 1936, the sociologist Richard. A. Schermerhorn (1903–1991) even described him as the "Dean of American Social Psychiatry."[62] Dunham would spend most of his career (1940–1976) at Wayne State University in Detroit, where he taught both in the department of sociology and the faculty of medicine. After leaving Detroit, he worked until his death at SUNY Stony Brook, where he was a professor of sociology and psychiatry, further emphasizing his social psychiatry credentials.[63]

The project's starting point was simple: Where did adults admitted to Chicago psychiatric hospitals live before admission? Faris and Dunham admitted that they were not the first to tackle this question, citing attempts to plot the geographical distribution of mental disorder earlier in the twentieth century.[64] These included studies published in 1901 by Scotland's deputy commissioner for lunacy John Francis Sutherland (1854–1912) and in 1903 by William A. White, who became superintendent of

St. Elizabeth's Hospital in Washington, DC, that same year.[65] Sutherland asserted that while "indigency, pauperism, destitution, and delinquency" only afflicted 10 percent of the Scottish population, 80 percent of those in asylums were classified as "pauper lunatics." Among the reasons Sutherland cited for the apparent increase in lunacy were "modern life, with its unparalleled competition in every walk, abuse of alcohol and tea, errors of diet, &c."[66] For his part, White began his article by discussing how aspects of the physical environment, such as climate and weather conditions, had historically been considered to be important factors in mental health. As he described, "the 'depressing effects of heat' and the 'stimulating effects of cold' are common in our everyday conversation, and I believe the physical and mental characteristics of the different races of men are to some extent an expression of the effects of the climatic and geographic conditions under which they live." Continuing, White explained that his study was originally intended to investigate this relationship between the physical environment (including elevation, latitude, temperature, and humidity) and insanity. What he found, however, discounted such factors and instead pointed to the role of "mental stress, the results of the contact of man with man in the struggle for existence; in short, the results of that struggle itself as exemplified in civilization."[67] In particular, his study revealed that insanity was more common in regions of the United States that had been settled by Europeans for longer and, therefore, were more "civilized," crowded, and competitive, thus reflecting contemporary concerns about disorders such as neurasthenia.[68] White also echoed contemporary concerns about the high rates of "foreign born" people in asylums. In addition, he found that rates of insanity for Black Americans were higher in the North than in the South because when "the negro goes north and enters into active competition with the white, who is mentally his superior, he succumbs in the unequal struggle."[69] On occasion, Faris and Dunham also interpreted the rates of certain mental disorders using racialist assumptions, though typically the explanations they provided focused more on socioeconomic factors.

Although their methodology was similar to that of Sutherland and White, the influence of Burgess, Park, and other Chicago School sociologists would steer Faris and Dunham clear of explanations that were rooted in concerns about civilization, urbanization per se, racism, immigration, or, indeed, meteorology and the physical environment (despite Chicago being known as the Windy City).[70] Faris and Dunham began by examining admissions data in both public and private psychiatric hospitals in Chicago over the period 1922 to 1934. This amounted to 34,864 individuals (or approximately three thousand per year), of which 27,863 were admitted to state hospitals and 6,101 were admitted to eight of Chicago's largest private hospitals.[71] When the overall "rates of insanity" (both state and private hospitals) were plotted onto a map of Chicago that had been divided into sixty-eight communities, clear patterns emerged: the highest rates of insanity were to be found in Zone 1, the city's central business district (or Loop); the rates became lower toward the outskirts of the city.[72] During 1930–1931, for example, the Loop had a rate of 1,757 admissions per 100,000 adult population. In contrast, Kenwood, "a high class residential area" situated south of downtown on Lake Michigan, had a rate of 110/100,000.[73] The only exception to this pattern was the Lake Calumet region to the far south of Chicago, which had slightly higher rates, owing to the "deteriorated condition of that region."[74]

In an additional chapter, Faris and Dunham compared Chicago's distribution with that of Providence, Rhode Island.[75] Providence had been settled two hundred years before Chicago and was a much smaller city that had experienced slower rates of growth. It lacked the tremendous influx of Black Americans and European immigrants experienced by other northern cities but did have settled populations of French Canadians and Italians. Overall, Providence was "smaller, more stable, slower growing, and more orderly than Chicago" and experienced less "crime, vice, family disorganization, political corruption." Nevertheless, Providence demonstrated a similar, though less pronounced, geographical pattern of social disorganization to that of Chicago: poverty, low rents, delinquency, divorce, crime, and suicide were highest in the deteriorating city center and decreased toward the periphery. Similarly, Providence's rates of insanity—just like Chicago's—were highest in these disorganized neighborhoods, "the central business district and industrial, hobo, and rooming house area[s]."[76] While the authors admitted that more work on Providence was required, the initial findings supported the idea that mental disorder was most commonly found in deprived urban areas.

There was one crucial difference, however, in the raw data collected for Providence and Chicago. While the rates for Providence relied solely on state hospitals, Faris and Dunham relied on both state *and* private hospitals for their study of Chicago. When the rates for private and state hospitals were separated out, the picture became more complicated. Since state hospital admissions accounted for approximately 83 percent of all admissions (which was on par with the rest of the country), the distribution of state hospital admissions did not vary too much from that of the total. The geographical distribution changed, however, when the rates for private hospitals were viewed in isolation. Communities with high rates of admission to private hospitals were more scattered across the city. While the highest rates of admission to private hospitals were still in the Loop, further analysis revealed that the addresses recorded tended to be for "high-rent transient" hotels, rather than for rooming houses. This suggested—unsurprisingly—that patients admitted to private psychiatric facilities tended to be wealthier.[77]

The other major difference between the state and private hospitals emerged when Faris and Dunham examined the disorders with which patients were diagnosed. Despite the fact that private hospitals accounted for only 17 percent of the total number of patients, they took in half of the total number of patients who would be diagnosed with manic-depressive psychosis. Because of this, the prevalence of specific diagnoses varied considerably between the state and private hospitals, with manic-depressive patients accounting for only 4 percent of the patients in state hospitals but 20 percent of patients in private hospitals. In addition, the percentage of patients diagnosed with "true paranoia, psychoneuroses, and without psychosis" tended to be higher in private hospitals. In turn, state hospitals had a higher percentage of patients with "organic and toxic psychoses," that is, where there was (respectively) evidence of brain abnormality (such as tertiary syphilis, brain injury, or pellagra) or drug or alcohol abuse.[78] To dig deeper into these diagnostic discrepancies, Faris and Dunham examined the geographical distribution of specific diagnoses. These included schizophrenia (which was further broken up into the following types: paranoid, hebephrenic, catatonic, simple, and unclassified), manic-depressive psychosis, alcoholic psychosis, drug addiction, general paralysis (tertiary syphilis), and old-age psychosis. When the distribution of these specific disorders was plotted, intriguing patterns emerged.

Faris and Dunham began their discussion of schizophrenia by noting that there was "little agreement as to its nature and causes."[79] This was highly problematic, since schizophrenia accounted for between 25 and 40 percent of first admissions in U.S. psychiatric hospitals. Their findings suggested, however, that more attention should be paid to socioeconomic factors. When the rates of schizophrenia were geographically distributed, it became clear that it, as with the overall rate of mental disorder, was most likely to be found in the most socially disorganized regions of the city. In these communities, the rates peaked at 1,195/100,000 in the Loop and 1,125/100,000 in Hobohemia. In contrast, Rogers Park, a "high rent apartment district" on the banks of Lake Michigan in the far northeast of the city, had a rate of 110/100,000, and the Gold Coast, the upscale neighborhood of luxury apartments and mansions to the north of downtown, had a rate of 119/100,000.[80] The mean and median rates for the entire city of 289/100,000 and 322/100,000, respectively, underlined how schizophrenia was clustered densely in a small number of deprived communities and not common elsewhere. These schizophrenia hotspots included the Loop and the rooming house districts that surrounded it, as well as "the first-settlement immigrant communities near the center of the city and in the deteriorated parts of the Negro area immediately south of the central business district."[81] Overall, foreign-born and Black Chicagoans had the highest rates of schizophrenia. But while the rate in this Black area was 662/100,000, the rates found in the two other predominantly Black communities were much lower, at 470/100,000 and 410/100,000. Moreover, the highest rates in predominantly Black areas were not found in Black Americans but in white foreign-born residents. Native-born whites also had high rates of schizophrenia in these areas. In turn, Black Americans had higher rates if they did not reside in Black areas. This suggested that some other explanation than "racial tendency" was responsible.[82] Such an interpretation went against a prevailing view that the Black psyche somehow differed from that of white Americans.[83] Overall, the data demonstrated constantly "high rates in the extremely disorganized parts of the city."

Faris and Dunham were cognizant, however, that psychiatric hospitals also differentiated schizophrenia into separate subtypes.[84] Paranoid schizophrenia, which was described as being characterized by "delusions of persecution and grandeur" as well as auditory hallucinations, accounted for nearly 60 percent of all schizophrenia cases. As such, its geographical distribution was similar to that of the total for all cases, with the most cases occurring in the deteriorated regions of the city. The difference in rates was starkest in the Loop (522/100,000) and the adjacent Gold Coast (22/100,000).[85] While the rates for the Gold Coast slightly complicated Burgess's concentric zone theory (in that social disorganization became less pronounced toward the outskirts of the city), they nevertheless strengthened the argument connecting mental disorder with deteriorating communities.

The distribution of hebephrenic schizophrenia, which was described as being typified by more random hallucinations and delusions; "silly, manneristic, and untidy" behavior; and "absurd and bizarre ideas," resembled that of paranoid schizophrenia. The lowest rates were found in Rogers Park in the far northeast of the city (36/100,000) and the highest in the Loop (568/100,000). The numbers of simple (marked by "gradual falling off of interest in the external world") and unclassified schizophrenia were much smaller than the other subtypes but also followed the same geographical distribution. There was, however, a pronounced difference in the distribution of the final subtype: catatonic schizophrenia. Patients with catatonic schizophrenia, which consisted of about 10 percent of total cases, were described as often being in a state of "excitement or stupor." Unlike the other subtypes, the Loop did not have the highest rates of catatonic schizophrenia. In fact, its rate for the subtype was among the lowest (24/100,000).[86] By comparison, the rate for the Gold Coast was 15/100,000. The highest rates were in the immigrant areas, peaking at 177/100,000 in a community in the southern part of the Near West Side, but not always in communities closest to the center, thus bucking the overall trend for schizophrenia and mental disorder more generally.

The demographic profile of catatonic schizophrenia patients provided clues for these discrepancies. Unlike the other subtypes of schizophrenia, catatonic patients were more likely to be female than male (at a ratio of 100:82). Those with catatonic schizophrenia were also younger than those diagnosed with the other subtypes; only 9 percent of males and 12 percent of females so diagnosed were over forty. Compared to patients diagnosed with the other schizophrenic subtypes, they enjoyed more stable lifestyles, for example, being more likely to own their own home and less likely to live in a rooming house or a hotel. Black Americans were more likely to develop catatonic schizophrenia than other subtypes, especially the paranoid subtype. Faris and Dunham suspected that their "culturally impoverished backgrounds as compared to the whites" prevented them from having "the heritage and experience in order to construct the elaborate mental system which characterizes the paranoid reaction."[87] This instance of disregarding the cultural value of the Black experience is one of the few explicitly racist assumptions present in *Mental Disorders in Urban Areas*.[88] Overall, however, they could not explain precisely why catatonic schizophrenia had a different geographical distribution than other subtypes. The rates became even more confusing with manic-depressive psychosis.

The distribution of most of the other mental disorders mapped out by Faris and Dunham would share the same pattern as noncatatonic schizophrenia. Admissions for alcohol psychoses,

drug-related psychoses, and tertiary syphilis all tended to clus-
ter around the Loop. The cases of senile psychoses were somewhat more varied in distribution, but the highest rates still clustered near Chicago's downtown and were associated with
poverty. With manic-depressive psychosis, however, this pattern broke down significantly. Whereas most of the maps in
Mental Disorders in Urban Areas shared the same pattern of a
black patch (representing high admissions) around the downtown radiating out in ever-lighter shades toward the edges of
the city, the map for manic-depressive psychosis showed no dis-
cernible pattern. Overall, rates throughout the city were low,
with less skewing toward the rooming-house districts than as
was the case for other psychoses. There were high rates in a few
of the communities in the center of the city, but some peripheral
areas also had high rates, despite other psychoses not being
commonly found there. Moreover, no pattern was found when
the cases were split into predominantly manic and depressive
types. For the manic type, the rates were highest in the Loop
(10.23/100,000), much like other psychoses, but the community
with the third-highest rate was Rogers Park (6.23/100,000),
which had the lowest rates for other psychoses.[89] The distribution was even more random for depressed cases: high rates
could be found throughout the city. While the highest rate
(7.4/100,000) was to be found in the Near West Side, just to the
west of the Chicago River, Garfield Ridge, in the west of the
city, had the second-highest rate (7.05/100,000).

As with catatonic schizrenia, patients diagnosed with
manic-depressive psychosis tended to have different demographic
and socioeconomic characteristics from those diagnosed with
other psychoses. Women were more likely to be diagnosed
with manic-depressive psychosis, at a ratio of 100:68, which was
typical for the United States generally. Those diagnosed were

also more likely to come from neighborhoods where there were higher levels of educational achievement and that had a "higher cultural level." They were equally likely, as noted earlier, to have been admitted to a private hospital as to a public one, also indicative of a higher income. Overall, according to the investigators, there was "a definite tendency for manic-depressive cases to be drawn from higher economic and social levels of the city."[90] Why was this the case?

It was one thing to map mental illness according to admission data. It was quite another to explain what lay underneath these rates. This was, as Faris and Dunham suggested, not only a "complicated task" but also "a separate problem" requiring different methods.[91] In his introduction, Burgess also warned that it was important to distinguish between the "factual findings" of the study and "interpretations of these findings."[92] Nevertheless, Faris and Dunham did attempt to explain why manic-depressive psychoses tended to be found in more socioeconomically stable communities. So long as the classification and diagnoses of such disorders were accurate (they were not, but this was put aside),[93] the rates suggested that "biological inheritance" was more significant than social factors. Faris and Dunham argued that precipitating social factors were present, but they were to be found across "all social and economic levels of life." These had to do with the "interplay of personality and psychological factors of family relationships and intimate personal contacts."[94] Since schizophrenia was associated with communities where individuals were more socially isolated, there was less opportunity for such relationships to develop. Beyond these initial hypotheses, however, the "random" pattern of manic-depressive psychosis remained a mystery.

Faris and Dunham were in more comfortable territory in explaining the geographical distribution of schizophrenia. With the partial exception of catatonic schizophrenia, its distribution mapped onto Burgess's zonal depiction of the city. Moreover, Burgess's description of the socioeconomic features of Zones I–V helped explain why this was the case. Essentially, "extended isolation of the person produces the abnormal traits of behavior and mentality."[95] Hobohemia, the rooming-house district, and the most deteriorated slum areas, as Faris had explained in an earlier article, were characterized by heterogeneity and mobility, factors that "greatly increase the cultural isolation of the person, and . . . produce breeding grounds for schizophrenia."[96] To illustrate, at the end of *Mental Disorders in Urban Areas* Faris briefly discussed three individuals diagnosed with schizophrenia and subsequently hospitalized. These three were among 101 patients Faris interviewed.[97] They included a Jewish boy whose neighborhood was "invaded" by Black Americans; a young Czechoslovakian woman who failed to learn English; and a "chubby, pink-cheeked boy with reddish hair worn in curls" who was "teased as a 'sissy.'"[98] It is worth emphasizing that Faris and Dunham argued that it was the capacity of the slum to isolate individuals that was paramount.[99] As Faris would stress elsewhere, the concentrations of mental illness in certain communities could not be explained alone by "density of population near the centers, poverty of the people, [or] racial and national characteristics."[100] Within these disorganized sections of the city, however, social isolation meant that "many persons are unable to derive sufficient mental nourishment from the normal sources to achieve a satisfactorily conventional organization of their world . . . resulting in a confused, frustrated, and chaotic personality. . . . It is just this type of unintelligible behavior which becomes recognized as mental disorder."[101]

So what was to be done about this pathological isolation? What steps could be taken to *prevent* such disorders? Despite the disturbing picture they—and their maps—depicted of pathological inner-city communities, Faris and Dunham refrained from making anything resembling policy recommendations. As the next three chapters demonstrate, other social psychiatrists—both social scientists and psychiatrists—would similarly stay silent. Part of their hesitation was likely because psychiatric reviewers had criticized early drafts of their monograph and, in particular, its social isolation theory.[102] It also, however, reflected one side of a debate within sociology at the time about the degree to which sociologists should become politically active or even involved in a "humanitarian" way with their subjects. On the one hand were those sociologists, starting with Albion Small, who stressed the need for objectivity. These included Robert Park, who according to Faris's history of the Chicago School, "directly attacked the humanitarian attitude when it appeared in sociologists. More than once he drove students to anger or tears by growling such reproofs as 'You're another one of those damned do-gooders.'"[103] On the other hand were Louis Wirth and Ernest Burgess, who were both involved in the mental hygiene and child guidance movements, with Wirth advocating for the development of a "clinical sociology."[104] In his introduction, for example, Burgess argued that if *Mental Disorders in Urban Areas* demonstrated that "if social conditions are actually precipitating factors in causation, control of conditions making for stress and strain in industry and society will become a chief objective of a constructive program of mental hygiene."[105] These words suggested that sociology had the potential to and, indeed, should inform public policy and, potentially, political change.

Faris and Dunham, however, did not discuss their study's practical implications. For Faris, the more senior of the pair, "an essential element of the discipline of sociology was keeping it as clear as possible away from emotion and politics."[106] As such, according to his son, Jack, sociologists should "avoid topics in which they had a particular personal passion."[107] Moreover, Faris expressed privately the need to be "careful" and "tentative" about what could be inferred from both the data on manic-depressive psychosis *and* schizophrenia. An example of this can be found in a 1964 interview in *US News and World Report* that was undertaken when he was serving on a Johnson administration advisory board. Answering a question about "population improvement," Faris warned that the rapid technological advancement underway would require higher levels of education. There was a need for "much change unless we want to tolerate a very large, miserable, and useless population at the bottom."[108] When asked what was to be done, however, Faris argued that, while social scientists had been examining the issue in detail, they were not ready to articulate the "formulation of a specific program." The population was "improvable," but how this was to be achieved was unknown. This was despite the fact that Faris had been researching the sociology of ability for thirty years and was of the opinion that, much like mental illness, genius was made, not born.[109] Faris's own work, in other words, indicated that it was possible to change society for the better, but he was reluctant to say how.

Dunham continued to research the ecology of mental disorder, focusing in particular on schizophrenia, delinquency, war neuroses, and methodological issues related to the subject. But in his subsequent publications he was also unwilling to explore the policy implications of social psychiatry and, in addition, expressed some skepticism about the relationship between social factors and mental disorder. In a 1948 article entitled "Social Psychiatry," for example, he did not make any mention of how sociological investigations could help prevent mental illness or inform policy in any other way.[110] Dunham was much more concerned about the methods used by researchers to explore mental illness, rather than the implications of such studies. An example of this can be found in a 1961 article where he lampooned the way in which the sociologist Robert M. Frumkin interpreted his findings related to occupation and mental disorder in Ohio.[111] After describing Frumkin's conclusion that "low prestige occupations have the highest rates of first admissions for the major mental disorders" as "hardly startling," Dunham criticized him for "barg[ing] joyously ahead . . . [and] proceed[ing] to all kinds of generalizations about man in American society which are not only dubious in general but also . . . should be boxed in by many qualifications."[112] In the same article, Dunham criticized an extended review of Hollingshead and Redlich's *Social Class and Mental Illness* (1958) that began by stating that the study "may well have a marked effect on the future practice of psychiatry."[113] The review, Dunham suggested, should have focused more on the study's shortcomings. He concluded his article by inferring that the link between social structure and mental disorder was "highly inconclusive."[114] At the heart of these doubts was a "sixty-four thousand dollar question": Were the differences in the geographical distribution of mental disorder attributable to "differences in the very texture of social life" or other factors, such as the selection of cases in particular studies, the mobility of patients, "statistical manipulations of the data," or a combination of these factors?[115] If this question could be definitively answered, a path to prevention could be forged. But, for Dunham at least, it had not been answered yet.

SOCIOLOGY AND BEYOND

As Dunham's concerns suggested, both he and Faris were aware that their study was open to criticism. Potential weaknesses included the possibility that the distribution patterns were attributable to chance, that wealthier individuals with mental disorders were being cared for in their homes and were not included in the hospital statistics, that the transient nature of some areas (for example, Hobohemia) undermined the validity of their findings, and—most importantly—that the mentally disordered were not "made" in disorganized communities but merely had drifted there.[116] But was this enough to undermine their study's influence among psychiatrists, sociologists, and others researching psychiatric epidemiology? Dunham reflected later that psychiatrists were not initially enthusiastic about *Mental Disorders in Urban Areas*. In a 1953 *AJP* article, he claimed that the study was "subject to violent attack by the psychiatrists and every possible objection was raised in order to explain the findings."[117] An analysis of the book's reviews, however, reveals more of a polarizing effect. While some reviewers were dismissive, others—including some psychiatrists—were fulsome in their praise. All reviewers agreed that the project was highly novel, including the sociologist John H. Mueller (1895–1965), who stated that "this little study, painstaking in its execution but modest in its conclusions, is the first serious attempt to take the patient out of the clinic and study him in the full light of day in his natural habitat."[118]

In terms of hostile psychiatrists, Dunham might have been thinking of the *AJP* review by the neurologist and psychiatrist Abraham Myerson (1881–1948), then working at Boston State Hospital. It would be inaccurate describe Myerson's review as particularly scathing, however. Indeed, he ended it by stating that any "psychiatrist who is eager for the advancement of psychiatry will make this book a part of his library and will welcome these sociologists and the discipline they represent as his allies in the campaign for the conquest of mental disease."[119] But

Myerson did reject that the book had much etiological significance. In examining rates of schizophrenia in Hobohemia, he stated bluntly that "there was no etiologic relationship." Hobos were simply disproportionately likely to be schizophrenic, and they congregated in Hobohemia. In other words, "Flies congregate where there is molasses, but the molasses does not create the flies." Similarly, he argued that a paranoid schizophrenic, in seeking isolation, would choose to live in rooming house districts in order to be "as isolated as a great city will permit him to be. . . . On his way to the hospital for mental diseases, the paranoid reaches the rooming house as his next to last stop."[120] Although Myerson did not use the term, he was effectively describing "downward drift," the most common criticism of Faris and Dunham's work.

Another psychiatrist, who was interestingly commissioned to review the book for *AJS*, wondered what was lost from the authors' statistical approach. After admitting that "no psychiatrist is competent to assay such a piece of work," James S. Plant (1890–1947), director of the Essex County Juvenile Clinic in Newark, New Jersey, stated that he would have liked to have seen more mention of the patients represented in the book's graphs and tables. As he described, "It hardly seems possible that such a painstaking piece of work could be done on so many people and yet yield so little knowledge about any one of them."[121] Plant's charge was slightly unfair, as Faris and Dunham had included a few pages at the end of their book describing the 101 patients that Faris had interviewed. Possibly with Plant's comments in mind, Faris would also write an article focusing in depth on one individual patient a few years later.[122] More generally, however, Plant's concern about the individual patient reflected a growing trend in psychiatric literature, influenced especially by the emergence of psychoanalysis, to focus on extended case studies exploring the life histories of a small number of patients. This style of psychiatric reportage would endure well into the 1970s before receding in the face of the statistical approach favored by biological psychiatrists. Within social psychiatry, however, efforts were made to balance the presentation of statistical data with case studies of individual patients. As discussed in chapter 5, this was particularly so with the Stirling County Study but can also be seen in other projects.

Other reviewers touched more squarely on heredity. The University of Rochester psychologist James D. Page (1910–1984) acknowledged that the book was the "first extensive ecological study of mental disease in an urban area," before downplaying its significance. After questioning the validity of their statistics, Page charged Faris and Dunham with being "either completely unacquainted with or conveniently forgetful of basic psychiatric facts," namely, that the "strong hereditary basis of schizophrenia and manic depressive psychoses" had been "definitely established."[123] In closing, he hoped that subsequent studies would be "founded on psychiatric facts rather than sociological bias." Such comments demonstrated that, although mental hygiene, child guidance, and the social sciences had done much to emphasize the social origins of mental disorder, many clinicians and researchers stressed heredity nonetheless.

Still others, however, were full of praise. The Hungarian-French ethnologist and psychoanalyst Georges Devereux (1908–1985), who worked for many years in the United States, was almost embarrassing in his acclaim:

> This superlatively brilliant book bids fair to set a new standard for research . . . in the field of sociological-psychiatric correlations. It is not a book to be reviewed, but read and re-read. For

the first time perhaps a *professional* insight into sociological factors has been drawn upon to investigate ecological factors in psychiatry. Not one sociological lead has been omitted or slighted.
Even in this day of torrential output in this field the authors must
be commended for their solid grounding in psychiatry. . . . Their
conclusions seem fully justified . . . if anything they are too
restrained.[124]

Devereux went on to dismiss the suggestion that psychotics had
"drifted" into poor areas and stated that the book amounted to
a "warning to certain champions of eugenics . . . [and to] serve
as further proof of the theories of Professor Franz Boas on the
influence of environment on physical constitution." And if that
was not enough, he concluded by stating that anyone who had
not read the book had "missed one of the significant contributions to psychiatry and sociology published in recent years."
Other physicians echoed—though not so vociferously—that
both sociologists *and* psychiatrists would gain much from the
book and the new approach it represented.[125]

More important than the initial response found in reviews was
the longer-term impact of *Mental Disorders in Urban Areas* on
subsequent interdisciplinary epidemiological research. As early
as 1940, for instance, mental hygiene, psychology, psychiatry, and
sociology textbooks were all mentioning the importance of Faris
and Dunham's research.[126] In research terms, the most immediate response was spurred by Burgess and took the form of follow-up studies in other Midwestern cities, including Kansas
City, Milwaukee, Omaha, Peoria, and St. Louis, that followed
Faris and Dunham's approach. On the one hand, the findings
of these studies tended to support what Faris and Dunham had
found. On the other, they also faced some of the challenges that

Faris and Dunham had faced regarding the accuracy of diagnosis, the adequacy of using only hospitalized patients, and the fact that the lives and experiences of individual patients got somewhat lost in the mass of statistical data.[127] And, as with Faris and Dunham, little was said in these projects about how to translate their conclusions into mental health policy.

Downward drift was also mentioned in these studies. Faris and Dunham had largely dismissed the possibility that schizophrenics "drifted" into deteriorated areas of the city because many of the patients they studied were too young to have done so. In a 1946 article, Dunham argued that the drift theory was "analogous to an earlier biological explanation for city slums: namely, that it is not the slums that make slum people but slum people that make the slums." He then contended that downward drift could not apply to immigrant communities with high rates of mental disorder because they did not drift there "because of personal instability." Taking the case of those who developed catatonic schizophrenia, Dunham argued that they represented "sensitive, self-conscious, and timid personalities who find it difficult to come to terms with a type of social life that is terrifically harsh, intensely individualistic, highly competitive, extremely crude, and often violently brutal." In other words, the conditions in these communities were not pathological to all, but they could potentially be damaging to vulnerable individuals. Dunham admitted that downward drift might apply more to Hobohemia and rooming house districts but stressed that other socioeconomic factors played a key role. Overall, he dismissed drift theory as "an attempt to annihilate the significance of ecological findings in much the same fashion as certain persons during the thirties tried to dismiss the depression by explaining the loss of a job on the basis of a person's neurotic makeup or emotional instability."[128] Such thinking supported the theory that mental illness was "born" and not "made," thus implying that preventive interventions would be ineffective. It also drew on President Herbert Hoover's conception of "rugged individualism" and the notion that success in life was purely down to the individual. Society could not, nor should not, play a significant role.[129] Whether one gravitated to such explanations, therefore, depended significantly on one's political leanings.

Discussions of downward drift continued nonetheless, and subsequent projects investigated its possibility more thoroughly.[130] Dunham would also reverse his position on the subject somewhat by the 1960s.[131] Although some of these studies provided evidence for downward drift, other high-profile studies, including Hollingshead and Redlich's study of New Haven, downplayed the theory.[132] One focusing on Buffalo, for instance, drew attention instead to the "psychologic strains imposed by low income with the concomitant struggle to obtain the necessities of living, the fear of unemployment, the lack of job satisfaction, the overcrowded and inadequate housing, the restricted educational and recreational opportunities, and the low social status." The authors also suggested that "relative drift" might also have resulted in a concentration of schizophrenic patients in certain areas; in other words, "schizophrenics remain in the lower quartiles while the rest of the population moves upwards."[133] It was also likely that in places like Hobohemia both social causation and downward drift occurred. Nevertheless, by the 1970s and 1980s, epidemiological evidence indicated that, even if downward drift did exist, socioeconomic conditions were a major factor in both causing and exacerbating mental illness.[134] By this time, however, most of the momentum behind social psychiatry and preventive mental health had disappeared.

CONCLUSION: A FITFUL START

In 1948, Dunham described how links between sociologists and psychiatrists, as represented by the field of "social psychiatry," had thus far emerged "fitfully."[135] As discussed in chapter 1, social scientists and psychiatrists, as well as those involved in mental hygiene and child guidance, gradually became aware of how they might work together to better understand mental illness. Although this courtship could be described as somewhat coy during the first part of the twentieth century, it would not take long for major, well-funded, and genuinely interdisciplinary projects to emerge. These studies, influenced by Faris and Dunham, would contribute to the community mental health movement and the end of the asylum era. But they would also be adversely affected by some of the problems that bedeviled Faris and Dunham and were subsequently highlighted by their critics.

By the 1950s, for example, heredity was less likely to be suggested as an explanation for mental illness. But by then there was also even more skepticism about the accuracy of psychiatric diagnoses. This was especially important given the different geographical distributions that Faris and Dunham had found for different psychoses. The overall pattern might have shown that mental disorder was associated with deprived communities, but the data for specific disorders, especially manic depression, complicated matters. Underlying these figures was the assumption that the diagnoses were accurate. Whereas Faris and Dunham admitted that their findings were weakened by diagnostic unreliability, by the late 1950s, the borderland between madness and sanity itself, influenced by radical thinkers ranging from R. D. Laing (1927–1989) to Thomas Szasz (1920–2012), had become blurry.[136] As the NIMH psychiatrist Leonard J. Duhl (1926–2019) would explain at a meeting of the "Space Cadets" (see chapter 4) in 1956, the definition of mental health was "a thing that is very, very difficult to answer and I would suppose that if we went around the room that we would get many, many different definitions of what mental health is and most of them, I think, would be based upon our own personal prejudices and beliefs and attitudes and the way we were brought up."[137] Determining a baseline for what was considered mental illness, therefore, posed a challenge that subsequent investigators attempted to overcome in various ways and to varying degrees of success.

Similarly, and much like Faris and Dunham, later social psychiatry projects would also focus intensively on the methodological strengths and weaknesses of their research. Given the methodological debates that surrounded Faris and Dunham's study, this inclination was understandable. It is possible, however, that this propensity to overanalyze the inner workings of their studies prevented such social psychiatrists from spending sufficient time contemplating the policy and, indeed, societal implications of their findings. Certainly, a delicate balance had to be struck between admitting that more research was needed and taking what was broadly understood to be accurate from the research and formulating preventive mental health strategies. Faris and Dunham refrained from making any such recommendations whatsoever, and the social psychiatrists that followed them were also tentative. As Faris's son Jack suggested, other, more "reckless" researchers might have made more of the data produced by his father and Dunham.[138] But that was neither Faris's nor Dunham's style. They, as with many of their successors, opted instead for a cautious, systematic, and stepwise approach, expecting that the slow accretion of evidence over time would make their case for them. The unexpected findings that their research had thrown up likely reinforced this reticence even further.

Seventy years after the publication of *Mental Disorders in Urban Areas*, not all that much had changed in this regard. In 2010, I traveled to Chicago to a conference entitled "The Social Determinants of Mental Health: From Awareness to Action" and hosted by the Adler School of Professional Psychology (now called Adler University).[139] That the conference was described as the first of its kind instantly betrayed a distinct lack of awareness of how "ecological" or social explorations of mental health had deep, historical roots that had could be traced to Chicago itself, the first "case study" of U.S. social science.[140] Historical understanding, however, was not the only thing lacking. Although there was considerable discussion of how social factors could affect mental health (the "Awareness" bit) and the need to gather more such evidence, there was scant attention to the "Action" dimension, in other words, what should be done about these social determinants. This was even though the conference occurred at the height of the credit crunch, when the socioeconomic and psychological damage caused by reckless bankers was being intensely felt not only in the United States but around the world.

On the final day of the conference, there was a roundtable featuring—among others—David Satcher, the former surgeon general. While there was a great deal of agreement that *something* should be done, there was precious little discussion of *what* this was to be. Toward the end of the session, a Black social worker stood up and spoke. She praised the august panel for their words but said that when she returned to work on Monday, nothing would have changed. Moreover, she doubted that politicians or policy makers would have the courage to enact the sort of political and social changes that would make a difference. She was warmly applauded as she headed back to her seat, but there was an underlying tension. Was she right? Would anything ever be done? Hobohemia and the rooming house districts that featured so prominently in the work of the Chicago School may have disappeared, but the social problems affecting the city's residents—especially the city's Black residents—had not.

3

SWAMP YANKEES AND PROPER
NEW HAVENERS

I can't pay no doctor bill.
(but Whitey's on the Moon)
—Gil Scott-Heron

On February 5, 1963, President John F. Kennedy gave a speech that would transform the provision of mental health care in the United States.[1] His "Special Message to the Congress on Mental Illness and Mental Retardation" began by heralding the progress made in tackling "the major diseases of the body." Although physical diseases were "beginning to give ground," "the public understanding, treatment and prevention of mental disabilities have not made comparable progress." This was despite the enormous financial, social, and emotional burden mental disorders placed on individuals, families, and society. At any moment, eight hundred thousand Americans were committed to "social quarantine" in "antiquated, vastly overcrowded," and "unhappy mental hospitals," where 1.5 million were treated annually at a cost of $2.4 billion. "A bold new approach" was required, one that prioritized prevention. The first step was to "seek out the causes of mental illness and retardation and eradicate them. Here, more than any other area, 'an ounce of prevention is worth more than a pound of cure.'" It was especially important "to eliminate or correct the harsh environmental conditions which are often associated with mental retardation and illness."[2]

Kennedy's speech was described as the "Magna Carta" of community mental health.[3] It spearheaded the passage of the Community Mental Health Act on October 31, 1963, three weeks before his assassination. As its formal title—the Mental Retardation Facilities and Community Mental Health Center Construction Act—specified, the act paid for the construction of nearly eight hundred of such centers between 1963 and 1980. After his death, an amendment was passed to pay also for the staffing of CMHCs. As with mental hygiene and child guidance clinics, CMHCs were staffed by multidisciplinary teams, including psychiatrists, social workers, psychiatric nurses, psychologists, and sometimes—as discussed in the second half of this chapter—indigenous paraprofessionals or nonprofessional mental health aides. In comparison to the hierarchical structure of an asylum, CMHCs were meant to be more democratic in terms of how power and knowledge were held and exercised. Such thinking was fueled in part by the findings of the JCMIH, a six-year project that spurred the 1963 act.[4] One recommendation found in the JCMIH's final report, *Action for Mental Health* (1961), was that different disciplines and professions (ranging from nurses and social workers to clergy and teachers) could perform therapeutic roles.[5] An important rationale for this suggestion was simply to meet the staffing needs of CMHCs, which, according to *Action for Mental Health*, should serve catchment areas of fifty thousand people.[6] But it also reflected an emerging notion that not only psychiatrists could contribute to the fight against mental illness.

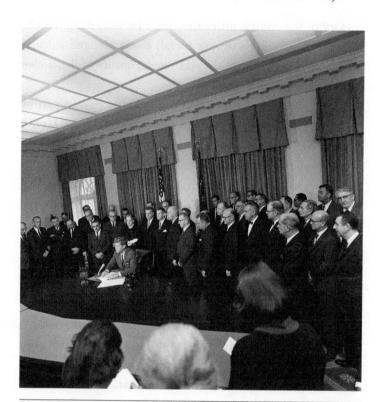

FIGURE 3.1 Kennedy signing the Community Mental Health Act.

Source: John F. Kennedy Library, ST-490-2-63, Stoughton, Cecil W. (Cecil William), 1920–2008, White House Photographs, John F. Kennedy Presidential Library and Museum.

Kennedy's emphasis on prevention was heavily influenced by social psychiatry. After World War II, a series of groundbreaking studies emerged that explored the relationship between socioeconomic factors and mental illness. Such projects often involved large interdisciplinary research teams consisting of both social scientists and psychiatrists and employing innovative methodologies. Their approach included digging deeply into the history of the communities they were investigating, resulting in rich portrayals of how social, economic, and cultural change affected community cohesiveness, quality of life, and— ultimately—mental health.

Many of these projects would be funded at least in part by NIMH, which was created as part of the National Mental Health Act of 1946 (it commenced operations in 1949) and in the wake of the momentum psychiatry had built during World War II. The Community Mental Health Act signified the first time that the federal government would intervene significantly in mental health, which had previously been left to individual states.[7] One of the act's chief objectives was prevention, but it was evident that significantly more research was required in order to inform the creation of preventive mental health policies. According to a 1948 article by NIMH's founding director, Robert H. Felix, and the sociologist Raymond V. Bowers (1907–1998), the research program would be "a fifty-year quest" geared toward discovering "the most economical and efficient methods of preventing the wasting of human resources."[8] This quest, Felix and Bowers stressed, would also be an interdisciplinary one, involving both psychiatrists and social scientists.

Felix and Bowers explained that while the relevance of the social environment to mental illness was "no longer in serious question," more work was needed to show how these "socioenvironmental factors" affected "the symptomology and psychodynamics of mental disorders."[9] The epidemiology of mental illness, in other words, remained poorly understood, especially as it related to socioenvironmental factors. They suggested that the social sciences were already yielding some hypotheses, leading on from Faris and Dunham's pioneering research, but these were often speculative. Fortunately, psychiatrists were increasingly willing to collaborate with social scientists, taking advantage of NIMH funding to do so.

With regards to etiology, Felix and Bowers argued that clinicians had been "too busy looking at the 'trees,'" while "social scientists have been primarily interested in the 'forest.'"[10] What was required were "socio-clinical studies" of both the mentally ill and healthy, studies of personality and its breakdown in different cultural groups, analyses of data found in pediatric and psychiatric clinics, studies of trauma and adjustment, and laboratory studies of "specific personality mechanisms."[11] Social scientists could also contribute to treatment, especially with respect to the social conditions in mental hospitals.[12] They were also crucial in achieving the "ultimate" yet "difficult objective" of prevention.[13] For instance, social scientists could help design and evaluate community-centered social programs, such as Chicago's Back of the Yards Neighborhood Council, founded by Joseph Meegan (1911–1994) and Saul Alinsky (1909–1972) in 1939.[14] Such programs were thought to promote mental health by reducing social problems and improving social integration, outcomes that were crucial to the "large-scale attack" on mental illness.[15]

Felix and Bowers's article effectively amounted to a call for NIMH-funded social psychiatry studies. One of the first such projects was a ten-year study focusing on New Haven, Connecticut, that initially involved the psychiatrists Frederick C. Redlich and Bertram H. Roberts (1921–1955) and the sociologists August B. Hollingshead and Jerome K. Myers (1921–2001), all based at Yale.[16] The project would culminate in two books: *Social Class and Mental Illness: A Community Study* (1958), by Hollingshead and Redlich (the senior researchers on the project), and *Family and Class Dynamics in Mental Illness* (1959), by Roberts and Myers.[17] As the volumes' titles indicated, the study's focus was on the role of class in the epidemiology and treatment of mental illness.

The first half of this chapter explores the development, methodology, and interpretations of the New Haven Study. In particular, I address how the concepts of class and inequality functioned on multiple levels within the study. On the one hand, the project used class as the primary lens through which mental illness in New Haven was analyzed. Hollingshead and Redlich fleshed out what they meant by class in detail, using two chapters to chart the evolution of the class structure in the city from 1638 (when it was founded by English Puritans) to the 1950s. Central to their analysis was their Index of Social Position, which divided New Haveners into five levels. Their overarching conclusion was that those at the lower end of the class structure were more likely to succumb to mental illness. On the other hand, it is evident that the privileged class status of the researchers (white, highly educated, and working at an Ivy League university) also influenced how the findings were interpreted. Those occupying the lower tiers of the index were often "othered," not merely representing members of a lower class but a different type of people altogether.[18] The findings, interpretations, and recommendations of the New Haven Study with respect to inequality and mental health, therefore, need to be assessed with the class dynamics of the study itself in mind.

The second half of the chapter demonstrates how similar issues of inequality affected the functioning of the CMHCs. Using Lincoln Hospital Mental Health Services (LHMHS) in the South Bronx as a case study, I examine how tensions related to class, race, and ethnicity hampered attempts to democratize mental health services and foster a more preventive approach to community mental health care.[19] As with many other CMHCs, LHMHS employed so-called indigenous mental health workers.

Such workers were from the local community and lacked formal training in mental health. What they offered, however, was local knowledge of housing, welfare, education, and other facets of community life, as well as the ability to translate (often literally) what the center's psychiatrists were attempting to communicate to patients and their families. Over time, however, disputes emerged between the indigenous paraprofessionals and the psychiatrists at LHMHS about working conditions, role delineation, decision making, and whose expertise really mattered.

The issue of inequality within social psychiatry theory and practice, therefore, was complex. The creation of CMHCs was in part an attempt to deal with inequalities identified by social psychiatrists in both the epidemiology and treatment of mental illness. But conflicts related to class, race, and ethnicity within the structure of the CMHCs themselves showed how such ideals only stretched so far when actually applied. If psychiatrists—even those choosing to work in community psychiatry—were unwilling to facilitate the development of more egalitarian working environments within CMHCs, how could they argue for less inequality in U.S. society more generally?

TWO FACTS OF LIFE

Hollingshead and Redlich began *Social Class and Mental Illness* by claiming that "Americans prefer to avoid the two facts of life studied in this book: social class and mental illness." Social class, they argued, was "inconsistent with the American ideal of a society composed of free and equal individuals living in a society where they have identical opportunities to realize their inborn potentialities."[20] But while Americans liked to talk about this ideal publicly, in private, inequality was practiced invidiously on an everyday basis. Efforts to redress inequality through school desegregation or fair employment practices, for example, were "resisted mightily" on the basis of "the traditional conviction that some men are socially superior to others."[21] Although it was harder to deny mental illness, Americans nevertheless abhorred the idea of it, stigmatizing those diagnosed with it and ridiculing psychiatrists as "head shrinkers" and "nutcrackers."[22] The idea that social class could have something to do with mental illness, therefore, was anathema not only to Americans but also American psychiatrists. The New Haven Study presented an opportunity to test whether these deeply held assumptions were in fact correct.

The New Haven Study can be seen as a part of a longstanding tradition at Yale to investigate mental illness innovatively.[23] As discussed in chapter 1, Yale was one of a small number of universities to experiment with providing a mental hygiene clinic to its students, and, with the generous support of the Rockefeller Foundation, it founded IHR in 1929, charging it to explore "the basic problems of human nature" and "train a skilled personnel for work in these fields."[24] As the pioneering medical sociologist Samuel W. Bloom has described, Yale would be central in the development of medical sociology, with Hollingshead playing a leading role.[25]

August de Belmont "Sandy" Hollingshead was born in Lyman, Wyoming, in 1907, the son of a stockbreeder.[26] He and his family moved to California with his family when he was young. He began his university education at Berkeley, proceeding to the University of Nebraska for his doctoral work, which he completed in 1935. Following teaching roles at many universities, postdoctoral work at the University of Chicago (with W. Lloyd Warner, who supervised Leo Srole's doctoral research), and military service during World War II, he was appointed

associate professor at Yale in 1947.[27] Although the four monographs Hollingshead would produce all touched on somewhat
different topics, the theme of class and social stratification ran
through them all.[28] Indeed, according to Bloom, it was this topic
that galvanized research at Yale in medical sociology.[29] Hollingshead became interested in class and social stratification during
a field trip to British Columbia in 1931, where he observed both
vertical stratification between the Doukhobor and non-
Doukhobor communities and horizontal stratification, particularly among the non-Doukhobors, on the basis of income, education, occupation, and ethnicity.[30] He would then turn to
studying small, Midwestern communities, culminating in *Elmtown's Youth* (1949), using a combination of participant observation and interviews. Hollingshead's interest in the relationship
between sociology and medicine was sparked while serving at
Randolph Air Force Base during World War II, where he got to
know many physicians. He did not act upon this interest, however, until he met Frederick "Fritz" Redlich in 1948.[31]

Redlich's path to Yale was also peripatetic but also very different. Born in Vienna in 1910, Redlich received his MD from
the University of Vienna in 1935, where he also completed his
medical internship and residency. He had visited Ohio as part
of an exchange program in 1931 and immigrated to the United
States as a refugee scholar in 1938 following the Anschluss. After
some time at a psychiatric institute in the Midwest, Redlich
worked as a psychiatric resident at Boston City Hospital from
1940 to 1942 before moving to New Haven in 1942 for another
residency. He joined Yale Medical School that year and would
stay until 1977, serving as dean from 1967 to 1972. He also served
in the U.S. Army Medical Corps in 1944 to 1945 and thereafter
completed psychoanalytical training at the New York Psychoanalytical Institute.[32] Redlich's psychoanalytical training was

reflected in some of his publications, which included coauthored texts on psychotherapy.[33] He was also interested in the social sciences, however, having studied in Vienna with the highly influential Austrian-American sociologist Paul Lazarsfeld (1901–1976), who founded Columbia University's Bureau of Applied Social Research.[34]

Eager to collaborate with social scientists, Redlich quickly sought out Hollingshead when the latter arrived in New Haven in 1947. The partnership would be productive but sometimes difficult. In addition to having disparate backgrounds, Hollingshead and Redlich differed in other respects. Redlich described himself as "an idea man," whereas Hollingshead was more of a "methodologist," an empirically oriented sociologist in the Chicago School tradition. While these two academic orientations complemented each other, the pair's political differences were more problematic. Despite Hollingshead's interests in class, politically he was "very conservative," a "Goldwater Republican," and anti-Semitic.[35] When chair of sociology between 1959 and 1965, for instance, he failed to repeal the department's anti-Semitic hiring practices.[36] According to Redlich, this put "a considerable strain on our relationship, because I was an immigrant and came from Nazi persecution. But we reached sort of a modus vivendi, where we didn't talk about these matters. But it was there." Much like Faris and Dunham, the pair would not collaborate after *Social Class and Mental Illness*. Redlich also described how he experienced friction from his fellow psychiatrists at Yale, who "had no use whatsoever for social science," believing its ideas to be "alien" and even "dangerous."[37] Still, he persevered, serving to bridge the "social, biological, and psychoanalytical streams in the department."[38]

Hollingshead and Redlich began planning their study in 1948 and applied to NIMH for funding in 1949. Initially rejected, they reapplied successfully in 1950. They were joined in the project by the sociologist Jerome Myers and the psychiatrist Bertram Roberts. Myers was born in Pennsylvania and, after attending Franklin and Marshall College and serving during World War II, undertook doctoral studies at Yale, where he graduated in 1950 and remained for his entire career. Roberts, much like Alexander Leighton (discussed in chapters 4 and 5), was dually qualified in both medicine and the social sciences, in his case an MD from the University of Toronto and a master's degree in sociology from Columbia. Before his untimely death in a yachting accident in 1955, Roberts had published widely in both medical and social science journals, including an article that discussed the challenges of interdisciplinary research.[39]

Of the two books published as part of the New Haven Study, *Social Class and Mental Illness* was the more prominent and influential. It was published first, was written by the two study leads, and would be one of the first winners of the ASA's MacIver Award, now its Distinguished Scholarly Book Award. It also provided an overarching introduction to the project as a whole. In contrast, the writing of *Family and Class Dynamics in Mental Illness* was undermined early on by Roberts's untimely death. Myers, however, would persist in completing the project with the support of Hollingshead, Redlich, and the psychiatrist Jay Katz (1922–2008). He would also cowrite a follow-up of the New Haven Study in 1968.[40] This chapter focuses mainly on *Social Class and Mental Illness* but also draws on *Family and Class Dynamics in Mental Illness*.

Central to both books was the five-tier Index of Social Position devised by Hollingshead and Myers.[41] Hollingshead and Myers began by taking a random sample of 552 New Haven families, each of which were subjected to a two-to-three-hour interview consisting of two hundred questions pertaining to ethnic, religious, economic, educational, social, and residential factors. The interview was supplemented by the interviewer's impressions of the family members and how they were adjusted to the community and to one another. In addition to basic socio-economic and cultural facts, the interviews revealed insights about "values, attitudes, aspirations, standard of living, ideas of the future, and . . . frustrations, desires, hopes, and fears."[42] After agreeing that New Haven society could be accurately divided into five social strata, Hollingshead and Myers independently divided the 552 families into the five tiers.[43]

Also feeding into the index was an in-depth analysis of how New Haven's history had contributed to its social structure.[44] As Hollingshead and Redlich explained, "cultural values and prac-tices from a past age [were] reflected in the behavior of people today." They divided their study of New Haven's history into "the Colonial Epoch" (1838–1818), "the Age of Industrialization and Immigration" (1818–1914), and "the Acculturation of the Immi-grants" (1914–present).[45]

The Puritans who founded New Haven came from the mer-chant and professional classes and established a class structure that was based mainly on religion. Although everyone was expected to attend the Congregational Church, only landhold-ers were able to become members and, thus, attain political rights. By 1700, the status structure had "crystallized" along hereditary lines. Since the community remained small (only six thousand residents by 1760) and consisted chiefly of the descen-dants of the original settlers, the status of every individual was known. Wealth could help one move up the social ladder, but official rank mattered more. During the early nineteenth cen-tury, challenges to this "Standing Order" began to emerge, par-ticularly with the formation of the Toleration Party in 1817, which succeeded in extending the franchise and reducing the power of the Congregational Church. After this, the official privileges of the forty to fifty old aristocratic families (known as the "quality") declined, but they still maintained significant power through their social status, economic might, and legal influence. Beneath them were "the better sort" (consisting of Yale professors, Congregational clergymen, doctors, and lawyers), "the middle sort" (shop owners and farm owners), artisans, and "the lower sort" (day laborers, fishermen, and sailors).[46]

As immigration and industrialization increased New Haven's population during the nineteenth century, another division emerged between immigrants and "Yankees," who could trace their ancestry back to well before the Revolutionary War. While the Yankees tended to own the manufacturing enterprises before the Civil War, German, Irish, Jewish, Swedish, and Italian immigrants began to find their own commercial niches and enter the professions. Their rise in status strained the existing social structure. In addition, because these new ethnic groups tended not to mix, a series of subcultures and social stratification also developed within ethnic groups. This was partly caused by the recognition that the Yankees "looked down upon them" and that as outsiders they could never truly aspire toward reaching the pinnacle of New Haven society.[47]

By 1920, approximately two-thirds of New Haven residents were either immigrants or the children of immigrants. By 1950, when the study commenced, only 12 percent of the city were of British American heritage; the rest of the population was of Italian (30 percent), Irish (25 percent), Jewish (11 percent), German (7 percent), Polish (5 percent), Scandinavian (3 percent), other European heritage (3 percent), and Black American (4 percent) ethnicity.[48] Although acculturation did occur to varying degrees, these New Haveners maintained a clear sense of their ethnicity. Moreover, they were also aware, through being "rebuffed by the

Yankees . . . of the American status dilemma: the public profession of equality and the private practice of inequality."[49] Overall—and despite their declining proportion in the population—individuals of British American origin continued to maintain their elite status. For instance, approximately two-thirds of people in professional and executive occupations were of British American extraction, despite this ethnic group consisting of 12 percent of the population. In contrast, only 4.5 percent of people in such occupations were of Italian origin, despite comprising nearly a third of the city's population.[50] The primary exception to this trend could be found in those of British American origin who may have been able to trace their ancestry to the colonial era but whose ancestors had always existed on the lower tiers of society. These so-called Swamp Yankees nevertheless held themselves "aloof" from the other immigrant groups.[51]

This social history of New Haven was mirrored in the index, onto which the epidemiology and treatment of mental illness was mapped. Its five tiers were broken down accordingly. Class I constituted 3.4 percent of New Haven's population. The bulk of this class (59 percent) consisted of "Proper New Haveners" who could often trace their ancestry to the seventeenth century. Wealth was important to this group, but family background was essential. One matriarch described another family as "not really being old New Haveners" because, while they had settled in Connecticut in the 1640s, they did not come to New Haven until 1772. In addition to this core group, other class I members consisted of wealthy business owners and professionals of Irish, German, Jewish, and Italian ethnicity. Given their high levels of education, income, and residential preferences, 95 percent of New Haven's psychiatrists were a member of this class, with the remainder in class II. These psychiatrists were then divided into those who were psychoanalytically oriented and those who were organically or biologically oriented. The analytically oriented psychiatrists tended to be of Jewish heritage (83 percent) and were well aware of social stratification. In contrast, the organically oriented psychiatrists were more likely to be of Protestant origin (75 percent) and to deny the existence of class-based prejudices.[52]

Class II (9 percent) consisted of aspirational families of mixed ethnic origin who valued career and financial success. They tended to be business managers (rather than owners) and worked in "lesser ranking" professions, such as engineering, accountancy, pharmacy, and teaching. Since these families did not tend to inherit considerable wealth, they had to balance the desire "to present a 'good front'" with saving for retirement or a rainy day.[53]

Class III (21.4 percent) consisted primarily of employees working in administrative, clerical, semiprofessional, or technical capacities, along with some small business owners, who could trace their ancestry to the first wave of European immigration (1830–1870). The income of class III had not increased with inflation, but most members enjoyed job security. Maintaining a home in a "good" area was a priority, and many feared that the influx of Black Americans would make this more difficult.[54]

Class IV constituted the largest proportion of the population (48.5 percent). Most male members worked in skilled or semiskilled trades, with women employed in manufacturing, clerical, and sales positions. The skilled workers in this class (many of whom were unionized) felt relatively satisfied and secure, as did many of the semiskilled workers. It was difficult, however, for class IV members to save money. Nearly half traced their roots to southern or eastern Europe, with the remainder being relatively recent immigrants from elsewhere in Europe. Class IV families were more likely to be broken, to be larger, and to include grandparents and/or boarders.[55]

Class V (17.7 percent) members tended to work in un-unionized, semiskilled, or unskilled occupations that were characterized by low pay, long hours, and periods of unemployment. Economic insecurity was widespread, and few expressed much hope that this would change, not least because of their low education levels (over half of men left school before the seventh grade). While 80 percent admitted to intractable money problems, 35 percent were "overwhelmed by the economic demands [of] society." Although Swamp Yankees were found in class V, 70 percent were recent immigrants from eastern and southern Europe.[56]

Overall, the index presented New Haven as having a rigid and historically rooted class structure that infiltrated most aspects of an individual's life (see table 3.1). This included mental health. Classes IV and V made up the bulk of psychiatric patients, contributing 78.3 percent of the total number, despite constituting 66.2 percent of the overall population.[57] But the ratio of patients to population was much higher for class V: whereas the 40.1 percent of patients representing class IV was less than class IV's

TABLE 3.1   Prevalence of total mental disorder
adjusted for sex and age

Class	Adjusted rate of total mental disorder per 100,000
I and II	554
III	528
IV	665
V	1,668

Source: August B. Hollingshead and Frederick C. Redlich, *Social Class and Mental Illness* (New York: John Wiley, 1958), 210.

48.5 percent share of the population, 38.2 percent of patients were from class V, despite that class making up only 17.7 percent of the population. Indeed, class V was the only class that had a higher share of patients than their share of the overall population. This was despite the fact that class V individuals were judged to be the wariest of a psychiatric diagnosis, not least because they feared ending up indefinitely in the "bughouse."[58]

When the rates for different types of mental disorder (psychoses and neuroses) were calculated, more striking patterns emerged. Whereas psychoses tended to be diagnosed in those at the bottom of New Haven's class ladder, people from classes I and II (much like those in wealthier Chicago neighborhoods) were more likely to be diagnosed with neuroses (see table 3.2).[59]

Specific disorders were even more differentiated according to class. While Faris and Dunham found that manic-depressive psychoses were commonly associated with wealthy parts of the city, Hollingshead and Redlich's data showed that such disorders (which they called affective psychoses) were over 2.5 times more common in class V than in classes I and II. Schizophrenia,

TABLE 3.2 Prevalence of psychotic and neurotic disorders

Class	Prevalence of psychotic disorder per 100,000	Prevalence of neurotic disorder per 100,000
I & II	200	390
III	291	237
IV	518	146
V	1,504	163

Note: Hollingshead and Redlich listed precise figures for classes III, IV, and V but not for classes I and II. I have approximated the latter figures from their graph.
Source: Hollingshead and Redlich, *Social Class and Mental Illness*, 230.

the most common disorder, was eight times more common in class V than in classes I and II, and organic psychoses (traced to mental deficiency and infectious diseases) were nearly thirty times more likely to be found in class V than in classes I and II. Most neuroses were only somewhat more prevalent in classes I and II than in the other classes, but so-called character neuroses (a contemporary catchall for patients who did not match the more specific types) were six times more likely in classes I and II than in class V.

Referral and treatment also divided along class lines. In terms of referral, class V members were far more likely to be referred by social agencies or the police/courts than people from classes I and II, who were more likely to be referred by private physicians or family/friends. In the case of schizophrenia, all class I and II cases were referred by either private physicians or family/friends, and none were referred by the police/courts. In contrast, over half of the class V cases were referred by the police/courts, with social agencies being the next most common form of referral (17.6 percent). Hollingshead and Redlich speculated that police (rather than family/friends) were involved more in class IV and V referrals because the family and friends of such patients were typically ignorant of their mental health problems and viewed them instead as "difficult," "ornery," "abusive," or "profane." They also noted that, while class I and II patients were usually induced gently into psychiatric treatment, the path taken by class V patients was characterized by "direct, authoritative, compulsory, and, at times, coercively brutal methods." As they described, "the goddess of justice may be blind, but she smells differences, particularly class differences."[60]

Class V patients were also far more likely to be treated in state hospitals and in public clinics than patients from classes I and II, who tended to be treated by private psychiatrists or in private hospitals. The specific treatment offered to lower-class patients and the duration of custodial treatment also differed. Lower-class patients were more likely to receive electroconvulsive therapy (ECT), lobotomy, or drugs than higher-class patients, who were more likely to receive psychoanalysis. When psychotherapy was offered to lower-class patients, it tended not to be analytic in nature but consisted of changing the "attitudes, opinions, and behavior of the patient by means of directive and supportive methods such as assertion, suggestion, reassurance, advice, manipulation, and even coercion."[61]

Why was this the case? In terms of referral and treatment, the cost of treatment was an obvious factor. Psychoanalysis, in particular, was more expensive than organic therapies, partly because of the time involved. Social barriers also posed a problem.[62] Hollingshead and Redlich assumed that it was possible for lower-class patients to benefit from psychotherapy but that "deeply rooted" attitudes and "value differences" on the part of both patient and therapist impaired its efficacy. Psychiatrists, they argued, were often ignorant of "lower class psychodynamics." But they also believed that the lower classes could simply not benefit from the same psychotherapeutic techniques offered to higher-class patients and that "new approaches are indicated to bring psychotherapy to lower class patients." Given that some of these "new approaches" included group therapy and "the use of less expensive personnel, such as social workers and clinical psychologists," it seems likely that some of the obstacles related to attitudes or values were actually proxies for financial barriers.[63]

Despite these findings, Hollingshead and Redlich—as with many other social psychiatrists—emphasized the limitations of their research and were reluctant to assume that the higher prevalence of mental illness in class V had etiological significance.[64]

On the one hand, they suspected that the high prevalence rates for people in the lower classes were attributable to the fact that they tended to stay in state hospitals for longer. On the other hand, since Hollingshead and Redlich only assessed *treated* mental illness, it could also have been that the reluctance of class V individuals to seek psychiatric diagnoses meant that its incidence in class V was actually higher.[65] The pair also struggled to assess the relative importance of hereditary, organic, and social factors in mental illness. While their study showed that sociocultural factors were "important in the prevalence of treated disorders," they could not conclude that "they are the essential and necessary conditions in the etiology of mental disorders. Reflecting Redlich's psychoanalytic orientation, the "tentative inferences" they did provide focused on the influence of class on different phases in the life cycle (from early infancy to old age). This discussion speculated in particular on how conditions in class V homes could be problematic. A "loveless infancy," for example, "was more likely in a class V family than in a class II family," producing "catastrophic consequences." Similarly, lower-class children were more likely to suffer from a "defective superego," resulting in poor educational attainment, "intensive sexualization," and juvenile delinquency. Whereas adolescents from classes I–III engaged in "petting, necking, and masturbation," those in classes IV–V engaged in "actual intercourse." Adult behavior was also analyzed along class lines. Since class V adults were inclined to physical violence, the instance of a class I husband beating his wife should be "evaluated quite differently from similar occurrences in class V."[66] Hollingshead and Redlich also suggested that while upper-class people were more vulnerable to stresses (which they defined as internal in nature: fears, guilt, and conflict), lower-class individuals were more afflicted by external "presses" of an economic, social, or physical nature.

Overall, however, the New Haven Study appeared less concerned with the pathological impact of these "presses" on class
V individuals than, for example, how failed social mobility could
affect those in class II. Hollingshead and Redlich acknowledged
that psychiatrists should be more aware of the class dynamics in
the communities they served, as well as where they themselves
fitted into the social structure, but the objective of such knowledge was less to break such a system down than to slot individuals into particular class categories and judge them accordingly.
Rather than prescribing prevention, the authors concentrated on
improving treatment, for example, making psychotherapy
shorter, cheaper, and more accessible by allowing nonmedical
professionals to practice it. They also expressed hope that drugs
could democratize psychiatric treatment.[67] But the resounding
message of the New Haven Study was one of caution, rather than
optimism.[68]

A CLASS APART

Hollingshead and Redlich concluded their book by asking if
American society was ready to meet the challenge posed by mental illness, which it had heretofore ignored. Judging by the
stated implications of their study, the authors intimated that this
challenge would be best met by throwing support behind psychiatry. Little was said, however, about how to address the other
factor that Americans were said to avoid: class, or to be more
precise, inequality. There was scant discussion of the structural
forces that ensured that people stayed in their place, let alone how
to overcome such forces. Likewise, the authors did not spend
much time contemplating the relationship between the social
inequities class V members faced and their high rates of mental

illness. Instead, the notion that class divisions were inevitable and that class V members were a different sort of people altogether lingered throughout the book. For the white, middle-class, and educated members of the research team, the members of class V represented an "other" that might be worthy of pity but not redemption.

In order to illustrate these attitudes, it is worth returning to how the "cultural characteristics" of class V, in particular, were portrayed. Of all the five classes, class V was described in the most detail, including lengthy descriptions of living conditions and quotations from class members. Over two-thirds lived in "crowded old tenements" that tended to be

> built on the sidewalk leaving no space for a front yard . . . so close to the house next door that the residents . . . can almost reach across to touch its begrimed clapboards. If there is a backyard, grass will have been succeeded by gravel, mud, broken bottles, and rusty bits of old metal. An old car with the tires cracked away from the rims may be gradually disintegrating as is the whole neighborhood. The approach to the building is up some broken wooden steps. The door which is gouged and defaced . . . and which has lost great slivers of its wood is swinging on its hinges so that it cannot be fully closed. . . . There has been glass in the door, but it has been replaced by plywood roughly tacked on. . . . The linoleum on the entrance floor is worn through to the scuffed wood beneath and littering it are scraps of newspapers and cigarette butts.[69]

Superficially, this field worker's description conveyed impoverishment, but it also indicated a disdain for the tenement's residents and their apparent inability to take pride in or improve their living space. Rather than emphasizing that the landlord has failed to maintain the building, attention was drawn to discarded cigarette butts and broken bottles.

A similar tone was present in the description of the apartment:

> From the ceiling hangs an old light fixture from which one bare bulb is burning. In other sockets are extension cords. One leading to a radio which is blaring. . . . Flies are buzzing around even in late fall. Prominent in the living room will be the ever-present huge television set. The floors are often covered with odd pieces of linoleum on which the design has been completely defaced. . . . The walls are bare except for the presence of a picture the size of a postcard. These pictures may be framed in carved wood frames and some, at least, were purchased or won during tours of the local carnival center. Nailed to the walls will be cheap crucifixes or religious statuettes in Catholic homes. There are few exceptions to this pattern.[70]

Again, here the squalor of flies and defaced linoleum was presented in order to set the people who lived in such tenements as a class apart. The possibility that they lacked the resources to replace their flooring or that the landlord had refused to pay for fumigation was not suggested. A passage concerning sanitation also highlighted residents' moral failings:

> Sanitation is a chronic problem for there may be only two toilets in a twenty-family tenement. . . . A serious sanitary problem associated with living in these tenements was brought to our attention by a respondent who told, much to the interviewer's belief, that "the —— piss out the windows." Near the end of the interview, the man slapped the interviewer on the knee and said, "Look, there's one of the bastards doing it now." The interviewer saw the respondent's story come to life before his eyes.[71]

Rather than highlighting the lack of toilets, the field worker's comments suggested that the residents were so uncivilized that they urinated out of window.

The passage concerning the typical class V living space also gravitated toward another factor deemed to differentiate class V members, specifically, cultural practices, including media consumption. An entire appendix was dedicated to "Social Stratification and Mass Communication," which further reinforced the validity of the five class divisions. Class V members were described as people who purchased (or won) art from carnivals, kept their radios blaring, and despite lacking the money for a lampshade, managed to own large television sets. In total, 76 percent of class V homes "boasted" a television set (possibly rented), even though only 9 percent of American families in 1950 would have had owned one, costing about $300 at the time (a decade later, 90 percent of families would possess one).[72] They did not tend to read. Televisions were kept on constantly at high volume during waking hours, creating

> bedlam as the thin partitions carry the sound from apartment to apartment. One disgusted man who worked an early morning shift and wanted to sleep in the evening said: "I can listen to the wrestling matches every Saturday night from the fellow next door on this side. I can listen to the fights with the fellow on the other side of me on Friday night. We live too close down here. Their bedroom joins ours. We practically live in the same room. Down here that leads to trouble. Everyone is spatting all the time."[73]

Although the participant's point was more about the crowded living conditions and the thin walls, the interviewer focused on how much class V members enjoyed television. Notably, this quotation was included in the section on "leisure time activities," rather than the state of housing.

Class V members were also described as "individualistic, self-centered, suspicious, and hostile to formal institutional controls" (including those related to health care), believing that the authorities took advantage of them. They lived for the day and gave into "impulse gratification," which "frequently leads to trouble for men and women in this stratum as police, teachers, and neighbors know."[74] Such traits—not the social system itself—led to "further isolation and discrimination" and "brittle, often transitory, and emotionally unsatisfactory" social relations. This, however, did not have to be the case. Tellingly, Hollingshead and Redlich provided a more suitable attitude in the last quotation supplied to represent class V members. The interviewee was a tenth-generation Swamp Yankee who asserted that it was perfectly possible not to be envious of the more fortunate and, thus, risk giving into one's impulses. He described how he went fishing in the same place as "a Jewish lawyer who's worth about a million bucks." This lawyer, however, did not "get any more out of his fishing than I do. I could lose an awful lot of sleep and an awful lot of happiness because he has the million bucks and I don't. By his rules, I can't afford to go fishing, but I can."[75] In presenting this alternative interpretation, Hollingshead and Redlich intimated that those on the lowest rungs of the social ladder were better off rationalizing their inequitable position, rather than challenging it or the system. Lower-class status might have been closely linked to poor mental health outcomes and more invasive treatment, but the researchers were not willing to criticize the class system explicitly. As discussed in the next section, such sentiments were also mirrored in the CMHCs that would be created shortly after the publication of *Social Class and Mental Illness*.

"A MASSIVE COMMUNITY
PSYCHIATRY ATTACK"

The New Haven Study, as with other post–World War II social psychiatry studies, influenced the Community Mental Health Act of 1963 and the CMHCs that would soon be constructed and staffed. The class V dwellings described in *Social Class and Mental Illness* were but one example of the "harsh environmental conditions" that President Kennedy described and that had to be addressed in order to prevent mental illness. CMHCs could not do much to address the structural factors that contributed to poverty, inequality, and racism in American society, but they were designed with some of these issues in mind. Specifically, CMHCs were structured to break down the class, racial, and ethnic barriers that divided the professional staff from the patients they served and interfered with service delivery. One of the ways this was done was by hiring indigenous paraprofessionals to serve as a link between it and the community.[76] Unlike many of the social workers, psychologists and, especially, psychiatrists who worked at CMHCs, indigenous paraprofessionals were from the local community and shared its racial, ethnic, and socioeconomic characteristics. As the psychiatrist Werner I. Halpern (1924–1997), who directed the Children and Youth Division of the Rochester Mental Health Center, described in 1969:

> The professional's confidence in his adequacy as the steward of psychologic or case work skills quickly wanes as he deals with the poor. Usually he does not get the positive feedback that assures him that he is in on the right track. He may easily become dismayed by what appears to him a chaotic or intransigent life style. . . . These and other factors cause him to turn away from

the needs of the poor, with the rationalization that his efforts will not be appreciated. The non-professional aide, who, in a sense, is also a representative of the poor, not only acts as a bridge between two worlds, but also seeks to modify both in order to bring a better rapprochement.[77]

Paraprofessionals, among everything else, helped professionals connect more effectively with the poor. As one of Halpern's paraprofessionals explained, it was best to provide services "in a way that people feel is most conducive to them. . . . We have to keep in mind . . . these people have been exploited and . . . are resentful and suspicious of agencies' offers to help them. They are used to telling these people and agencies all of their personal business and getting nothing in return."[78] Indigenous paraprofessionals were also hired for a more basic purpose: to provide inexpensive staff for CMHCs. It was difficult to find enough professionals to staff the hundreds of anticipated CMHCs, and indigenous paraprofessionals provided a cost-effective solution. In turn, such positions provided jobs for members of the local community, as well as the promise of future career opportunities in mental health.

Unfortunately, however, the experience of some indigenous paraprofessionals also showed how inequality within CMHCs could undermine such good intensions. As the case of LHMHS demonstrates, when indigenous paraprofessionals attempted to gain more authority and responsibility within the CMHC structure, they encountered resistance from professional staff, especially psychiatrists serving in managerial and directorial capacities. Although the JCMIH had warned in *Action for Mental Health* that "the quest for status must not be permitted to stand in the way of progress in mental health care," not all psychiatrists were willing to give up their authority.[79]

LHMHS, based in the South Bronx, was one of the first CMHCs to employ indigenous paraprofessionals. It was founded in 1964 as a partnership between Lincoln Hospital and the Division of Community and Social Psychiatry at Yeshiva University's Albert Einstein College of Medicine (AECM), which ran Lincoln Hospital.[80] Indigenous paraprofessionals were recruited for LHMHS as part of a three-year demonstration project funded by the Office of Economic Opportunity in 1965, the body tasked with administering most of President Johnson's War on Poverty programs.[81] A further NIMH grant was awarded to study the program's effectiveness. Three neighborhood service centers were established and staffed by indigenous paraprofessionals under the supervision of a center director and assistant director (both professionals).[82] Indigenous paraprofessionals were also employed at LHMHS's larger multiservice center, where they were in the minority compared to professional staff.[83] According to the child psychiatrist Robert Shaw (1926–2009) and the psychologist Carol J. Eagle, who were the director and assistant director, respectively, of the adjacent Children's Mental Health Services at Lincoln Hospital, the project was intended "to launch a massive community psychiatry attack on the fragmentation, apathy, and social pathology of the South Bronx."[84] As their quotation suggested, during the 1960s, the South Bronx was one of the most impoverished slums in the United States, characterized by deteriorated housing, high levels of crime and addiction, low levels of education, and poor health outcomes, including high infant mortality. In terms of health provision, there was one hospital bed per 4,500 people in the South Bronx, compared to one bed per ninety-three people in wealthy Westchester County, twenty-five miles to the north. All these beds were in Lincoln Hospital, the area's sole hospital. By contrast, Westchester County boasted one public hospital and twenty-eight private hospitals.[85] Moreover, families in the area around Lincoln Hospital had the lowest incomes in the Bronx.[86] The racial composition of the population had changed enormously during the postwar period because of white flight. In 1950 it had been two-thirds white, but by the late 1960s, the population was 55 percent Puerto Rican and 25 percent Black American.[87] The indigenous paraprofessionals employed to spearhead this "attack" on mental illness were a mix of these backgrounds; the "professional" staff was predominantly white.[88]

The contrast between the enthusiasm that initially greeted the use of indigenous paraprofessionals at LHMHS and the tensions that would emerge is best illustrated by comparing a series of papers written or cowritten by the LHMHS social worker Emanuel Hallowitz (1921–2001) between 1966 and 1968.[89] In the first two papers, Hallowitz described the role of the paraprofessionals positively. Their primary role in the three neighborhood service centers was to run the "psychosocial first-aid stations," which served as clearinghouses for problems that "ran the *gamut of human misery* from helping a resident make application for public housing to requests for assistance in more complex and stressful situations," including "helping a resident accept and obtain psychiatric services." Indigenous paraprofessionals interpreted for Spanish-speaking patients, negotiated with landlords and court officials, advocated for patients' welfare benefits, and coordinated communications with various agencies, dealing with over one thousand cases per month.[90]

The article showcased the paraprofessionals' effectiveness in the case of Mrs. Garcia. She was initially an emergency room patient at Lincoln Hospital, having attempted suicide by taking an aspirin overdose. The staff psychiatrist enlisted the support of the paraprofessionals to find out more about her situation and help calm her down. The paraprofessional determined that

Mrs. Garcia's husband had been beating her and had recently thrown her out of the house, thus preventing her from seeing her children. After consulting his supervisor, the paraprofessional suggested having a "long, informal talk" with the husband. At this point, "the supervisor grew a little anxious and said to the aide, 'How do you feel about going there?' The aide, a short, stout man responded, 'How do you mean?' The supervisor was a little embarrassed, but said, 'Well, Mr. Garcia sounds fairly tough.' Whereupon, the aide said rather simply, 'Well, I can protect myself, can't I?' and the supervisor responded, 'Oh, yes, of course.'"[91]

Regardless of how the paraprofessional intended to "protect" himself, it is clear from this passage that indigenous paraprofessionals were both willing and able to cut to the heart of matters affecting the mental health of community members in ways that professional CMHC staff were not. The paraprofessional and Mr. Garcia "sat until late in the night," talking about their mutual roots in Puerto Rico. After explaining to Mr. Garcia that police and court involvement could follow, the two arrived at a solution: Mr. Garcia "firmly agreed" to give Mrs. Garcia her children on the condition that she return to Puerto Rico. When the supervisor objected that Mrs. Garcia did not want to return to Puerto Rico, the paraprofessional replied: "One thing at a time." Shortly after, Mr. Garcia gave up his apartment to his wife and their children, and the paraprofessional helped him find a room of his own.[92]

Mrs. Garcia's case showed how effective the paraprofessionals could be in resolving the problems at the root of many emotional problems. It demonstrated how the paraprofessional was far more resourceful, creative, and, indeed, courageous in tackling Mrs. Garcia's problem than the timid supervisor. Other cases cited by Hallowitz and the social psychologist Frank Riessman (1904–2004) also showcased how paraprofessionals could liaise effectively with social services and the police, serve as a "friend in need" in times of difficulty, sustain the hope of patients, and—crucially—teach them how to assert themselves, make their needs known, and "maneuver within the labyrinth of agencies" upon which they had to rely.[93] Indigenous paraprofessionals may not be "sophisticated" in terms of mental health knowledge, according to Hallowitz and Riessman, but they were "savvy."[94]

Despite these advantages, however, Hallowitz and Riessman did recognize that the social, racial, and economic gulf between them and those running LHMHS caused tensions. Coming from "a disadvantaged population," they brought to the job the same "strong feelings toward the power structure" that their fellow community members held:

> On the one hand, there is fear, suspicion and distrust that they will be exploited, fired out of hand, discriminated against because of color, ethnic background or religion. On the other hand, supervisors and administrative personnel are invested with an omnipotence and omniscience. . . . The feeling that the professionals know everything and they know nothing is often balanced by counter feelings that it is only they who really care about the poor; that it is only they, the nonprofessionals, who really know what is going on; that they, the nonprofessionals, are down to earth while the professionals are on cloud nine. . . . Though the aides are delighted when they are initially "accepted in to the system," and revel in their new status as mental health aides, they soon discover they are still low man on the totem pole. Struggle ensues to define their role more clearly and to attain a higher status than they are originally assigned.[95]

Professionals could also find their relationship with paraprofessionals difficult. Although a professional may be "eager to see the nonprofessional develop his skills and to take on more complex tasks . . . he is reluctant to give responsibility to the non-professional and to allow him much independence of action or judgment." Thus far, however, such struggles had been "kept to a minimum," and the benefits of using paraprofessionals "far outweigh the difficulties enumerated."[96] The broader psychiatric community echoed this view when the APA awarded LHMHS a Silver Achievement Award for its innovations.[97]

This enthusiastic tone had evaporated in a subsequent unpublished paper that Hallowitz presented to the National Association of Social Workers conference in May 1968. Hallowitz began by stating that there had been "a spate of books and papers extolling the virtues of the 'indigenous nonprofessional.'"[98] In contrast to what he had written previously, he then stated that contrary to "myth,"

> the poor do not necessarily have special knowledge, insight, or intuitions not available to the more affluent; neither is the poor person . . . more sympathetic to others in the same plight; neither does his poverty give him special knowledge about effective administration, program planning, interviewing skills, community action. . . . He does not necessarily, despite the common assumption, understand his community or culture better than could the professional from the outside. On the whole, we found the poor and disadvantaged no more free of prejudice and snobbery than any other group in our society. The one clear advantage of the nonprofessional drawn from his community is that he understands the language, style, and customs of his neighbor.[99]

Moreover, "a good sociologist or anthropologist who has gained community acceptance can understand the dynamics of the community much better than the nonprofessionals."

Paraprofessionals were hired, Hallowitz contended, "for their survival characteristics: aggressiveness, assertiveness, and manipulativeness. We are delighted when these abilities are used effectively in working with other institutions, but we tend to react with anger when these same qualities are directed against us." Similarly, the message that paraprofessionals could "teach the professional" led to a "sense of grandiosity" on their part; any attempts to provide constructive criticism or supervision were perceived as a "threat." It was difficult to fire "incompetent" paraprofessionals, partly because it meant sending such an individual "to the welfare rolls" but also because it "may reactivate the other workers' fears of being discriminated against or fired and produce a good deal of hostility."[100] The local knowledge possessed by paraprofessionals could be useful, but it had its limits.

Although Hallowitz directed most of his invective at the paraprofessionals, he recognized that the paternalistic attitude of the professionals was also somewhat responsible. When a conflict arose, the professionals often responded with "hurt, disappointment, or counter-hostility." Feeling unappreciated, the professional staff asked: "Don't they realize how much we've done for them? Don't they realize that we were the first to hire nonprofessionals in the Bronx? Don't they realize what a battle we had with the medical school and the university to get permission to hire nonprofessionals, to get their wages raised, their working conditions improved?"[101] Moreover, Hallowitz admitted that "although on an intellectual level, we do want to have the nonprofessionals participate in the decision-making and policy and program direction, we still have the unconscious conviction that we know better."[102]

What caused Hallowitz's newfound pessimism? Essentially, what Hallowitz found irksome was the paraprofessionals' increasing willingness to speak out about their working conditions and the management of LHMHS. Although he did not mention it, one grievance involved payment delays. Yeshiva University struggled to manage the paperwork for the multifunded center early in its history, which stalled payment for days or weeks. Paraprofessionals felt the shortfall in their income acutely and were often threatened with eviction as a result. Although a sit-in by the paraprofessionals in 1968 helped resolve the situation, this—according to the LHMHS directors—merely gave the paraprofessionals the confidence to issue new demands. The instance that Hallowitz did cite involved a plan to send a team of both professional and paraprofessional workers to a poverty conference: "Feeling virtuous, we were astonished when our Community Mental Health Workers demanded to know why we were sending professionals at all, and why we felt we had the right to select the nonprofessional delegate."[103] The supervisors relented and allowed the paraprofessionals to select their delegates, despite fears that a "popularity contest" would ensue. Another row erupted over a plan presented by the paraprofessionals to have a monthly meeting "on agency time" and without a professional present. Again, the supervisors relented.

Alongside Hallowitz's disillusionment, his paper was notable for its condescending attitude toward the paraprofessionals, described as irrational, childish, naïve, defensive, suspicious, belligerent, unorthodox, and requiring constant coercion and manipulation. Given the racial and ethnic composition of the paraprofessionals (100 percent Black or Puerto Rican), it is impossible to ignore the racist and ethnocentric overtones in such characterizations. Moreover, Hallowitz argued that professionals had "greater knowledge, self-awareness, and professional discipline" than paraprofessionals. They had "better verbal facility" and could "always out-argue the nonprofessional." As such, it

was difficult for professionals to stand by and allow the paraprofessionals to learn from the inevitable mistakes that they
would make. The fact that paraprofessionals, according to Hallowitz, often failed to do a "quality job" "impels the professional
to find ways of controlling and directing the worker's activity."
Since paraprofessionals were likely to make "unreasonable, if
not irrational demands," professionals had to employ "extreme
patience and flexibility," prompting Hallowitz to ask, "How
much deviance can we tolerate?" It was best, therefore, to give
paraprofessionals control over relatively superficial decisions concerning décor, furniture, opening hours, and waiting room procedures to give them the illusion of power. For more substantive
decisions, it was vital to ensure "that the workers are not under
the misapprehension that *they will decide.*"[104]

These portrayals reveal how, despite the unique and useful
attributes and insights paraprofessionals brought to CMHCs, it
was difficult for some professionals, such as Hallowitz (a social
worker, not a psychiatrist), to yield their authority. A clear hierarchy based on racial, ethnocentric, and classist prejudices per-
sisted, placing paraprofessionals at the bottom. Another example of inequality was mentioned in an article by the psychiatrist
John Talbott and colleagues. After being accused by a professional of theft, the paraprofessional retorted that the professional
stole "time." This took the form of "leaving early for private practice, conducting stock business over the phone, and taking long
lunches." The difference was that the professional could get
away with such "theft."[105] Furthermore, paraprofessionals were
aware of how they were perceived by professionals: "Yeshiva
and selfish white power structure works on the premise that
Puerto Rican, blacks and radical whites are simple, ignorant
animals without functioning minds. Feed them by providing
a job, but do their thinking for them."[106] This was despite the

fact that paraprofessionals, according to some mental health professionals, "knew what the issues were . . . [and] didn't bullshit around . . . so they had a lot more success than the professionals."[107]

Despite Hallowitz's misgivings, the paraprofessionals would persist in demanding a greater say in how LHMHS operated. Matters escalated in March 1969, when 70 percent of LHMHS staff (including over one hundred paraprofessionals and sixty-seven AECM faculty members) undertook a work action, locking out LHMHS Director Harris B. Peck and others.[108] The specific trigger was the decision not to rehire four paraprofessionals who were thought to be improperly dismissed, but there were also concerns about "personnel practices, inefficient management, inept program coordination, failure to develop . . . programs," and the "racist . . . orientation" of management.[109] One of the chief catalysts was the awarding to LHMHS of a NIMH staffing grant, which required the establishment of a more rigid and vertical administrative structure that disempowered the paraprofessionals.[110] As the paraprofessional Cleo Silvers recalled, the workers demanded an end to the use of psychotropic drugs (because of side effects), training to upgrade their status (not least because "the workers actually did more contact with the patients than the doctors"), and an end to the use of any therapy "that didn't include . . . a recognition of the economic and social conditions in the community."[111]

Many of these grievances were showcased in a documentary produced in 1970, which presented the paraprofessionals' perspective. Their frustration with what they saw as an overreliance on medication, for example, was illustrated in this exchange between a female worker and one of the LHMHS directors: "Why after four years of this program have you got the same people, sick people, coming back and forth going to Bronx

State . . . walking round like zombies because they're full of dope. And I'm talking about medicine, if you don't know. Now you tell me why it is like that." Other workers felt that AECM undermined the broad array of social support they provided to patients. One male paraprofessional explained how: "When I first came here, we dealt with people's needs. If a man was depressed and he lived in a rathole, we went out and helped him and we carried his bed on our backs. In other cases, we started putting pressure on the landlords. And then word came down from The Man: 'We don't move patients anymore. Cool it.' We found out later that one of the landlords was a big contributor to Einstein." He added that home visits were stymied by the lack of funding for taxis, which meant that they often had to take public transportation for hours at a time to reach patients. All of this created the impression "that most of the programs were paper, designed to pull in private and federal grants. . . . We were just window dressing for Albert Einstein's liberal reputation."[112]

Other paraprofessionals stressed the underlying socioeconomic problems that made their preventive work so difficult, with one stating that "even if we could move all of our patients out of the ratholes, the ratholes would stay and new patients would move into them." Overall, the paraprofessionals demanded "a different definition of medicine. Health isn't anything mysterious. It isn't a drug company's financial report or research on the masses. It's strong bodies, good minds, and people being treated as people."[113] LHMHS had been envisioned as an innovative, community-led service but had retrogressed into a more traditional and hierarchical model where preventive mental health was sidelined. All of this undermined the morale of the paraprofessionals. As they articulated their newsletter, *Tell It Like It Is*: in 1968, "you whites are crying that we don't respect authority, we won't compromise. Damn right. Your authority is wrong and we have been compromising too long so now we hear what the Workers are saying loud and clear and you better listen: We are no longer employees OF but we and the people of the community ARE the program."[114]

The ensuing work action (described by LHMHS directors as a "palace revolt") saw the paraprofessionals and some of their professional colleagues take over the running of LHMHS from its directors for over two weeks. During this time, the paraprofessionals maintained the outpatient services with the support of the professionals who supported them and introduced new policies and programs. Although they were supported in their efforts by the Black Panther Party, who helped them organize and brought them food and water, and by the local community, they were not supported by their union (Hospital Workers' Union, Local 1199).[115] The paraprofessionals continued to run LHMHS until they were forcibly evicted, resulting in twenty-three arrests and sixty-seven dismissals.[116] Eventually, however, the administration capitulated in the face of community pressure. All workers were reinstated, the ties to Lincoln Hospital and AECM were severed, and eventually a new director was hired.[117]

To the LHMHS administrators and New York City Health and Hospitals Corporation officials, the situation was a "disaster."[118] NIMH inspectors were also critical, charging that the developments would "ordinarily warrant suspension of the grant."[119] Such views were articulated at length in a monograph by the former LHMHS associate directors Seymour R. Kaplan (1922–1988) and Melvin Roman. Kaplan and Roman generally treated the paraprofessionals in a patronizing manner, as Hallowitz had done. They saw them as "insular and self-absorbed," which was a somewhat ironic characterization, given that the paraprofessionals saw themselves as representing the interests of the community at large.[120] The Black paraprofessionals, in particular, were described as militant, hostile, vulgar, and abusive. To prove the point, Kaplan and Roman included excerpts from *Tell It Like It Is*, which, among other things, described a particular administrator as a "sly pig." Such characterizations, claimed the authors, caused personal and professional harm. While this may well have been the case, the authors displayed little willingness to put themselves into the position of the paraprofessionals, living in one of the poorest neighborhoods in New York City and enduring substandard healthcare amid race riots and the assassinations of those who had promised change. Instead, Kaplan and Roman compared the paraprofessionals' actions as absurd, tragicomic, surreal, and reminiscent of *Alice in Wonderland*. Such characterizations demonstrated the lack of willingness of CMHC professionals to implement substantive changes and downplayed the vital work paraprofessionals had already demonstrated.[121]

The activist work of the LHMHS paraprofessionals, however, was not finished. Their actions led to the formation of Health Revolutionary Unity Movement and Think Lincoln, which focused on the perilous state of Lincoln Hospital, sometimes referred to as the Butcher Shop. Its reputation was so bad that locals joked that if you were stabbed on one side of the street, you crawled to the other to avoid being picked up by the ambulance that would take you to the hospital. Fitzhugh Mullan, a pediatrician who worked at Lincoln, credited the LHMHS paraprofessionals as providing "the most significant input" for the subsequent Lincoln Hospital action and reforms.[122] Collaborating with the Blank Panther Party and the Puerto Rican liberation organization the Young Lords, these groups occupied Lincoln Hospital in 1970, instigating a series of innovations, including introducing a heroin detoxification program and acupuncture therapy.[123] Building on these developments, a new hospital was built in 1976 that would enjoy a much better reputation, though the neighborhood's problems remained.[124]

LHMHS's story and aftermath demonstrates how racial, ethnic, and classist prejudices held by some—but not all— professional mental health workers in CMHCs undermined the ambitions of community mental health more generally. Paraprofessionals brought insights, skills, and experiences to CMHCs that were indispensable to their operation, especially as places of preventive mental health. In the South Bronx and similar neighborhoods, they served as a bridge between the highly educated and typically white professional staff and the surrounding community at a time of heightened racial tension. They helped mitigate some of the mistrust bred out of the inequalities articulated so eloquently in Gill Scott-Heron's (1949–2011) contemporary spoken-word poem "Whitey on the Moon" (1970).[125] If those running CMHCs had been willing to give paraprofessionals a more central role in such centers' planning and operation, it is likely that more progress in tackling the inequalities that were thought to contribute to mental illness would have been made. In the face of managerial intransigence and conservatism, however, paraprofessionals were more likely to symbolize the structural inequalities that social psychiatry and community mental health were meant to overcome.

CONCLUSION: TOGETHER, NOT EQUAL

In order to summarize how social psychiatrists' findings about inequality factored into CMHC operations, it is helpful to turn briefly to how psychiatrists viewed their role within community mental health. Although some were in favor of making CMHCs more egalitarian spaces and turning management over to the communities, others feared the blurring of roles in CMHCs and believed that psychiatrists should maintain their place at the top of the mental health hierarchy. Still others simply felt that the quality of medical care would deteriorate if psychiatrists were not in charge. CMHCs, they thought, would quickly transform from psychiatric clinics into social service centers, leaving patients with serious mental illnesses at risk.

Such attitudes can be found in the development of the American Association for Community Psychiatry (AACP), founded in 1984 in response to the perception that the role of psychiatrists within CMHCs was being downgraded. Although the initial CMHC legislation intended that psychiatrists would be in charge of CMHCs, this eroded over time as the number and authority of psychiatric social workers and other nonmedical mental health workers increased.[126] According to AACP's founder Gordon H. Clark Jr. (b. 1947), as the percentage of CMHCs led by psychiatrists dropped from 56 percent to 3 percent between 1971 and 1985, psychiatrists felt increasingly "marginalised . . . they didn't feel adequately valued, they didn't feel that they had authority commensurate with their medical-legal responsibility. So . . . their position was very tenuous and they persistently seemed to be under threat, so they often left for greener pastures, such as private practice or working for hospitals."[127] Partly responsible for these trends were the financial realities affecting CMHCs. JCMIH had indicated in their 1961 report that a multidisciplinary approach to running CMHCs involving paraprofessionals was necessary not only for reasons of efficacy but also because of staffing and funding pressures. As Clark described, "When funding cuts, endorsed by non-psychiatric government officials, are combined with an anti-professional community bias . . . centers often simplistically conclude that money can best be saved by eliminating the higher priced personnel and substituting less expensive mental health workers."[128] In this way, paraprofessionals and other nonmedical mental health workers were used by some psychiatrists as scapegoats for insufficient funding of community mental health.

It is also clear, however, that some community psychiatrists thought that CMHCs had gone too far in emphasizing what paraprofessionals and nonmedical professionals could offer, at the expense of psychiatric authority. The hierarchy within CMHCs, in other words, had to be maintained. As Clark stated elsewhere, "CMHCs developed in an era marked by tremendous social pressures toward equality as evidenced by the civil rights and women's rights movements. This undoubtedly contributed to role-blurring in these centers."[129] Others went further in criticizing the "expedient deprofessionalization" or "pseudo-egalitarianism" that had emanated out of "the notion that everyone can do almost everything—all it takes is a warm heart and an extended hand."[130] These views diminished the significant role paraprofessionals (as well as other nonmedical mental health workers) played in liaising between patients and psychiatrists, various agencies, and estranged family members, educating patients about available municipal services, translating (often literally) obscure psychiatric concepts for patients, providing lay counseling, and being the "friend in need" when patients were in despair and needed hope.

Overarching the situation was a perceived tension related to the two primary goals of community mental health, namely, reducing inequities in treatment and preventing mental illness. While I shall discuss this issue in more depth in chapter 5, it is worth noting how the difficulty in achieving these two goals affected paraprofessionals and the broader notion of equality within mental health and society more generally. Often psychiatrists and historians have assumed that the preventive aspects of CMHCs were quickly ignored and that CMHCs resorted to being merely treatment centers.[131] To an extent, this is true: CMHCs could undertake some types of preventive work, but they could only do so much about making society as a whole more equitable and, therefore, better for mental health. They could do even less when, as in the case of LHMHS in the mid-1970s, their budgets were drastically cut. In 1975, $750,000 was cut from LHMHS's $4,000,000 budget, followed by a $500,000 cut the following year. The paraprofessionals bore the brunt of the redundancies.[132]

It is also true, however, that this supposed division between prevention and treatment was something of a false dichotomy, as the research of Hollingshead and Redlich demonstrated. Those on the lowest rungs of New Haven's social ladder not only had higher rates of mental illness but also struggled to access the best treatment. Inequality cut across *both* prevention and treatment. Tackling it in innovative ways could, therefore, serve both purposes. This is where indigenous paraprofessionals were invaluable. As the people of the South Bronx and elsewhere awaited the enormous structural changes required to tackle intransigent social problems, paraprofessionals could support the mental health of their communities via both prevention *and* treatment. In terms of prevention, they had the insights, experience, and contacts to help community members avoid the worst privations of poverty, such as malnutrition, homelessness, and despair. As the case of Mrs. Garcia illustrates, they could also intervene in cases of domestic violence and support children living in chaotic environments. But through these preventive efforts, they could also encourage community members to access psychiatric treatment at CMHCs when necessary or provide lay counseling themselves. All of this helped reduce the inequities related to mental health services that Hollingshead and Redlich had identified. If inequality is defined in part as unequal access to opportunity (including opportunities to access healthcare), indigenous paraprofessionals were clearly helping alleviate it.

Hollingshead and Redlich's compelling case study of New Haven was pivotal in establishing the connection between inequality and mental health. Subsequent work has solidified the link, but—much like Hollingshead and Redlich—has offered few concrete suggestions about how to address the problem.[133] Indigenous paraprofessionals could do little to transform society, but they did make a significant difference within impoverished communities in terms of reducing mental health inequalities. The case of LHMHS also demonstrates, however, that highlighting the role of inequality in mental health through academic social psychiatry research was one thing; dismantling the system that gave rise to such inequalities was quite another. Even within community mental health it was difficult to flatten the hierarchy, share power more equitably, and—perhaps most importantly—recognize the value of lay insights and experiences regarding mental health.[134]

4

MADNESS IN THE METROPOLIS

I look out the window and I see the lights and the skyline and the people on the street rushing around looking for action, love, and the world's greatest chocolate chip cookie, and my heart does a little dance.

—Nora Ephron

New York was a city where you could be frozen to death in the midst of a busy street and nobody would notice.

—Bob Dylan

In April 1962, alarming headlines flashed across U.S. newspapers about mental illness in New York City. Entitled "New York Living for Nuts Only," "Scratch a New Yorker, and What Do You Find?" and "City Gets Mental Test, Results Are Real Crazy," the stories highlighted the shocking and possibly incredible figure that 81.5 percent of Manhattanites had "'mild, moderate, or impairing' symptoms of mental disturbance."[1] A quarter of participants were effectively incapacitated by their mental state, unable to work or function socially.[2] Were cities that bad for mental health?

These stories were spurred by *Mental Health in the Metropolis: The Midtown Manhattan Study* (*MHM*).[3] The Midtown Manhattan Study was a large-scale, interdisciplinary project that ran from 1952 to 1960 and investigated the relationship between environmental factors and mental health in a residential neighborhood in New York City's Upper East Side. In addition to *MHM*, the project would ultimately produce three other monographs, although one of these was merely a revision and enlargement of the initial volume.[4] None of these other volumes, however, would match the first's notoriety or influence. As with other social psychiatry studies, Midtown was generously funded, in its case, through grants from NIMH, the Millbank Memorial Fund, the Rockefeller Foundation, and other benefactors.

Of the four studies analyzed in this book, Midtown was the most momentous, given its combination of size, complexity, novelty, and interdisciplinarity. In addition to over a dozen senior investigators, the study utilized twenty-three predoctoral research aides, twenty-three social scientists and social workers, and ninety-nine volunteers (fourteen of whom contributed over five hundred hours).[5] It would become well known, especially within the social sciences, where it was regarded as a landmark study.[6] In 1987, *MHM* was named a "Citation Classic" by the Institute of Scientific Information, indicating its ongoing significance to sociology.[7] The ASA noted that while the study had been "greeted by a storm of controversy," it was also "a milestone of social research." Midtown introduced novel methodologies, including probability sampling, the use of standardized forms, and machine technology, that would become standard practice. Unlike Faris and Dunham's Chicago study and Hollingshead and Redlich's New Haven study, Midtown did not rely primarily on hospital admissions data but instead conducted an extensive examination of how socioeconomic and cultural factors affected an entire cross-section of people in an ethnically, socially, and economically diverse area of New York City.[8]

The media's focus on the apparently rampant madness in New York reflected prominent twentieth-century views that cities were bad for mental health.[9] But this was not the project's most important insight. Published in the same year as Michael Harrington's *The Other America*, *MHM*'s fundamental finding was that mental illness was strongly associated with poverty, inequality, and community disintegration, socioeconomic factors that could be found in both urban and rural environments.[10] In this chapter I explore how Midtown was developed and carried out, before turning to its findings and legacy. Thanks to the availability of archival sources and oral histories, it is possible to get a unique insight into the challenges involved in bringing such a complex project to fruition.[11] Midtown's large, multidisciplinary project team included a handful of opinionated, stubborn characters who often disagreed about many aspects of the project. A host of personnel changes during the course of the project, not least the unexpected death of the project's founder, Thomas Rennie, were also disruptive. Although Midtown was intended to produce knowledge of interest and importance to both academics and policy makers, a tension ran through the project about exactly how to translate its findings into practice. When were epidemiological findings definitive enough to inform policy? How much did society have to change in order for psychiatry to become truly preventive? And where should researchers draw the line between mental health and illness? Midtown demonstrates that while those involved in social psychiatry might have been united in their goal of preventing mental illness, they also debated vigorously about how to achieve this elusive ambition.

CRAZY CITIES?

In a recent chapter on urban mental illness, Edward Shorter discusses how the idea of the "toxic city" emerged during the mid-to-late nineteenth century, concluding that "cities have had a bad rap in psychiatry."[12] Shorter argues that given the sheer variety of cities and their combination of "risk and protective factors," it is "meaningless" to ask whether cities are good or bad for mental health.[13] Nevertheless, many have tried to do just that, including the Midtown researchers. And while it might be "meaningless" to judge cities as a homogenous category, identifying factors specific to certain cities, or even to cities more generally, has been and continues to be helpful in terms of determining both the risk factors and protective factors that Shorter describes.[14] Chapters 2 and 3, for example, have already showcased two drastically different cities. While Chicago in 1930 was characterized by its relative newness, size, sky-scraping architecture, rapid population growth, and ethnic and racial diversity, New Haven in 1950 was much older, smaller, less ethnically and racially diverse, and had a much more established and rigid class structure. It makes sense, therefore, that while Faris and Dunham gravitated toward studying poverty and community disintegration, Hollingshead and Redlich investigated class. Such factors are not unique to cities, as the Stirling County Study would demonstrate (see chapter 5), but they could be exacerbated or compounded by factors present in cities, ranging from the style and condition of housing to the often transient or changeable nature of the population.

U.S. concerns about urban mental health grew alongside cities themselves, as they expanded both up and out during the late nineteenth and early twentieth centuries and in concert with increased industrialization and immigration. The ideal U.S.

community, according to many, was not situated in a city with towering skyscrapers and streets teeming with traffic, noise, and commotion but in a bucolic rural setting or small town.[15] Concerns about urban mental health were also reflected in the neurological condition neurasthenia, which became widely diagnosed between 1869, when it was popularized by the American neurologist George Miller Beard (1839–1883), and the 1920s.[16] Neurasthenia, as David Schuster describes, was a response to the rapid pace of living in advanced, industrial, urban environments; in other words, it was a "pathology of progress."[17] Although it was diagnosed in many countries, neurasthenia was often portrayed as a particularly American disorder. It was called "American Nervousness" by Beard and was nicknamed "Americanitis" by others.[18] Unlike twentieth-century psychiatrists and sociologists, who were often concerned with the impact of urbanization on the mental health of the poor, however, neurasthenia's proponents believed that the nerves of the upper classes were more vulnerable to the sensory overload triggered by modern living. This may also have been because poorer people were unable to afford the rest cures, nature-based holidays, and electrotherapeutic remedies prescribed to neurasthenics.

By the 1900s, American sociologists began to build on the work of their European counterparts regarding cities and mental health. Particularly influential was Georg Simmel's "The Metropolis and Mental Life" (1903).[19] Much like the American neurologists who diagnosed neurasthenia, Simmel noted how "the intensification of nervous stimulation" typical of urban environments could affect the psyche of individuals: "With each crossing of the street, with the tempo and multiplicity of economic, occupational and social life, the city sets up a deep contrast with small town and rural life with reference to the sensory foundations of psychic life."[20] Such nervous stimuli resulted in a "blasé attitude," which "reduced everything, and everyone, to an exchange value in the market."[21] Exacerbating the situation was the prevalence of the "money economy" in urban environments, which transformed "intimate emotional relations between persons" into anonymous, reserved, and rational exchanges characterized by "unmerciful matter-of-factness."[22] This contrasted with the warmer and more intimate relationships found in rural settings, an observation also made by the pioneering German sociologist Ferdinand Tönnies (1855–1936).[23] Simmel observed that this "reserve" meant that city residents (including himself) "frequently do not even know by sight those who have been our neighbors for years." Personal reserve often went beyond mere indifference and could be manifested in "a slight aversion, a mutual strangeness and repulsion, which will break into hatred."[24] The resulting social disintegration and individuation, according to Durkheim, led to anomie and in extreme cases, suicide.[25] The counterpoint to the antipathy produced in the metropolis was that individuals were also afforded a great deal of personal freedom, sometimes to the point of eccentricity. The motivation for asserting one's uniqueness, however, was nonetheless driven by the city's propensity to make individuals feel anonymous, unimportant, and merely a "cog in an enormous organization of things."[26]

For Simmel, therefore, cities had an ambivalent impact on the personalities of their inhabitants: they gave people freedom, but they also made them feel detached, impersonal, and unimportant.[27] While the first Chicago School sociologists also emphasized both the positive and negative aspects of cities on personality, their successors stressed the latter. Robert E. Park, representing the first generation, acknowledged the damaging effects of social disintegration in certain neighborhoods but also stressed how the city offered transformative opportunities for migrants from rural parts of the United States and Europe to forgo old cultural patterns and create new ones with migrants from other backgrounds.[28] Louis Wirth, representing the next generation, also noted how cities could foster the development of social solidarity through the involvement of individuals in voluntary associations.[29] But Wirth also described how cities bred "impersonal, superficial, transitory, and segmental" relationships and considered urban environments likely to produce "personal disorganization, mental breakdown, suicide, delinquency, crime, corruption, and disorder."[30] Wirth's contemporaries would tend to agree.[31]

Following World War II, interest in urban mental health grew, buoyed by intensive interest in psychiatric epidemiology more generally, the adoption of new methodologies (especially quantitative and statistical approaches), and rapid changes to the urban environment.[32] American cities were being transformed through suburbanization, ghettoization, and urban renewal projects that had a mixed record of creating living environments that were better than what they replaced.[33] Underlying these developments were racial tensions (as white middle-class Americans left city centers for the suburbs), the emergence of car culture (which made suburbs possible and drew populations away from cities), and ongoing research into the effects of city living on mental and physical health.[34]

Some of this research included animal experiments, most notably using rats. Edmund Ramsden has described how the work of the ecologist and psychologist John B. Calhoun (1917–1995) helped establish the rat as the ideal model for exploring the relationship between living in crowded, urban environments and mental health.[35] Calhoun's "rat cities" appeared to demonstrate how crowded, urban environments resulted in increased levels of stress and, subsequently, pathology.[36] Lacking only space in their "rat utopias," they bred uncontrollably, resulting in ever-crowded conditions. While male rats formed gangs and attacked females and the young, females would abandon their offspring; other rats became homosexual, then still regarded as a mental disorder by many psychiatrists.[37] Rat utopia became "rat hell," a "behavioral sink."[38] These rat experiments reinforced the notion that cities were bad for mental health, with Calhoun's *Scientific American* article on the subject in 1962 becoming one of the best-known and oft-cited psychology articles of the twentieth century.[39] Later, however, Calhoun and others emphasized that the relationship between population density and pathology was more nuanced than his rat cities suggested. Strategies could be employed to mitigate stress in urban environments.[40]

Along with the psychiatrist Leonard Duhl, who pioneered the "Healthy Cities" movement, Calhoun formed an interdisciplinary group called the "Space Cadets" in 1956 to further explore environmental factors and mental health. Consisting of a core group of about twenty researchers from backgrounds ranging from psychiatry and sociology to mathematics and physics, the Space Cadets met twice per year from the mid-1950s to the mid-1960s. They discussed a wide array of topics, including the degree to which Calhoun's rat cities could predict or explain what occurred in human cities.[41] Other topics debated by the Space Cadets included noise, privacy, race and ethnicity, and the quality and type of housing.

During Space Cadets' initial meetings, slum housing—defined as crowded, decaying, unplanned, and populated by poor residents—was typically depicted as being bad for both physical and mental health. Slums, such as those that the Space Cadet Daniel Wilner studied in Baltimore, were also described as being "a good deal worse" than the subsidized housing projects that were being constructed.[42] But contrasting views were also emerging, influenced by urban renewal critics such as Jane Jacobs (1916–2006).[43] The urban renewal of Boston's West End, a predominantly Italian-American neighborhood, was a flashpoint.[44] The Boston Redevelopment Authority, along with many wealthy Bostonians, had long considered the West End to be an essentially unhealthy space. Empowered by the Housing Act of 1949, the authority recommended that the West End be razed to the ground and replaced with residential high-rise apartments, a fate that occurred in 1958. But the work of the Space Cadet and Massachusetts General Hospital psychiatrist Erich Lindemann (1900–1974) and his colleagues at the Center for Community Studies would cast doubt on whether such urban renewal would improve mental health. Lindemann employed the sociologist Herbert Gans (b. 1927) and the social psychologist Marc Fried (1922–2008) to investigate how West End residents viewed their community and its impending destruction.[45]

Living in the West End for eight months, Gans found that, far from perceiving their neighborhood as in decline, West Enders saw it as "by and large, a good place to live," with decent and clean—if old—housing, little crime, and minimal drug abuse.[46] Although largely Italian-American, it also welcomed other immigrants. Above all, it was not a slum. Moreover, Fried determined that it was the West End's demolition that proved to be pathological, not the place itself. In his essay "Grieving for a Lost Home," Fried outlined how a high proportion of West End residents had feelings of sadness and depression, with some declaring that they had contemplated suicide, or "taking the gaspipe." Not all West Enders felt the same, however. While members of the Figella family "suffered" from the move and felt isolated in their new home, the Giuliano family was more positive about it. With these complexities present, urban renewal, according to Fried, could not just be about "bricks and mortar."[47]

Midtown, therefore, was conducted in the midst of ongoing debates about urban renewal and the relationship between urban life and mental health. None of Midtown's major contributors, however, were experts on the urban environment to the extent of Duhl, Calhoun, or Gans. Yet they were tasked with investigating New York City, then the most emblematic of cities. It might have been anticipated that what Midtown would reveal about mental health in the Big Apple would prove highly significant in resolving these debates. But, despite the headlines that greeted the publication of *MHM*, this was not to be the case.

MIDTOWN'S ORIGINS

In Midtown, there was certainly an epidemiological puzzle to be solved, but there was also the pressure to formulate mental health policy. The necessity to determine how, when, where, and why people suffered from mental illness was also intensified by World War II, which convinced psychiatrists that such problems were much more common than previously thought. These pressures were expressed by *MHM*'s lead author, the anthropologist Leo Srole (1908–1993), in his introduction to the book's second chapter:

> By measure only of calculable dollar costs drained from national income, mental illness stands charged as the gravest public health liability of our time. By duration of its creeping blight over the victim's life span, mental illness must additionally be arraigned as the most insidious of human afflictions. It is ironical, in this light, that in magnitude of the research counterattack mounted against it, mental disorder remains one of the most neglected of our public health problems. These observations may suggest something of

the pressures upon science to engage the problem on an all-out alarm basis. The Midtown Manhattan study . . . represents one among many research responses to those pressures.[48]

Midtown's goal was to "test the general hypothesis that biosocial and sociocultural factors leave imprints on mental health which are discernable when viewed from the panoramic perspective provided by a large population."[49] To do so, the project combined the expertise of clinical psychiatry, medical epidemiology, and the social sciences. This required a large, interdisciplinary team of researchers who would have to figure out, often on the fly, how to translate and understand one another's terminology and methods.

The person who envisioned, designed, and initially led this complex operation was Thomas Rennie, who founded the project and directed it until his death in 1956, at the age of fifty-two. Possibly because of his untimely death, Rennie is not as well known as some of the others involved in Midtown, yet the project was largely his brainchild, and the project team would often debate how best to ensure that his vision came to fruition. Born in Motherwell, Scotland, Rennie immigrated to Pittsburgh with his family in 1910. After graduating from the University of Pittsburgh and Harvard Medical School, Rennie spent 1931 through 1941 at Baltimore's Henry Phipps Psychiatric Clinic with Adolf Meyer, becoming "an outspoken Meyerian."[50] He espoused Meyer's concept of psychobiology, which conceptualized mental disorder as an adaptive personality disorder, not as the symptoms of a diseased brain, and that psychiatrists had to consider the biological, psychological, and social context of the patient. For Rennie, "the principles of psychobiology were simple: to determine why and how the patient's mental disorder developed." Essentially, this was Midtown's ultimate goal. Rennie also followed Meyer in his belief that it was important to analyze case histories, his advocacy for occupational therapy, and, crucially, his respect for the social sciences.[51] Rennie left the Phipps Clinic in 1941 for Cornell, where, in 1950, he became the first professor of social psychiatry in the United States. Before Midtown, Rennie cowrote a book on parergasia (a Meyerian term for dementia praecox) and also wrote about psychiatric social work, psychiatric education, vocational rehabilitation, and mental hygiene.[52] These publications hinted at Rennie's Meyerian roots, his diverse interests, willingness to collaborate, propensity for research innovation, and concern that psychiatry move beyond the hospital and become a more active force in society. A review of *Analysis of Parergasia* by the schizophrenia expert Jacob S. Kasanin (1897–1946), for instance, praised it for being "imaginative" and highlighted that the "most important" implications of the study were for mental hygiene. It provided a "program of prevention which seems to be of great value."[53] This focus on creative approaches and preventive psychiatry would foreshadow Rennie's plans for Midtown.

Rennie's use of Meyer's term "parergasia" (meaning incongruity of behavior) provides another indication of his dedication and debt to his mentor. Meyer can be considered a kind of grandfather to the Midtown Study. Not only did Meyer mentor Rennie, but he also taught Alexander Leighton, who succeeded Rennie as Midtown's director.[54] Significantly for Midtown, Meyer impressed upon his protégés the value of the social sciences. While Rennie was very much a psychoanalyst in a psychoanalytical department, Meyer instilled in him the idea that social factors were central to understanding mental health and that to understand these factors it was necessary to learn from sociology, anthropology, and related disciplines.

Although the archival record left behind by Rennie is limited, a glimpse into his personality and character is made possible through his correspondence with Meyer. Rennie wrote to Meyer in 1931 to inquire about psychiatry internship possibilities at the Phipps Clinic.[55] His approach to Meyer, who was at the height of his career, was rather forward. In his first letter he asked if his previous medical training would forgo the need for an internship and lead directly to an assistant residency. Following Meyer's reply in the negative, Rennie asked more questions, including a request to start six months earlier than the advertised start date if offered the position. The reference letters provided to Meyer on Rennie's behalf described him as a "delightful," imaginative individual who was "industrious" and had skill in music, as well as medicine.[56] He was said to have "an unusual personality which appeals to many sorts of people," but, unfortunately, no more details about what made Rennie's personality "unusual" were provided.[57] Meyer offered Rennie the position on April 7, 1931, a day after the latter prompted the former for a response.[58]

Rennie would stay at the Phipps Clinic for a decade, joining Cornell (where Meyer had been employed between 1904 and 1909) in 1941. In 1940, Rennie wrote to Meyer to explain the reasons for his departure, stating that, while he regretted leaving, he looked forward to the added status, latitude, extra responsibility, and salary that came with his new position. Given his failed promotion bid (which had caused some embarrassment to both himself and Meyer), he would have remained the "fourth ranking person in the department" indefinitely had he stayed at Phipps. At Cornell and the larger Payne Whitney Clinic, there was "a real job to be done" where he could "be of more value."[59] Rennie's desire to do something meaningful with his training is also evident in his attempt to "get into Army service" during World War II.[60] Although he was "very eager," he also desired an assignment that would make use of his psychiatric experience; he did not want to confine his duties to general medical practice. Ultimately, Rennie found his role working at a Veterans Administration hospital rehabilitating returning veterans and serving on the Army Advisory Committee of Greater New York.[61] He would also work on a variety of mental hygiene and mental health charities, most notably becoming the first chair of the New York City Community Mental Health Board. Rennie's work with veterans, social services, and mental health charities gave him a "community orientation" and convinced him that, along with psychiatric treatment, patients need "the help of social agencies, pastors, general practitioners, their families and their friends."[62] All of this, though somewhat fragmentary, paints the picture of a pleasant yet determined and fairly ambitious psychiatrist whose personality and experiences made him a good leader; who brought an imaginative, innovative, and open-minded style to research; and who was dedicated to a preventive and community-based approach to psychiatry.

These characteristics also help explain Rennie's vision for Midtown. In his introductory chapter for *MHM* (written shortly before his death, six years before the book's publication), Rennie described how psychiatrists "feel deeply impelled to turn their interest outward from the individual patient to the family, the community, and the total cultural scene." While part of this work included raising mental health awareness, it also included preventive initiatives. Midtown would help determine how to develop such a "truly preventive program." In order to discover "the forces within the social environment which contribute to the personal dilemma . . . a working relationship between the social scientist and the psychiatrist" had to be forged. The "forces" to be investigated by Midtown's social scientists included "cultural background, socioeconomic status, ethnic identification . . . and many variables imposed by urbanism itself—density, heterogeneity, secularism, isolation, anonymity, and spatial, vocational, and social mobility, as well as . . . exogenous disease and physical malfunction."[63] These factors would be investigated in both people already diagnosed with mental health problems and—importantly—those who were well. Overall, Rennie's plans for Midtown were both bold and far-reaching, both in terms of forging an interdisciplinary psychiatric epidemiology and in informing preventive mental health policy.

MIDTOWN'S METHODS

The investigators charged to carry out Rennie's vision were an eclectic mix of mental health professionals and social scientists. The interdisciplinary nature of the project was mirrored in the variety of academic positions held by the core project members. These included Leo Srole, a professor of sociology and psychiatry at the State University of New York Medical Center (previously at Cornell); Thomas S. Langner, an assistant professor of sociology (psychiatry) at Cornell; Stanley T. Michael (1912–1986), a research associate in psychiatry at Columbia; the anthropologist Marvin K. Opler (1914–1981), a professor of social psychiatry at the University of Buffalo School of Medicine (previously at Cornell); and Alexander Leighton, a professor of sociology and anthropology at Cornell and head of its Program in Social Psychiatry. This core team was also supported by psychiatric social workers, clinical psychologists, psychiatrists, and the anthropologists Eleanor Leacock (1922–1987) and Vera Rubin (1911–1985), who worked on the project from 1952 to 1955 and 1953 to 1955, respectively.

This rich combination of expertise was matched in the array of methodologies devised for the project. Rennie stressed that one of *MHM*'s goals was "to give a picture of our struggles to arrive at the appropriate methodologies" required to investigate mental health in New York City. The finished product achieved just that, providing more than fifty pages detailing the methods used to undertake the project, as well as a series of methodological appendices. One of these was appendix H, which summarized the "errors, artifacts, and biases" that might have influenced how the mental health ratings were determined. A potential source of bias was that even though the interviewers were "all professionals highly trained in the interviewing art," they might interpret the mental health of upper-class respondents as being better than it actually was and do the opposite for lower-class respondents.[64] This was despite the fact that an attempt was made to pair interviewers up with respondents from similar ethnic and class backgrounds. In this case, the risk of such bias was deemed to be small; however, drawing attention to it indicates how the researchers often questioned their own approaches and spent considerable amounts of time anticipating and addressing the critiques that they suspected would emerge.

Although its lead author, Leo Srole, invited the "general reader" to skim over this "shoptalk," these pages are helpful in terms of assessing how the project team set about their work and why—to use Rennie's word—"struggles" emerged.[65] They also help explain some of the hesitancies the contributors had about articulating Midtown's policy implications, which amounted to not much more than fifty words, let alone fifty pages. It suggests that, while guiding mental health policy might have been one of

Midtown's aims, the project team was more comfortable with conducting, describing, and debating thorny academic details. This is despite the fact that many of the researchers had been politically active and outspoken in the past. It also indicates the challenges inherent in synthesizing the views of numerous researchers from disparate disciplines. As much as Midtown was devised as an interdisciplinary enterprise, this was difficult to achieve in practice. Finally, it provides a reminder of the fact that Midtown was conducted in the first—and ultimately only—wave of postwar social psychiatry research. Its authors were counting on many more large, interdisciplinary epidemiological studies being conducted in the future. Midtown was conceived of as merely the first of a long succession of studies that would gradually provide a firm foundation for both psychiatric epidemiology and mental health policy. This, however, was not to be the case.

Overall, the Midtown Study was supported by four primary methods:

1. A home interview survey of 1,660 residents of Yorkville, a neighborhood of approximately 175,000 people (as of 1954) on Manhattan's Upper East Side

2. A "Treatment Census," providing a snapshot of the 2,240 Yorkville residents who were psychiatric inpatients or outpatients during a set period

3. A "Community Sociography," providing the social and historical context of Midtown

4. An "Ethnic Family Operation" led by Marvin Opler and meant to be the subject of the third, unpublished Midtown volume[66]

Midtown investigated the mental health of both patients and nonpatients, the suspicion being that those in treatment merely represented "the visible portion of an iceberg."[67] The "keystone" and largest element of Midtown's study design, therefore, was the Home Interview Survey, which was administered to 1,660 white residents between the ages of twenty and fifty-nine years of age.[68] The survey focused on individuals not currently receiving psychiatric treatment and provided an estimate of the total frequency of mental illness.

One initial balancing act, described by Srole as "The Crucial Decision," was weighing reliability of diagnosis against sample size. The study could either be based upon an intensive clinical examination to determine a reliable diagnosis of a *small* number of people or use survey methods to determine the mental health status of a *larger* number. Rennie had originally opted for the former option, recruiting a smaller cohort consisting of about one hundred households, which would be examined in great depth. In a team discussion, however, it was acknowledged that a sample of this size would not allow for "group-to-group comparisons of Midtown's cross-cutting demographic segments."[69] As comparing groups according to ethnicity, socioeconomic status, physical health, age, and gender was central to the study, Rennie and his team unanimously opted to utilize a larger sample size of at least 1,500 individuals.

This decision would lead to "many inexorable consequences" regarding the interpretation of findings, but it also represented how balances between the methods of psychiatrists and those of social scientists had to be struck. The psychiatrists working on Midtown may have been interested in population health, but their inclination, especially given the psychoanalytical training most American psychiatrists received at the time, was to focus on the individual or, at most, the family as the subject of analysis. They were keen to get the diagnosis or mental health assessment *correct*, as was their clinical duty. The social scientists, in contrast, were less concerned about the accuracy of individual diagnoses or assessments, since a large enough sample size would reduce the significance of errors. As Srole would explain in a six-page letter to Rennie in June 1953, questionnaire items could not be designed "to elicit near-perfect reliability in responses."[70] Perfect reliability was not required to make conclusions and, moreover, progress was constantly being made toward *"optimal* reliability."[71] It is also worth noting that during the early 1950s, when the design for Midtown was being determined, psychiatric diagnosis was less reliant on the APA's *Diagnostic and Statistical Manual of Mental Disorders (DSM)* than it would become later. *DSM-I* was published in 1952, but *MHM* did not mention it or any other existing diagnostic manuals. Instead, "the primary basis for the psychiatrists' choice and decision was clinical experience."[72]

Regardless, the purpose of the survey was not to measure mental *illness* but mental *health*. This distinction also bemused the psychiatrists. As Kirkpatrick and Michael noted, "Rennie was fully aware that the special preoccupation of the physician is primarily with pathology and secondarily with health, that the medical man is trained and tends almost unthinkingly to describe health in terms of pathology."[73] In order to help the project team focus on mental *health*, therefore, Rennie wrote his own definition of it on a chalkboard in the team's conference room. This blackboard definition would remain a reference for the team while the survey was developed:

1. Ease of social interaction

2. Capacity for pursuit of realistic goals

3. Fulfillment of biological needs, such as child bearing and rearing

4. Satisfying sense of social belonging: sensitivity to the needs of others

5. Feeling of adequacy in social roles (especially sexual)

6. Optimal balance between interdependency-dependency, rigidity-plasticity needs

7. Capacity for utilization of essential creativity

8. Capacity to accept deprivations and individual differences

9. Conservative handling of hostilities and aggressions

10. Identification with ethical and moral values

11. Adaptability to homeostasis (stress)

12. Healthy acceptance of self (e.g., body image and ego image)[74]

The psychiatrists were advised to remember these points when they made their ratings.

Ultimately, the survey would comprise an in-person interview lasting two hours. It was designed to be "less fluid than a psychotherapy session" but "more freewheeling" than a medical intake interview.[75] The survey was guided by a two-hundred-item questionnaire designed by Rennie and the project psychiatrists Kirkpatrick and Michael.[76] Many questions were designed to tease out particular psychiatric symptoms, such as anxiety or depression. For example, respondents were asked to agree or disagree to the following statements: "You sometimes can't help wondering whether anything is worthwhile anymore"; "I am often bothered by nervousness (irritable, fidgety, tense)"; and "In general, would you say most of the time you are in low spirits?"[77] The interviewer would probe if the respondent answered "don't know" or kept quiet. These probes were anticipated to provoke "free association elaborations and asides" that would provide further insights into the interviewee's mental health. Often the comments that followed "were so revealing that the rating could have been made on the strength of these amplifications alone."[78]

The interviewers also noted respondents' behavior during the interview. This included whether they were "hostile," "suspicious," "friendly," or "solicitous" about being interviewed, as well as overall impressions about the interviewees and their homes. Interviewers made notes about respondents' "apparent ease or tension, affect or mood, appropriateness of replies, apparent level of intelligence, dress and grooming habits, the presence or absence of muscular tics, stutter or stammer in speech, memory difficulties, and physical deviations and disabilities."[79] One interviewer reported that "poverty, ignorance and neglect are the most striking features of R's home," proceeding to say that "R might drink ten beers in a tavern with friends on payday." Overall, the interviewer found R "contemptuous and suspicious," with the "boastful charm of an adolescent boy."[80]

All of these factors, along with data about previous psychiatric care and involvement of social services, would be weighed by Kirkpatrick and Michael, in their mental health ratings.[81] In other words, they made assessments based on the combined data from the survey instruments, rather than from any personal observations. The specific ratings were broken down accordingly: well, mild symptoms, moderate symptoms, and impaired, which was further broken down into marked symptoms, severe symptoms, and incapacitated. Kirkpatrick and Michael explained that the process of assigning these ratings "was something like diagnosis, and yet it was definitely not diagnosis, but rather an assessment of probability based on a kind of data that lacked much of the information upon which most clinicians usually rely." The two psychiatrists also had to be mindful of their "own biases and predilections," the different approaches taken by the interviewers, and the respondents' attitudes toward the interview itself. Even basic responses could be misleading. When a respondent stated that they did not enjoy their line of work, for instance, was that "an expression of many years of loathing or an expression of annoyance which arose today?" If an interviewer had not probed for more information, it would be difficult for the psychiatrists to tell. Kirkpatrick and Michael stressed that in such cases they would *"lean away* . . . from judgments of illness." In any case, the psychiatrists had to trust that the respondents were being honest and comprehensive in their answers. In time, however, the psychiatrists—and Rennie—grew more confident about their ratings and remarked that often they were easy to assign, especially with those "at the extremes of the mental health scale."[82] As the survey could not cover Yorkville residents who were in psychiatric hospitals, a Treatment Census was conducted by the psychiatric social workers Freeda Taran and Margaret Bailey. The measure of treated mental disorder could then be compared to the prevalence determined by the survey.

Alongside these assessments of Midtown's mental health were laid the Community Sociography and Ethnic Family Operation (EFO). Although the results of the EFO, led by Opler, would not be published as planned, it nevertheless comprised a considerable percentage of the Midtown project team, including (during the peak of its activity) five anthropologists, eight doctoral candidates, and numerous volunteers. The Anthropology Section, as it was described, provided an analysis of prominent ethnic communities in Midtown, including Italian, Czechoslovakian, Irish, Hungarian, Puerto Rican, German, and "American" populations, thus demonstrating how important questions of ethnicity were in terms of determining urban mental health.[83] An individual's cultural background was considered a vital reference point in determining their mental health. While the psychoanalytical orientation of Rennie instilled in the project team the notion that certain "universal psychologic processes," such as sublimation, repression, and projection, applied to all cultures, cultural differences with respect to religion, parent-child relationships, and acculturation, as well as how certain ethnic groups were regarded in society, all had effects upon personality. The EFO was not meant merely to provide "background information" but would illuminate "the process of individual adjustment itself."[84] Its work was meant not to reveal stereotyped characteristics but how the character and behavior of individuals was shaped by their cultural background.[85]

The Community Sociography was also portrayed as an essential component. In order to understand Midtown's mental health, it was crucial to grasp its history, geography, institutions, culture, and "its own pervading sociopsychological climate." By doing so, it became easier to compare Midtown with the rest of Manhattan, the other New York City boroughs, and other urban areas. The sociography operation was conducted by a group of research aides, sociology students, and community volunteers under Srole's direction, who employed a combination of secondary sources, interviews, and participant observation. Whereas the EFO was barely mentioned in *MHM* (likely because of frictions between Opler and Srole), the Community Sociography was covered in three chapters, in an attempt to encapsulate the heart of a city of "unspeakable complexity" and "extreme heterogeneity."[86] Although Midtown was predominantly white, it was ethnically and economically diverse, with residents living in housing ranging from "Gold Coast" apartments (a nickname borrowed from Chicago) to slum tenements.[87] Ethnicity and socioeconomic status were described as being "closely intertwined," with "Old Americans" representing the bulk of upperclass residents, second- and third-generation immigrants rising to the middle classes, and recent immigrants on the bottom tiers of the social ladder. Other observations included the fact that children were under-represented, comprising only 15 percent of the population (half the rate of other U.S. cities). This was because of the high number of "singleton" residences in Midtown (25 percent, compared to 11 percent in other U.S. cities) and the large numbers of childless couples and working women (women outnumbered men at a ratio of 125:100).[88] These discrepancies with other U.S. cities raised the question of how representative Midtown was. While it was different in many respects from other U.S. cities—and, indeed, other parts of New York City—it bore many similarities to neighborhoods in other cities that bordered the central business core and contained a mix of "Gold Coast and slum" residences.

Viewed in its entirety, Midtown was a massive undertaking with numerous moving parts and involving dozens of investigators from a range of disciplines. Many decisions about what methods to employ were discussed at length and required negotiation and compromise to determine. Many of the balances struck would not only alienate members of the project team at various times but also provide easy targets for critics and reviewers once *MHM* was published. While any project of the size, complexity, novelty, and ambition of Midtown was bound to encounter problems, the number of upheavals, disagreements, rivalries, and interdisciplinary divisions it experienced was remarkable, threatening the completion of the project and ultimately undermining its impact.

TENSIONS IN MIDTOWN

Many of Midtown's tensions can be traced to Rennie's death in 1956. As Midtown's architect and director, Rennie's vision and leadership abilities had held the project together. An episode before his death and involving the project's anthropologists, however, foreshadowed the issues that followed. Although the precise origin of the dispute that emerged is difficult to determine, it was related to the management structure of the project and the various roles and responsibilities held by the anthropologists. The first indication of the dispute can be found in a letter dated September 30, 1954, from the anthropologist Marvin Opler, director of the EFO, to Rennie.[89] The letter concerned the anthropologists Eleanor Leacock and Vera Rubin, both of whom had been invited onto the project by Opler, who knew them from Columbia. Both Leacock and Rubin would go on to prominence within their field. Leacock became well known as a Marxist-feminist cultural anthropologist with expertise in Canada's Innu population, feminist theory, and racism in American education and would eventually chair the City University of New York's anthropology department following a long period during which she was blacklisted. She was assistant director of the EFO in 1952, while she was completing her PhD at Columbia.[90] Rubin also graduated with a PhD from Columbia in 1952 and was a specialist in Caribbean studies, aging, and medical anthropology. She founded the Research Institute for the Study of Man in 1955 and cofounded the journal *Transcultural Psychiatry*. She joined Midtown as the other assistant director of the EFO in 1953.

The subject of Opler's letter to Rennie was a memo from Rubin and Leacock to Opler and Rennie, which had been sent earlier that day. This memo has not been preserved in the archival records, but it seems to have included an ultimatum and threat of resignation over the way the project was being handled.[91] Rubin and Leacock's memo, in turn, was spurred by one from Opler to all anthropology staff on September 24, 1954, which was "written to promote efficiency in the massive research ahead, to orient volunteer personnel, to indicate how the project is organized, and how its direction and supervision is best formulated." In what followed, Opler proceeded to set out a series of five "rules . . . made effective here and now" to ensure that the fieldwork "be productive and efficient, and that professional ethics, manners and careers be preserved and promoted to best effect in the future." These five "rules" concentrated on the leadership and direction of the project. Any mention of Midtown had to note that Rennie was study director. Opler insisted on being described as being "in charge of" the Anthropology Section; all the members of the section were to be described as "under [his] supervision." Moreover, changes to theses or fellowships connected to the project had to be approved by Opler and were subject to Rennie's approval. Finally, Opler proposed dropping the terms "senior anthropologist" and "core staff" from everyday communications, explaining that the term "senior" implied "invidious age distinctions" and "grated upon his ear." He concluded by stating:

> We all face large tasks, difficulties in them, and probably some difficulties in accomplishing goals of research. With efficient and mature judgment, and a modicum of trust and considered exchange of opinion, we can also have some real success in research. *As an anthropologist I hope we can make good use of an opportunity, developed in medical science, to benefit human beings.* Being also, like you, in the same profession and biological species, I will appreciate any attempts to reach consensus.[92]

Compared to some of Opler's other memos and letters, this directive was fairly measured in tone. The tenor, wording, and immediacy of his response to Rubin and Leacock's memo and subsequent correspondences reveal that Opler was not always so restrained.[93]

Opler began his response to Rubin and Leacock's memo by explaining that he had "specific reactions to this Memo," which he intended to explain without being "contentious, persistent, confusing, or boastful." He proceeded to state that he would convince his fellow anthropologists to "fully and wholeheartedly accede to *one* Director of the Study" (Rennie) and "*one* in charge and supervision [*sic*] of all anthropology work" (himself—Opler). This was to ensure "that we are doing *one type of study*, integrated and co-ordinated in character, in *one* project with *one* focus." With respect to his management of Rubin and Leacock, Opler stressed that he had "tried at all points to support as best I could the reputation and career of each of the two colleagues and to prevent any damage to either."[94]

Rennie responded to Opler's letter on October 4, 1954, with a brief memo to all relevant staff detailing the line management of the project. Specifically, the work of the six field teams "should be cleared through Drs. Rubin and Leacock . . . under Dr. Opler's overall guidance."[95] By the end of the month, however, the situation was again deteriorating. Opler wrote to Rennie on October 29, 1954, stating that while Rennie's memo had "solved admirably a then-current crisis carried to some lengths by two of my colleagues [Rubin and Leacock]," it had not resulted in "less work and smoother operations" but instead "more work, less accomplished, and continual clash," with many of his colleagues "acting out" in meetings, especially when Rennie was absent.[96] As well as Rubin and Leacock, Opler implicated that Srole had also been "acting out," foreshadowing future disputes.[97]

Opler sent another letter to Rennie on January 26, 1955, indicating that the situation had worsened, threatening the timely completion of the EFO. Rennie had been ill since September 1954 but had continued to provide Opler with "suggestions and directives." Opler explained that he had taken up Rennie's suggestion to "effect rapport" with Leacock, asking her "at her desk and with warmth and concern if we could discuss any matters she might have on her mind." Leacock responded negatively to Opler's overture, and, when he tried again the following week, she left the office "with something of a tirade including, 'I don't see that I have anything to discuss with you.'" Opler was convinced that Rubin and Leacock "had attempted, in effect, a serious and self-interested 'strike' against research," "had damaged morale," and "had gone into high gear to tear a carefully built structure down." The team was at an impasse, with Rubin and Leacock not willing to discuss matters with Opler, leaving him to conclude that "Old Humpty Dumpty cannot be put back together again."[98]

A month later, Rubin and Leacock issued another ultimatum, this time demanding that the anthropology projects be split into two independent studies with separate teams and publications. Opler wrote again to Rennie on February 18, 1955, stating that while the decision regarding the ultimatum was up to Rennie, he was "embarrassed by the fact that both [Rubin and Leacock] are anthropologists," described them as "hostile" and "unethical," and decried the idea of splitting up the study. This would not be the only time Opler would worry about Midtown's cohesiveness. One of Opler's lingering concerns after Rennie's death was that his vision of a unified, interdisciplinary study be realized. He also apologized for recommending Rubin and Leacock and stated that Leacock's "first remarks to him since the classic 'I have nothing to discuss with you' ... were 'Alright, Marvin, go and push the anthropologists around,'" remarks that Opler claimed had "no touch with any reality."[99] The next day (a Saturday), Opler continued with another letter to Rennie, this time describing Rubin and Leacock as "basically hostile individuals" who were "shallow and self-interested," ultimately recommending to Rennie that they be fired or their roles restricted.[100]

The records do not precisely describe the fate of Rubin and Leacock, though a letter exists from Leacock to Rennie requesting to be relieved of her fieldwork duties.[101] What they do indicate, however, is how large-scale social psychiatry projects, such as Midtown, were not just idealistic attempts to determine the causes of mental illness and the steps to prevent them. They were also, to use Opler's admittedly strong words, opportunities for "empire building, control of others, and STATUS."[102] In Opler's opinion, the efforts of Rubin, Leacock, and, indeed, Srole to split up the anthropology projects undermined the overall cohesion of the project and, crucially, Rennie's vision for it. To him, they were ultimately egotistical attempts by those involved to put their careers ahead of the project. Given the struggles many social scientists endured in trying to obtain tenure during the height of McCarthyism (including not only Leacock but also Opler), such efforts at self-preservation were somewhat understandable.

Opler's letters to Rennie were also full of effusive expressions of his praise and admiration for his director. In one letter, Opler claimed that there were "self-generated confusions that may operate in all people, including myself, the mentally disturbed, in Dr. Leacock or Dr. Rubin. I consciously exclude Dr. Rennie from the list. . . . Of all my colleagues on this Study, my deepest admiration for balance in personality, good sense in science, and accomplishment in the fields in which we are working goes to Dr. Rennie."[103]

These odd words, in a letter penned solely to Rennie, reveals insights into Opler and Rennie's close relationship and the broader political context of social science research during the early Cold War, which also helps explain some of the project's tensions.

Opler had graduated with a PhD from Columbia in 1938, having conducted research on the Ute and Paiute tribes in Colorado and Utah supervised by the pioneering anthropologist and folklorist Ruth Benedict (1887–1948). Benedict's *Patterns of Culture* (1934) heavily influenced Opler's views on culture and psychiatry, though he maintained that *Race: Science and Politics* (1940) was her "greatest book."[104] Opler would find a position in 1938 at Reed College in Oregon, where his elder brother, the anthropologist Morris Edward Opler (1907–1996), was working (Morris Opler would leave for Claremont College that year).[105] Marvin Opler excelled at Reed College, where he first became interested in psychiatry. He quickly became chair of the anthropology department but in 1943 was appointed to the War Labor Board. According to the historian David H. Price, the FBI was informed that Opler had been involved in a number of (to them) suspicious left-wing activities, including leading the University of Buffalo's National Student League (an organization deemed to be communist by the House Un-American Activities Committee) when he was a student in the 1930s.[106] Opler was soon assigned to a Japanese-American internment camp at Tule Lake, Oregon, to work as its chief community analyst.[107] At Tule Lake, he developed positive relationships with the detainees, setting up *senryu* (a type of Japanese poem) societies and using crepe paper to make rock gardens in the desert.[108] Believing he was a "wobbly," a "long-hair," and a "conscientious objector," the FBI continued to investigate Opler while he was at Tule Lake.[109] Their interest intensified after he began to criticize the War Office's policy of segregation in his daily reports to Washington, which he correctly predicted would lead to "low morale, anger, frustration . . . despair . . . [and] disloyalty" among the detainees.[110] Although Price notes that a final interview with Opler in December 1945 was the end of the FBI's interest until the 1960s, an oral history interview with Opler's son, Lewis Opler (1948–2018), reveals otherwise.

According to Lewis Opler, his father was awarded a Fulbright after World War II to do research in Burma and was given an endowed chair at Harvard at roughly the same time.[111] Then, disaster struck. First, the money for the endowed chair disappeared, and then the FBI told Opler that he would not be able to get a visa for Burma unless he spied for them. Refusing this, Opler found himself unemployed. After taking on a few temporary positions, Opler capitalized on his experience at Morningside Hospital in Portland, Oregon, in 1938, and began applying for positions in psychiatry departments.[112] He wrote letters to eighty-eight psychiatry departments across the United States, and one of them came to Rennie at Cornell, who was then planning Midtown.[113] Rennie was told by Clyde Kluckhohn (1905–1960) at Harvard that Opler had been blacklisted (thus explaining why the endowed chair had vanished), but Rennie hired Opler anyway. Rennie also hired Eleanor Leacock despite her Communist Party sympathies.[114] Lewis Opler described how his father believed Rennie "saved" his family and how his father "loved Rennie," who was always "very supportive" of him, sentiments that come through clearly in the archival record.[115] For Opler, Rennie's death was "a great tragedy"; for Midtown, it increased division and discord.

REPLACING RENNIE

Rennie died of a cerebral hemorrhage on May 21, 1956. He was replaced by Alexander Leighton, who wrote in *MHM*'s foreword that Rennie's death was "a loss from which the Midtown Manhattan Project could not fully recover."[116] As this section explains, these words carried more weight than the reader might have realized. The fact that Cornell asked Leighton, who was already directing the Stirling County Study (see chapter 5), to run Midtown hints that the university hoped that the project would soon finish. According to Lewis Opler, Cornell had never provided sufficient support for Midtown. Rennie was never given research leave to direct the project and had to do so on his own time.[117] When Leighton took over, his mission was effectively to "wind it down," and given that he was also running Stirling County, he was "heavily beset with his own prior research responsibilities."[118] Indeed, he would spend 1957 and 1958 at Stanford writing one of his Stirling County outputs and not managing Midtown in person.[119] Although Midtown's data had largely been collected by then, the task of analyzing and writing up its findings was only beginning. This difficult process would further disrupt an already divided team.

Opler and Leighton did not have a warm relationship.[120] There were a few potential explanations for this. For a start, Opler's devotion to Rennie and his vision for the project likely made it difficult to accept Leighton's accession to the directorship of Midtown. Leighton was also stationed at a Japanese internment camp during the war, specifically Poston, in Arizona. According to the anthropologist Peter T. Suzuki, Leighton held some different views from Opler concerning the mental health status of detainees and whether loyal and disloyal detainees should be segregated.[121] There is no evidence, however, to support that the two ever discussed the camps. A more certain source of Opler's coolness toward Leighton was the latter's review of Opler's *Culture, Society, and Human Values* (1956), published a few months after Rennie's death.[122] In a letter expressing his frustration at Midtown's progress, Opler described the contrast between Leighton's review and that of Clyde Kluckhohn, describing them "as different as night and day."[123] In the same letter, Opler "wondered if there is anything about me which suggests, even remotely, threat, deceit, formalism or lack of concern about your own valid interests and accomplishments, past, present, or future."[124] After Opler left Cornell in 1958, the two would also spar over the need to obtain departmental clearance for publications coming out of the Midtown research and other matters.

Even more animosity was evident between Opler and Srole. As indicated earlier, hints of this percolated throughout the Rubin and Leacock affair. A six-page letter from Srole to Rennie in mid-1953 demonstrates that, as with Opler, he had ardent opinions that he did not hesitate to share. The letter was spurred by an "unedifying" meeting that "dramatized anew the Tower of Babel potentialities in an interdisciplinary team with different scientific approaches and degrees."[125] Rennie was generally successful in managing these two strong personalities, or, as Lewis Opler put it, he at least "kept everybody from destroying each other." Leighton was not quite so successful.

Srole and Opler's antipathy toward each other masked similar backgrounds. Both emerged from relatively modest Jewish immigrant upbringings to excel academically. Srole's mother died when he was an infant, and he spent time in Chicago foster homes before his father's remarrying, a difficult experience that contributed to his becoming "a very sensitive guy."[126] Shy and withdrawn during high school, Srole would "force himself out of his shell" and join the debating team. After completing undergraduate studies at Harvard, he proceeded straight into doctoral studies at the University of Chicago, where he worked with W. Lloyd Warner (1898–1970) on the Yankee City Project, a sociohistorical study of Newburyport, Massachusetts. This project would help inspire the Community Sociography component of Midtown. Srole graduated in 1940 and found employment at

NYU and Hobart and William Smith Colleges during 1941 and 1942.[127] As with Opler, Srole had an eventful war. He became a military psychologist with the U.S. Air Force in 1943, conducting psychological assessments of personnel in a rehabilitation hospital. Later he became the UN director of Landsberg Jewish Displaced Persons Camp, where he would resign in 1945, protesting the poor conditions there.[128] His resignation was covered in the *New York Times*, and Srole lectured about his experience, heralded as "the portent of the new generation of leadership arising in American Jewry."[129] Srole's son, Ira Srole, has also described how his father managed to extract some of his family members who had been exiled by the Soviets to Siberia. Back in the United States, Srole worked for the Anti-Defamation League before joining Midtown in 1952.[130]

These experiences shaped Srole—much like Opler—into a forthright yet sensitive individual who had the willingness and ability to debate his point of view vigorously. According to his son—and similarly to Opler—Srole had "a fairly quick temper," "did not suffer fools gladly," was "not to be trifled with," and "was not at all shy about expressing his opinions. If he needed to make waves, well, so be it. He made waves."[131] In addition, according to Lewis Opler, both men "had big egos and couldn't be in the same room."[132] All this, after Rennie's death, combined to make an already tense situation even more volatile.

Much of the bitterness between Opler and Srole related to disagreements about the content and authorship of the three volumes planned for Midtown. The ghost of Rennie hovered over these debates. Concerned about how the research should be divided between volumes 1 through 3, Opler wrote a series of letters to Leighton in January 1957, one of which accused Srole of taking credit for some of Rennie's writing.[133] On March 27, 1957, Leighton attempted to settle the issue in a memo to Opler, Srole,

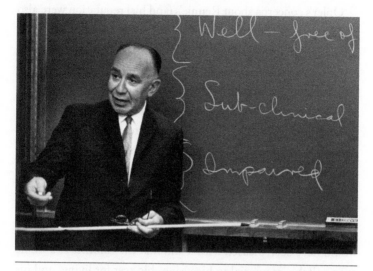

FIGURE 4.1 Leo Srole in front of blackboard.
Source: Photo courtesy of the Srole family.

and Thomas Langner. In it, he proposed that the project be divided into two teams, one led by Srole (supported by Langner) that would complete volumes 1 and 2, and one led by Opler and tasked with completing volume 3.[134] Although Opler eventually agreed to this division in a letter to Leighton written the following day, he warned that this "expeditious solution" might undermine the proposed volumes' "interdisciplinary strengths" and add to the "divisiveness and partial analysis that I have deplored for some time." It would result in an "inferior product" that would "fail to deliver the kind of scientific products for which we are responsible," thus "damaging" the reputations of all concerned, including the deceased Rennie.[135] In a marginal note, Opler reminded Leighton that "obviously, I am as concerned in March, 1957, about what my or Rennie's name is attached to, as I was in June, 1952, or will be in January, 1958."

Opler's concerns about Rennie's (and his) reputation were also bound up in Rennie's original vision for Midtown, namely, to produce an interdisciplinary, coherent, and integrated study that could be articulated with one unified voice. As the episode with Leacock and Rubin shows, Opler was eager to ensure that Midtown did not disintegrate into a series of disparate projects. It had to remain whole. Leighton's foreword to *MHM*, however, acknowledged that not all aspects of Rennie's vision had been realized: "The work bears the stamp of much that has transpired since Rennie's death. It probably differs in many respects from what he would have done, and undoubtedly lacks qualities which his genius would have contributed. We hope, however, that he would have been pleased with it and that the volumes as a whole are a suitable memorial to his vision, his zest for living, and his compassion for humanity."[136] At least some of these differences related to the unity of the project. The way *MHM* was written, with individual, rather than shared, chapter credits and with quite different conclusions expressed within them (see the following section), reiterates that this element of Rennie's vision was not achieved.

A few months later, Opler announced that he would be leaving Cornell for a position at the University of Buffalo.[137] Debates about the volumes, however, continued. One thorny issue concerned the volumes' authorship, which emerged in June 1960, when Srole and Langner consulted legal advice in order to change the original publication contract. Writing to the publisher, McGraw-Hill, Srole argued that Rennie's death had "changed matters drastically" since the initial contract was signed.[138] He contended that since Rennie had only written one chapter and had not survived to edit the volumes, it could not be assumed that he "would have accepted responsibility for the whole structure of assumptions, formulations, interpretations, and hypotheses that each volume has erected." Srole proposed instead that, while the series be named in Rennie's honor, he should not be listed as an author of volumes 2 and 3 and that Opler's name should not be listed for volume 1.

Opler mulled over his response in a letter to his elder brother, Morris. He described how Leighton and Cornell Department of Psychiatry Chair Oskar Diethelm (1897–1993) were possibly "acting behind the scenes in this maneuver," unless Srole was "lying in that detail as in others" or "using their names illicitly." Although Opler was "outraged," he was not certain that he could afford a legal battle, citing the costs of putting his children through university, and asked his brother for his advice "before plunging."[139] Correspondence between the various parties would continue until November 1960, when authorship was finally agreed: Opler's name would be added to volume 1, but Rennie's name would not appear on volumes 2 or 3. Opler's name, however, would not be associated with any of the chapters in volume 1, and volume 3, which he did draft, was never published.

MIDTOWN'S MESSAGE

Ultimately, the key finding of Midtown was that socioeconomic status (SES) had a major bearing on mental health. Specifically, "offspring of low SES-origin families at all age levels reflect maximum vulnerability to mental morbidity and minimum fulfillment of wellness." The gap between low and high SES was particularly striking with respect to the "well" and "impaired" categories. Whereas 30 percent of individuals currently in the highest SES strata were considered "well," only 4.6 percent of those in the lowest SES strata were considered "well."[140] Similarly, while 12.5 percent of those in the highest strata were considered "impaired" (with 0 percent "incapacitated"), 47.3 percent of those in the lowest strata were considered "impaired" (with 9.3 percent "incapacitated"). These findings, amplified by Midtown's innovative methodology, echoed those found in the studies of Chicago, New Haven, and Stirling County, Nova Scotia, which also emphasized the negative impact poverty, inequality, community disintegration, and social isolation had on mental health.[141]

Amid the debates and division that accompanied the production of *MHM*, however, the implications of this particular finding were underemphasized. In introducing the "Goals and Guidelines of the Study," Srole described how Midtown was intended to drive "*basic research* . . . about the still elusive mainsprings of most mental-disorder processes" and "*program research* to guide public and professional policy." As previously described, this focus on policy-relevant research was highly important to Rennie and, by extension, Opler. Ultimately, however, much more was written about Midtown's academic contribution than about its policy implications. Moreover, all of the book's conclusions were presented in a "restrained" manner.[142]

Some of this restraint was attributable to the interdisciplinary nature of Midtown and the "Tower of Babel" risks that Srole had expressed as early as 1953. In a 1967 interview, Srole described how "only selected investigators have the personality for multidisciplinary research. . . . Other individuals have their identity wrapped up in one discipline and cannot broaden it; they create friction on such projects."[143] Similarly, Leighton admitted in his foreword that "because of the differences in orientation stemming from their various disciplines, the authors had to spend much time in working through to mutual understanding and hammering out acceptable modifications."[144] Although Leighton added that "the completion of the volume is a testimony to their patience and determination," this did not mean that the authors were unified in their assessment of what Midtown ultimately meant. This is exemplified by the book's two epilogues—one written by the psychiatrist Stanley Michael and one written by Srole—which prevented the articulation a single set of interdisciplinary conclusions, an ambition of both Rennie and Opler. Michael began his epilogue (entitled "Psychiatrist's Commentary") by stating that *MHM* was "written by sociologists . . . based on sociological data." This was not entirely correct. Although Srole wrote or cowrote most of the chapters, Rennie had written the introduction, and Michael and his fellow psychiatrist Price Kirkpatrick had written chapter 4; moreover, the ratings made by Michael and Kirkpatrick were pivotal to the overall analysis. Nevertheless, Michael restated the dominance of the sociologists a few pages later, explaining that "the reader who is not mindful of the formulation and design of the report may be impressed with a sense of sociogenic overdeterminism. This impression is further strengthened by the fact that manuscript was written by sociologists." Michael would later stress that Midtown's findings should be treated with caution in terms of applying them more generally, which undermined the goal of using the study to "program research." Although Michael concluded by stating that Midtown would be "a springboard for future research in social psychiatry," his "Psychiatrist's Commentary" did not amount to a ringing endorsement and suggested that a disciplinary gap remained between psychiatry and the social sciences.[145]

Srole also qualified Midtown's findings in his epilogue (entitled "Sociologist's Sight Lines: Retrospective and Prospective"), suggesting that they would only serve as "temporary scaffolding for constructing new and more focused hypotheses."[146] His policy recommendations were articulated obliquely and were restricted to concepts, such as parent education, which had long been established.[147] In the 1967 interview previously mentioned, Srole admitted that "investigators who conduct a large scale undertaking like the Midtown Study, incorporate in their scientific roles neither responsibilities nor skills in conveying their findings to the lay community or in implementing their findings on the social policy level."[148] According to Srole, who also expressed disappointment that Midtown's impact had been "imperceptible," this "split between study and action" was unfortunate and argued that funders should support such "diffusion of knowledge." Srole was implying that had there been sufficient funding, the policy implications of Midtown would have been better articulated. In the end, however, it was only in the conclusion of chapter 12, cowritten by Srole and Langner, where any hint of policy implications was expressed, though not with much specificity: "Ultimately indicated here may be interventions into the downward spiral of compounded tragedy, wherein those handicapped in personality or social assets from childhood on are trapped as adults at or near the poverty level, there to find themselves enmeshed in a web of burdens that tend to precipitate (or intensify) mental and somatic morbidity; in turn, such precipitations propel the descent deeper into chronic, personality-crushing indigency."[149] Among the publications that would emerge out of Midtown, this statement came the closest to detailing what had to be done to prevent mental illness, the guiding mission of social psychiatry. The reader was left guessing, however, about what the actual "interventions" should be.

To a degree, such inconclusiveness was simply characteristic of Srole. Even in the posthumously published *Personal History and Mental Health* (1998), which represented "the late Leo Srole's final perspectives on adult mental health," he refrained from being conclusive: "As was characteristic of him, [*Personal History and Mental Health*] is exploratory, not confirmatory; it raises questions, and does not declare conclusions."[150] But, as the archives reveal, the paucity of policy recommendations in *MHM* also reflected deeper problems within the research team that had spanned the entire project. Some of these problems were interdisciplinary, some were personal, and some were simply born out of tragedy. In the end, what they really meant was that Rennie's ambition for "psychiatry to move into a vigorous period of real preventive work" was not realized.[151]

CONCLUSION: MIDTOWN'S LEGACY

Despite the hyperbolic press that greeted *MHM*, Midtown did not settle the debates about mental health in urban areas. Here, too, points of division can be identified. Srole tended to downplay the "1 in 5" statistic in the years that followed. He would later write that prominent sociologists, especially those of the Chicago School (as well as politicians and the general public), often had an "anti-city bias" and were overly nostalgic about rural America.[152] In 1972, he disputed the contention of the epidemiologists Linda Dohrenwend (1927–1982) and Bruce Dohrenwend (b. 1927) in the *American Handbook of Psychiatry* that rates of psychiatric disorder were higher in urban areas than in rural ones.[153] Srole argued that it was difficult to judge whether U.S. cities per se were pathological because of their transient nature.[154] Many of the "functionally impaired" individuals studied in Midtown "were largely escapees from smaller places, now at liberty in the metropolitan community rather than in an institution." Recalling Simmel, Srole suggested that "the semi-nomadicism of the American people, at least for adults discontented with their present community milieu, is in the service of therapeutic ends."

Rather than blaming the city, Srole contended that "parental psychopathology, economic poverty, and family disorganization . . . are psychologically disastrous for many children, white and black, in their midst. I am not sure, however, what part of this pathogenic combination is ultimately chargeable to the metropolis as such and what part to the smaller places that first berthed such crippled parents and then in effect extruded them by making life intolerable and insupportable for them."[155] Srole concluded by arguing that while children suffered from the "psychopathogenic" conditions in both "metropolitan and rural slums," for adults who found rural communities constrictive, cities could be a "therapeutic milieu."

Opler, in contrast, was more willing to discuss the "1 in 5" statistic and expressed more concern about the impact of city living on mental health. Although he had written none of *MHM*'s chapters, he was nonetheless interviewed about the study for a story entitled "Majority of New Yorkers Mentally Ill, Says Professor." Stating that Midtown "could be representative of every American city," Opler argued that the findings indicated the need for many more outpatient treatment facilities in metropolitan areas.[156] These clinics would soon be realized through the Community Mental Health Act of 1963 and subsequent amendments. Elsewhere, Opler pointed out that it was not the crowding found in cities that was problematic for mental health but rather how cities could alienate individuals from one another.[157] Increasing segregation on the basis of race, ethnicity, and socioeconomic status occurring in cities was making the situation worse, not better.[158] Such an assessment differed from Srole's more optimistic description of cities as potentially "therapeutic."

By the 1970s, Opler's concerns about the state of cities were proving true in New York City. Deinstitutionalization, which had seen sixty thousand patients released from hospital care in

New York City between 1965 and 1981, had occurred at a time of economic stagnation and urban decay, contributing to mass homelessness.[159] By the early 1980s, there were 36,000 homeless people in New York City; approximately 75 percent had spent time in a psychiatric hospital.[160] In Srole's archive, clippings from newspapers and academic journals detailing the increasing plight of the city's mentally ill and homeless indicate his concern about the situation. These included the work of Ellen Baxter and Kim Hopper, doctoral researchers who had conducted two hundred interviews with homeless New Yorkers, finding that mental illness was highly prevalent in such groups.[161] New York City would continue to see change and upheaval, experiencing a "cleanup" under Mayor Rudolph Giuliani during the 1990s, followed by the 9/11 terrorist attacks, Hurricane Sandy in 2012, and, most recently, the COVID-19 pandemic. These momentous changes occurred amid changing immigration patterns, increasing gentrification, and growing inequality. Although Srole, Opler, and the other members of the Midtown team would have undoubtedly bickered about the details, they all would have agreed that these factors would have affected the mental health of New Yorkers, too.

When set against the broader history of social psychiatry, Midtown provides three key contributions. First, with respect to debates about urban mental health, Midtown's findings suggested that it was not cities themselves that were pathological but rather factors such as poverty, community disintegration, and inequality. These socioeconomic problems were often concentrated in cities, but the degree to which they were present could differ from city to city and across time. Moreover, just as cities could decay and disintegrate, they could also renew and revitalize. While forced, top-down attempts at urban renewal tended not to succeed, cities could also create nurturing environments for grassroots community movements that could foment socially progressive change.

Second, Midtown provides an example of how, in seeking to grasp the rise and fall of social psychiatry, it is important to analyze not only the findings of landmark studies but also *how* these findings were produced. The archival and oral history sources required to reveal the inner workings of such studies are not always available. But when they are, they can present rich insights into how science—and social science—is conducted. Midtown shows how social psychiatry was never a unified, cohesive movement that spoke with one voice but rather a messy conglomeration of ideas that was derived through a complex and often tortuous process of negotiation and interdisciplinary translation. That does not mean, however, that such ideas should have been disregarded and dismissed. In contrast, it behooves us to work harder to tease out the many core messages that still have relevance today.

Finally, Midtown shows how social psychiatry researchers were often more comfortable developing the theory of social psychiatry than they were in applying it themselves or even suggesting how others might do so. Midtown did not deliver on Rennie's ambitions to conduct "program research" or produce a framework for "preventive psychiatry." Instead, its researchers spent their time fine-tuning their methods and analyzing their results in the hope of producing findings that were beyond reproach. Such a focus is understandable, especially in light of the highly competitive, cutthroat, and politically fraught academic context in which such researchers worked. But, amid all the concerns about mental illness during the postwar period and—more importantly—all the resources available to combat it, this tendency to amass ever more evidence before asserting unequivocally that a great deal of mental illness could be prevented or alleviated by eliminating poverty seems somewhat shortsighted and naïve. There would only be one Midtown, and once its legacy had begun to fade, that chance slipped away.

5

FROM COVE TO WOODLOT

They left 300 years buried by on the Bay
Where the whales make free in the harbour
—Stan Rogers

During the evening of September 20, 1950, Tom Young, a thirty-five-year-old farmer, settled into his rocking chair with a pipe, as a gale battered the spruce trees in his woodlot and rain clattered against the windows of his farmhouse in southwestern Nova Scotia. The storm paradoxically reminded him that his walls were solid and his animals were safe; if anything, the rain would be good for his crops. His wife and two young children were healthy, and, glancing at his rifle on the wall, he smiled at the thought of deer season in October. All was well. Moments later he was clutching at his chest and struggling to breathe as his heart palpitated erratically. A few days later, Tom had been referred to a psychiatric clinic and diagnosed with an anxiety attack. What was the matter with Tom?

This question provided the framework for *My Name Is Legion: Foundations for a Theory of Man in Relation to Culture*, the first monograph in the Stirling County Study of Psychiatric Disorder and the Sociocultural Environment.[1] Founded by the husband-and-wife team Alexander Leighton and Dorothea Cross Leighton in 1948, the Stirling County Study has been one of the most longstanding epidemiological studies ever conducted, only rivaled in longevity by the Framingham Heart Study, which also began in 1948, and the Lunby Study of psychiatric epidemiology in Sweden, which began a year earlier. Between the first publication based on the project in 1950 and most recent in 2019, dozens of others have emerged, including the three weighty monographs that are explored in this chapter: *My Name Is Legion* (1959), *People of Cove and Woodlot* (1960), and *The Character of Danger* (1963). One of the coauthors of the most recent article was Jane Murphy (1929–2021), who married Alexander Leighton after he and Dorothea Leighton divorced in 1965 (Dorothea Leighton would also leave the project that she cofounded at that point). Having joined the project in 1951 as an administrative assistant, Murphy then worked as an interviewer for the project, graduating with a PhD in 1960 from Cornell, where the study was institutionally based. She then took over the directorship of the study from her husband in 1975, though he continued to work on Stirling County for the remainder of his life. Murphy, too, worked on the project until her recent death. It remains to be seen whether the 2019 article will be the last publication produced by this most venerable of studies.[2]

In some ways, Stirling County bore many similarities to the other projects explored in this book, specifically, the New Haven and Midtown studies (the latter directed by Alexander Leighton after Thomas Rennie's death). Its goal was similarly to understand the epidemiology of mental health, specifically: "How much psychiatric disorder is there? What are the proportions of different varieties and kinds? How are these distributed in relation to sociocultural factors? In short: How much? Of what kinds? And where?"[3] Moreover, its "practical aim" was "to increase the effectiveness of preventive psychiatry."[4] In order to answer these questions, it employed a highly interdisciplinary approach, exemplified in the backgrounds of Alexander and Dorothea Leighton, who were both qualified in psychiatry and anthropology. Their large team (115 people were involved in total, including thirty-two medical consultants and thirteen secretaries) of both Canadians (including francophones and anglophones) and Americans included psychologists, statisticians, sociologists, photographers, administrators, and members of the local community, including the mayor.[5] Stirling County benefited from generous funding from NIMH, the Department of Health and Welfare Canada, the Nova Scotia Department of Public Health, the Carnegie Corporation of New York, the Millbank Memorial Fund, and the Ford Foundation.[6]

In other ways, however, Stirling County differed considerably from the other studies featured in this book. In addition to its durability, it focused on a rural, rather than an urban, environment, namely, southwestern Nova Scotia in Canada.[7] Here, there were no debates about the pathological nature of urban life. The economy still relied on fishing, logging, and farming, as it had for centuries. The ethnic composition of Stirling County had also remained comparably static, comprising primarily French Canadian (Acadian) and English Canadian communities, along with smaller numbers of indigenous Canadians and Black Canadians. Finally, Stirling County differed in that it incorporated a CMHC into its operations and research. The Bristol Mental Health Centre (BMHC—Bristol was a pseudonym, as was Stirling County) was founded in 1951 by the Leightons and their colleagues "to show that the great majority of people with mental illnesses could best be treated in their own communities, that preventing mental illnesses and promoting mental health were feasible goals, and that the involvement of community members . . . would not only strengthen the program but would also increase the ability of the community to recognize and cope more effectively with many of its psychological and social problems."[8]

In practical terms, BMHC supported the research objectives of Stirling in three ways: first, it enabled investigations into the distribution of mental illness in the community; second, it permitted the qualitative study of specific cases to achieve "a high-magnification picture of cause and effect in the relationship of environment and disorder"; and third, it allowed the researchers to explore how a rural CMHC could facilitate preventive psychiatry.[9] This third point is particularly important because CMHCs, which were just starting to emerge in 1951, would be expected to be places of preventive psychiatry. In this way, BMHC provided a preview of what CMHCs could be expected to achieve in terms of preventive mental health.

I begin this chapter by analyzing the origins, methods, and findings of the Stirling County Study, as well as the challenges it faced. Stirling County exemplified both the strengths and the weaknesses of other social psychiatry studies. On the one hand, it was a masterfully interdisciplinary and in-depth project that delved deeper than any other into the social, cultural, and economic environment of its target population. Whereas other studies would spend a chapter or two outlining historical and contemporary context, Stirling County devoted an entire tome (*People of Cove and Woodlot*, 574 pages) and created an archive of thousands of photographs, which are digitally accessible today.[10] It benefited especially from Dorothea and Alexander Leighton's previous anthropological research, as well as the latter's intimate familiarity with the geography and people of Stirling County. It also profited to an extent from the fact that Dorothea Leighton was a woman (one of the few prominent female social psychiatrists during the period), and she, according to Nancy J. Parezo, epitomized the patient, respectful, empathetic, grounded, and culturally relativistic approach to anthropology that was typical of other female anthropologists of the time.[11] Although the most deprived Stirling County residents were not perceived in such terms, generally speaking, most subjects of the study were regarded respectfully and at times almost reverently.

On the other hand, Stirling County also stubbornly insisted that its findings—which emphasized the pathological impact of social disintegration—were preliminary and required more study. As a result, it failed to articulate the structural problems that contributed to such disintegration, let alone discuss what to do about them. Such unwillingness often jarred with the case studies presented in the Stirling County publications. After heart trouble was ruled out, for example, Tom Young's attack was attributed primarily to his financial worries, how they might affect his young family, and how these problems would reflect on how he was perceived in the community: "It appeared that, no matter how he schemed and planned, he could not get on top of the situation and make life secure."[12] All of this was presented, however, in a highly provisional and speculative fashion. Alexander Leighton also mused about the role of other factors, ranging from the hereditary to the psychoanalytical, including a potentially traumatic episode Tom had experienced as a soldier. Eventually Leighton concluded that "it is inadvisable at present to accept any theory without reservation. It is equally inadvisable to reject them all." By the end of *My Name Is Legion*, Tom Young was left "dangling with the noose of his anxiety around his neck." Part of this was likely a rhetorical strategy that effectively set up the study's next two books. But it also reflected an equivocality that did not lend itself to policy application. Moreover, the belief that more research was required would not change decades after Stirling County had begun. Writing in 1982, Alexander Leighton insisted that "very little is known about how to prevent most mental illnesses." It remained a "major target" for psychiatry, but one that required significantly more research.[13] In addition, Stirling County's researchers often displayed classist and judgmental attitudes toward the residents of deprived communities, who were often portrayed as shiftless, lazy, and largely responsible for their situation in life. Given this mindset, it is not surprising that they did not argue that radical socioeconomic and structural changes were needed for preventive mental health.

What Stirling County's researchers did believe, however, was that CMHCs could play a role in preventive mental health. This is one of the reasons, after all, that they established BMHC in 1951. After sketching the history of BMHC, I then investigate the role prevention played in CMHCs built after the 1963 Community Mental Health Act. Prevention was meant to be fundamental to every CMHC, but this failed to be the case in practice. While some preventive innovations were introduced, such as the use of indigenous mental health workers (discussed in chapter 3) or parent and teacher education, the activities of CMHCs concentrated greatly on treating mental illness, not preventing it.

That this was so reveals one of the primary shortcomings inherent in the approach to preventive mental health that emerged after World War II. Social psychiatry research pointed to the role of deep-seated structural problems, such as poverty, inequality, and social disintegration. CMHCs were meant to be preventive institutions, but they could not meaningfully address the root causes of such issues. While the Johnson administration did attempt to deal with these issues through Great Society legislation, such as the Economic Opportunity Act (1964), the

Civil Rights Act (1964), and the Social Security Amendments of 1965, these initiatives either did not go far enough or were undermined by subsequent events and/or subsequent administrations. By the 1970s and 1980s, many of the social problems associated with mental illness, including the social disintegration highlighted by Stirling County, had worsened. In other words, if CMHCs really were to deliver preventive mental health, they needed to be supported by a sustained and transformative foundation of progressive policies tackling poverty, inequality, social isolation, and social disintegration. If this had been established, CMHCs might have become the preventive institutions they were intended to be, and social psychiatry might have lived up to its promise.

WELCOME TO STIRLING COUNTY

Before delving into the origins of the Stirling County Study, it might be useful to know where Stirling County is. Doing so, however, is tricky. Stirling County was a pseudonym chosen by the Leightons to protect the identity of its residents. Since Nova Scotia means "New Scotland," they thought it might be appropriate to use a Scottish place name and so selected Stirling, a small city in central Scotland that used to be its capital. The decision to disguise the true location of Stirling County was a response in part to concerns from residents, who were wary about being involved in a project investigating mental illness.[14] But while the importance of keeping Stirling County's true identity secret was stressed by Murphy as recently as 2015, sixty-seven years after the project began, it is easy to determine where it actually is.[15] The most obvious clue is a map of the county included in *People of Cove and Woodlot* (figure 5.1).[16] Since one of the study's

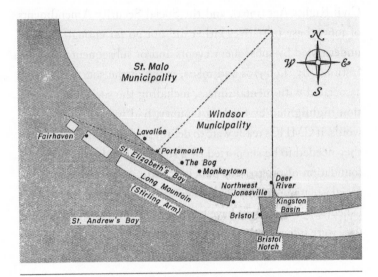

FIGURE 5.1 Map from *People of Cove and Woodlot.*

Source: Charles C. Hughes, Marc-Adelard Tremblay, Robert N. Rapoport, and Alexander H. Leighton, *People of Cove and Woodlot* (New York: Basic Books, 1960). Permission requested from Hachette.

objectives was to paint a detailed portrait of Stirling County's geography, history, and people, there were also broad hints elsewhere. I will, however, respect the wishes of the investigators and the people of Stirling County and not reveal the identity of the place here.

Perhaps more important than its precise location is how and why Alexander Leighton came to select it as a case study in psychiatric epidemiology. Leighton was born in Philadelphia in 1908, the son of Irish immigrants. His father was a structural engineer who cofounded a construction business. In 1916, a deadly polio epidemic struck Philadelphia and other East Coast cities, prompting the Leighton family to escape the city.[17] After receiving advice from some physicians, the family decided to relocate to Stirling County, Nova Scotia, for the duration of the epidemic and later summered there regularly.[18]

Ted Leighton (Dorothea and Alexander's son) has emphasized the impact these summers had on his father. Alexander Leighton quickly became fascinated by the natural environment of Stirling County and spent long days exploring the local woods, often with indigenous guides hired by his parents. These guides, some of whom became long-lasting friends, taught Leighton woodcraft and explained their worldview to him. This, according to Ted, was "absolutely formative with respect to his view of the world."[19] Leighton's fascination with the natural world spurred his early academic pursuits, including a short publication on porcupines in the *Journal of Mammalogy* in 1926, when he was just eighteen years old.[20] More significantly, his indigenous guides cultivated an abiding interest in Leighton about different cultures, foreshadowing his studies in anthropology. Finally, Leighton's knowledge of Stirling County helped confirm that it had all the cultural, social, and historical elements required for a comparative epidemiological study. There were two dominant cultural groups (represented by English Canadians and Acadians), three main economic activities (fishing, farming, and logging), and a considerable range of socioeconomic diversity.[21] But perhaps outweighing everything was the fact that Stirling County was simply somewhere Leighton enjoyed being. After taking up a position at Dalhousie University in nearby Halifax toward the end of his career in 1975, Leighton would spend the final decades of his life in the county that dominated his life's work.

The academic training and early careers of both Dorothea and Alexander Leighton also provide insights into the approach they used in the Stirling County Study. For his part, Alexander Leighton's fascination with ecology led him to Princeton, where he completed a BA in 1932. Becoming intrigued by the role of the nervous system in behavior, he then studied neurophysiology at Cambridge with Edgar Douglas Adrian (1889–1977), winner of the 1932 Nobel Prize for Physiology and, later, president of the Royal Society. Leighton's decision to go to Cambridge was based on both pragmatic and academic considerations. His father's previously thriving construction business was struggling amid the Great Depression, and Leighton determined that spending long years earning a PhD in biology might not be the most practical career choice, especially if he was called upon to support his family. His focus, therefore, gravitated toward medicine, which would give him the option of either continuing to pursue his research interests or clinical practice. After doing some premedical training at Cambridge, he returned to the United States and joined the third year of the MD degree at Johns Hopkins.[22]

Leighton's time at Johns Hopkins would be pivotal for two reasons. There he met Dorothea Cross, who was also studying medicine. They would marry in 1937, study psychiatry together, and both be drawn into anthropology. There the Leightons would meet Adolf Meyer, then chief of psychiatry. Meyer had also mentored Thomas Rennie, as well as other leading social psychiatrists. As with Rennie, Meyer instilled in the Leightons a deep appreciation for the role the social sciences could play in explaining human behavior. He encouraged self-reflection, problem solving, open-mindedness, and being empathic and respectful when interacting with and learning from other cultures.[23] Alexander Leighton later recalled how Meyer specifically suggested that he study anthropology. A member of the Social Science Research Council (SSRC), Meyer knew many leading social scientists and provided an introduction for Leighton to meet the Polish anthropologist Bronislaw Malinowski (1884–1942) when he visited Baltimore.[24] The Leightons soon met other leading anthropologists, including Margaret Mead, Ruth Benedict, Clyde Kluckhohn, and Ralph Linton (1893–1953). Illustrating their desire to pursue anthropology even further, the couple applied jointly for an SSRC fellowship in 1940, which gave them the opportunity to do coursework at Columbia and then complete six months of fieldwork among the Navajo and three months with the Yupik on St. Lawrence Island in the Bering Strait.

Dorothea Cross Leighton's path into social psychiatry was similarly indirect. She was born in Lunenburg, Massachusetts, in 1908 into a family of "decisive, strong-willed, well-educated men and women from propertied Protestant heritage." Her mother was a teacher who had opened one of the first nursery schools in the state when the health of Cross's father deteriorated following a bout of tuberculosis. According to Parezo, Cross was "humble" and "down-to-earth" and, though she was valedictorian of her high school, set her "career goals lower" than her family would have liked.[25] Her original plan was to be a nurse, which did not, at the time, require an advanced degree. Nevertheless, Cross's mother convinced her to attend Bryn Mawr, her alma mater, so that she could at least experience college. Majoring in biology and chemistry, she graduated in 1930 and found a job as a chemistry technician at Johns Hopkins Hospital but soon grew bored. She decided to become a general practitioner and enrolled at the Johns Hopkins School of Medicine, where she was given a full scholarship.[26] Upon graduating in 1936 near the top of her class, however, she "experienced career-stopping discrimination" when applying for internships in internal medicine. Her letters to prestigious medical schools were returned with the statement: "Sorry you are a woman." The only opportunity forthcoming was at the local Baltimore City Hospital, which proved to be a rewarding experience nonetheless.

By August 1937, the Leightons were married. With Alexander staying at Hopkins and specializing in psychiatry, Dorothea decided to join him, partly because it would be easier for them to start a family (something she desired alongside a career) and partly because doing different specialties "would be an awful mess."[27]

In 1939, during their psychiatric residencies, the Leightons paused to study anthropology in earnest, a hiatus that would transform their careers. Their goal was to understand "how different cultures viewed illness, how religion and medicine were culturally combined, and how biomedicine could be more useful to people."[28] Ultimately, they wanted to apply their anthropological insights to improve medicine and psychiatry in particular. By studying the Navajo and the Yupik, the Leightons were following Malinowski's dictum: "If you want to look at the earth you had better begin by going to the moon and looking back."[29] But, while applying what they learned during the course of their fieldwork remained important, learning about diverse cultures became an end in itself. As one reviewer later described Alexander Leighton, he was "a psychiatrist who has fallen under the spell of cultural anthropology."[30] While these field trips effectively proved to be the beginning of the end of both Leightons' medical careers, they did use their medical skills to develop rapport and trust with both the Navajo and the Yupik, which facilitated the life histories they would record.[31] Later, they criticized the ways in which the Office of Indian Affairs (OIA, renamed the Bureau of Indian Affairs in 1947) attempted to provide health services to the Navajo. Clinics were inaccessible for most Navajos and staffed by apathetic and ignorant physicians. Moreover, the Navajo medicine men were also "ignored . . . scorned and derided" and, therefore, underutilized.[32] They recommended that, rather than demanding that the Navajo adapt to Western medicine, the OIA should change its approach. Such insights were fleshed out in the Leightons' first monograph, *The Navajo Door* (primarily written by Dorothea Leighton, though Alexander Leighton was listed as first author), which was commissioned by the OIA commissioner and sociologist John Collier (1884–1968) and would help convince the OIA to work with indigenous groups regarding healthcare, rather than against them.[33]

During World War II, both Leightons continued to work at the intersection between anthropology and medicine. Dorothea Leighton worked as a researcher with OIA, during which time she would coauthor three highly influential books, including *The Navajo* (1946).[34] As mentioned in chapter 4, Alexander Leighton, a U.S. Navy Medical Corps reservist, was posted at a Japanese Relocation Center in Poston, Arizona, where he was tasked with studying how the detainees adapted to this artificial—and coercive—environment. His research resulted in *The Governing of Men* (1945), which, as its title suggested, represented something of a departure from the empathetic and collaborative approach that emerged from the Leightons' work on the Navajo.[35]

Leighton was then transferred to become chief of the Foreign Morale Analysis Division in the Office of War Information, which focused on understanding Japanese morale and attitudes toward surrender.[36] In addition to a number of Japanese American anthropologists, Leighton's team included Kluckhohn, Benedict, and Morris Opler, all of whom had far more seniority in terms of anthropology. Dorothea Leighton also spent time on the team. Among the team's findings was that the morale of the Japanese was rapidly waning in early 1945. These insights, however, were largely dismissed, as plans were already afoot to employ atomic weapons against the Japanese, of which Leighton's team was unaware.[37] After the bombing of Hiroshima and Nagasaki, Alexander Leighton served as research leader of the United

States Strategic Bombing Survey to assess survivors' psychological state. He described these two final assignments in *Human Relations in a Changing World* (1949), which implied that the use of atomic weapons had been unnecessary.[38]

Alexander Leighton's leadership responsibilities during World War II helped him when it came time to manage the very large, multicultural, and multidisciplinary team that made up Stirling County. They also further reinforced that the social sciences could and should inform policy but that effecting change was not always easy. Moreover, unlike Marvin Opler, whose wartime experience with the Japanese internment camps reinforced his left-wing views, Leighton remained attached to the establishment, finishing his military service as a commander in the U.S. Navy. Although soft-spoken and pleasant, he insisted on wearing his navy uniform throughout his time at Poston, even though it bred mistrust in the detainees.[39] He later expressed disdain for the antiauthoritarianism that emerged during the 1960s, blaming it for some of the problems that faced BMHC.[40] Politically, he may have been liberal and voted Democrat, but he was not a radical.[41]

Dorothea Leighton emerged during World War II as an innovative, pioneering, and influential anthropologist. But she was also torn between her research and her desire to have a family. After her husband found employment at Cornell in 1947, Dorothea Leighton was overlooked for positions in anthropology, despite having a far more impressive track record than the successful male candidates.[42] She would eventually find employment at Cornell in 1949, but by that time she had three children and often played hostess for her husband. Until the Leightons divorced in 1965 and she took up a professorship in public health at the University of North Carolina, she alternated between full- and part-time work. Although Dorothea Leighton was equally responsible for creating the Stirling County Study and would be first author of its third monograph, her role in the project would be unfairly overlooked, with Alexander Leighton and his second wife, Jane Murphy, receiving more credit.[43] Perhaps, given her modest and unambitious personality, as well as her dedication to her children, she did not mind that her contributions were overshadowed. Regardless, it is important to assert her equal role in conceiving of Stirling County and developing it during its most important phase.[44]

THE SEA, THE FOREST, THE FIELDS

All the social psychiatry studies featured in this book painted detailed portraits of the communities they investigated, taking historical, social, cultural, and economic factors into account. The Leightons, however, went further. Just as the people of Chicago, New Haven, and New York City were shaped by the urban geography of their cities, Stirling County's residents were shaped by the physical geography of their landscape. As *People of Cove and Woodlot* described, the "sociocultural map" and the "geographic map" shared "a high degree of coincidence."[45] As such, the natural environment, dominated by the sea, the forests, and the fields, had determined how people made a living for two hundred years and influenced their culture, attitudes, and personality.

The overriding presence of the Atlantic loomed largest, as most county residents lived within a few miles of the sea. Fishing had been a mainstay of the economy since Stirling County was settled in the mid-eighteenth century and continued to be so during the 1950s. In addition to supporting fishing villages, which tended to support a population of about five hundred people, fish processing employed people in larger centers. More generally, the life of people living along the coast was oriented toward the sea more than the land: "Daily work, home life, and social events are geared toward the rise and fall of the tide, the vagaries of weather, the movement of fish." Counterbalancing the subservience to the elements, a typical fisherman operated independently and "so far as human authority is concerned . . . defines his own tasks and sets his own hours."[46] Women rarely worked outside of the home, except occasionally working at a fish plant. In these tight-knit communities, the church played an important role, especially so in Acadian Roman Catholic villages but also in Protestant English villages. Younger generations, however, were beginning to abandon tradition for jobs in the cities, as the songs of Stan Rogers and other Canadian folk musicians would soon express.

Forests represented Stirling County's second most important physical feature. Over 70 percent of its landmass was covered by woods that often stretched all the way to the coast. Forestry and related occupations (including sawmill work, driving logging trucks, and selling Christmas trees), therefore, represented a significant proportion of the economy. Previously, much forestry work had been a winter activity, but the introduction of trucks, power saws, and new roads meant that it could now be done year-round.[47] Although some types of forestry work were not seen as desirable, the industry held a certain romantic appeal. As with fishing, it connected people intimately with the natural world, and even those who had forgone forest work still sought escape there via hunting. The woods were "becoming more avocation than vocation."[48]

Farmland represented Stirling County's final significant landscape, though the economic importance of farming was considerably less than fishing and forestry. Farms such as Tom Young's

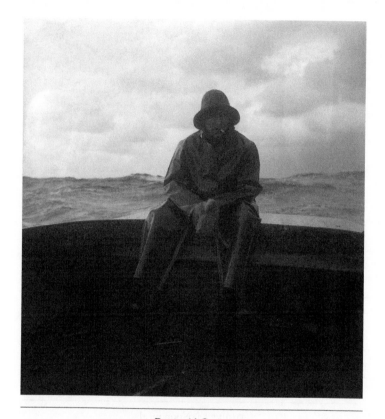

FIGURE 5.2   Reginald Comeau sets out.

Source: Alexander H. Leighton Nova Scotia Archives 1988-413/negative 2848-d,
Nova Scotia Archives. Photographer: John Collier Jr. Right to
reproduce purchased by Smith.

were scattered in between the coastline and the forest, with small
hamlets supporting these operations. Many of these farms were
mixed, with dairy cattle, sheep, and poultry being reared alongside the growing of crops, consisting primarily of fodder. Farmers often owned small woodlots, and people involved in fishing and forestry often did some farming themselves. Overall,

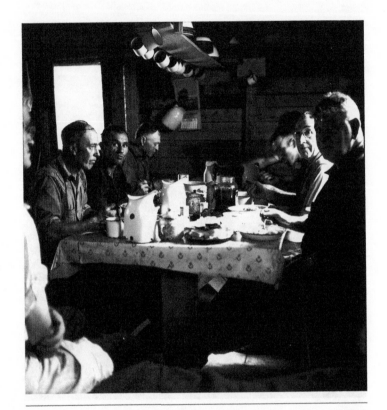

FIGURE 5.3 Noon meal.

Source: Alexander H. Leighton Nova Scotia Archives 1988-413/negative 375-d,
Nova Scotia Archives. Photographer: John Collier Jr. Right to
reproduce purchased by Smith.

farming tended to be a subsistence enterprise; it provided food
for the immediate community, rather than trade goods. Therefore, many individuals who owned a farm also had to work elsewhere for cash. Farming was perceived as "something to fall back
on" rather than something in which to invest. Compared to fishing and forestry, farming was "supplementary," and farmers stood

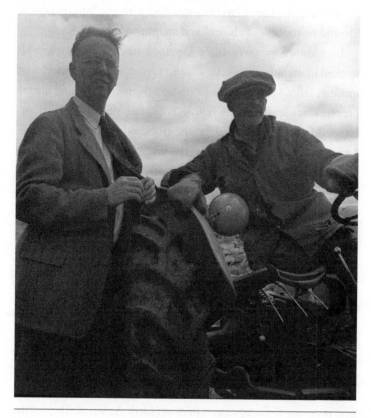

FIGURE 5.4 Leighton and farmer.

Source: Alexander H. Leighton Nova Scotia Archives 1988-413/negative 288-d,
Nova Scotia Archives. Photographer: John Collier Jr. Right to
reproduce purchased by Smith.

"poised between two infinities—the sea and forest." Despite
experiencing economic precariousness and fluidity, the Stirling
County researchers found that most farm residents enjoyed the
slow pace of life, the fellowship found in their communities, and
the independence of owning their own land and house. Others,

particularly the young, were dissatisfied with the "unevenness of life and restriction of choice" and sought to leave.[49]

In addition to these three keystone industries, people also worked in manufacturing, retail, and various services. In terms of income, large farm owners, professionals, managers, and entrepreneurs made up the wealthiest quarter of the population. Landed farmers, successful fishers, truckers, and service workers had moderate incomes. Finally, the lowest earners were woodlot owners and wageworkers in fish plants, lumber processing, and agriculture. Of this lowest quartile, approximately 8 percent lived in "shack-type houses" that lacked modern conveniences.[50]

Stirling County residents were also significantly molded by culture. The two main groups were Acadians, who spoke French and were predominantly Roman Catholic, and those of British origin, who tended to be Protestant, representing numerous denominations. Those of Black, Chinese, and indigenous Migm'aw origin made up a much smaller proportion of the population. Although Acadians and the English Canadians worked in the same primary industries, they usually lived in different communities. The Acadians were descended from among the first permanent European settlers in North America. Their early history was marked by the "Dispersal," or "Great Expulsion," which occurred between 1755 and 1764 and saw 11,500 Acadians from a population of 14,100 forcibly removed from what are now the Canadian maritime provinces (Nova Scotia, New Brunswick, and Prince Edward Island) and northern Maine and relocated them to the thirteen colonies, Britain, and France.[51] Some, however, escaped to live in the woods, including in sections of Stirling County. After the Treaty of Paris of 1763, which ended the Seven Years War, more Acadians returned to Stirling County. Partly because of this dramatic history, Acadians were considered "more militant about their ethnic identification than . . .

English-speakers."[52] The Roman Catholic Church was also pervasive. In turn, the majority of the first English speakers to come to Stirling were United Empire Loyalists from New England who opposed the American Revolution. Their towns and villages tended to be less homogenous than the Acadian ones, and the role of religion was less pronounced.

The presence of these two distinct cultures provided the researchers a unique opportunity to compare how sociocultural factors affected mental health. Using social disintegration as the basis for comparison, the researchers conducted an in-depth analysis of an Acadian and an English-speaking community ("L'Anse de Lavalée" and "Fairhaven," respectively), which were both socially integrated, as well as "Bristol," the largest town and the county seat. They also, however, examined communities that were socially disintegrated, namely, the culturally mixed and economically depressed neighborhoods of "Northwest Jonesville," "Monkeytown," and the "Bog."

Stirling County's better-off residents characterized these latter communities as being marked by "sexual promiscuity, laziness, untrustworthiness, drunkenness, fighting, family instability, poverty, Acadian-English interbreeding, [and] theft," many of the hallmarks of social disintegration.[53] While the researchers noted that such depictions were often exaggerated, their own depictions of these depressed communities were also predominantly negative. The anthropologist John Collier Jr. (1913–1992), whose photographs graced the book, described them in a judgmental style reminiscent of the New Haven researchers describing class V residents (see chapter 3). Here, "men often appear like little boys and boys as silent as old men." These "rejected" communities were "built on pride of exactly the opposite values of the surrounding communities . . . here, there is pride in the luxury of laziness and abandon. . . . They seem to accept the role put upon them, that of ne'er-do-well and loafer, a role that they have turned into a kind of royalty of the debased, who have nothing to lose and very little to gain."[54] He described residents as "resigned to their poverty and hopelessness . . . [and] miseries." They demonstrated "no embarrassment and no excuse for the debris and poverty scattered around, the rickety table with bits of food, the walls hung with sooted old prints and calendars of old years." Fieldworkers also noted the squalid conditions, describing utensils left on a stove as "black—greasy and encrusted with various old foods."[55] Despite these disapproving observations, Collier did allow himself a moment of self-reflection, rarely found in social psychiatry literature, stating that "it is a challenge to enter a home here. It is not they who rise to meet you; it is you who must brace yourself to meet them. No concessions are asked or given by these bedraggled people. You must like them or reject them on their own grounds. It is you who must sacrifice a part of your values to reach equality with them—and if you can do this, they will be your friends."[56] Although this hinted that it was possible for researchers to overcome their class prejudices, they were generally not sympathetic to the individuals living in these depressed communities. It also marked a contrast from how the Leightons engaged with indigenous communities, indicating that nineteenth-century notions of "deserving" and "undeserving" poor remained influential among social scientists.[57]

The Stirling County researchers used a variety of methods to understand how environmental factors and mental health interacted in these communities, including historical research, questionnaires, surveys, photography, economic reports, church records, newspapers, and extensive observation, interviewing, and descriptive analysis. The researchers also participated in numerous activities alongside residents, including hauling lobster pots, cutting timber, and attending weddings.[58] They assessed the degree of social disintegration by noting the amount of poverty, cultural confusion, violence and crime, broken homes, and similar factors in various communities.

The prevalence of mental illness in Stirling County was determined by examining institutional records (of hospitals, county homes, and almshouses); interviewing teachers, general practitioners, and community leaders about undiagnosed mental illness; and—most importantly—by conducting the county-wide Family Life Survey and Bristol Health Survey, which (similarly to Midtown) assessed mental illness in the general community by interviewing 10 percent of adults in Bristol. The researchers then used the first edition of *DSM* (1952) to determine how likely residents were to suffer from a mental disorder and rated the degree of impairment, ranging from none to severe. Overall, they determined that two-thirds of Stirling County's adult residents had suffered from a psychiatric disorder at some point in their life, though most were only mildly or moderately impaired. The researchers estimated, with several caveats, that half were currently suffering from a psychiatric disorder at any given time. One-third suffered "to an extent that constitutes a human problem calling for alleviation and prevention."[59] Such prevalence, though expressed differently, resembled what was found in Midtown, thus downplaying the idea that cities, per se, were bad for mental health. But what factors were most pathological in Stirling County?

In Stirling County, gender and age had a bearing on the prevalence of mental illness. Women were more likely to have a psychiatric disorder than men but tended to be less impaired.[60] They presented psychosomatic and neurotic symptoms more often, while men exhibited more sociopathy. The researchers believed that one of the reasons for this discrepancy was that attitudes regarding women and the expected roles in society were changing rapidly, even in Stirling County.[61] Age was also a factor in prevalence. Although the likelihood of mental illness increased between the ages of twenty and seventy (reducing thereafter), specific life stages were pivotal, for example, just after retirement for men and around the time of menopause for women.[62]

Overshadowing gender and age, however, was social disintegration. In the most disintegrated areas, both the rates and the nature of mental disorder for both genders were similar. Both men and women were equally subject to "the noxious influences of environment." Overall, the rates of mental disorder in the depressed areas were "outstandingly high." Nearly 90 percent of men in such communities were classified as "almost certainly psychiatric" or "probably psychiatric." This was double the rate for men in Stirling County as a whole. Moreover, when the severity of impairment was taken into consideration, both men and women in the depressed areas were far more afflicted by mental disorder than those in wealthier communities. Overall, less than 5 percent of the people in depressed areas of Stirling County were given a rating of "probably well."[63] All of this confirmed the project's overall hypothesis that mental disorder was associated with social disintegration. But why?

The researchers first downplayed downward drift. They acknowledged that "disordered individuals" could form "disintegrated groups" but that far more significant was how "disintegrated social systems produce disintegrated personalities." Although some of the causative factors were organic in nature, including higher rates of childhood infections and malnutrition, the authors stressed "that the psychological effects of disintegration were outstanding." For example, "If you were to introduce a random sample of symptomatically unimpaired people into the Disintegrated Areas . . . we think most of these individuals would become impaired. Conversely, if you were to take people out of the Disintegrated

Areas and make a place for them in a well-integrated community, we believe many would show marked reduction or disappearance of impairment."[64] Given the tentative and careful way that many social psychiatrists tended to phrase their conclusions, these two sentences are striking. Their implication was that by altering the sociocultural environment, it was possible to both reduce and, by extension, prevent a significant amount of mental disorder.

The authors determined that the most problematic aspects of social disintegration were those that affected an individual's ability to love and be loved, achieve recognition, be spontaneous in terms of pursuing cultural and educational opportunities (rather than physical gratification), and to feel as if they belonged to and knew their place in a moral order.[65] In contrast, lack of physical security and repression of sexual and aggressive impulses were not associated with mental disorder.[66] With respect to sexual and hostile urges, the situation was seemingly reversed: individuals unable to restrain sexual and aggressive impulses had the highest rates of mental disorder. Matters were more complicated regarding lack of physical security, not least because this was associated with poverty. The researchers found that within the depressed areas, an individual's risk of mental disorder was high regardless of their relative position of economic advantage.[67] Poverty was seen to be linked with the prevalence of psychiatric disorder only when it existed alongside other aspects of sociocultural disintegration. It was not thought to be a sufficient condition. It is possible here that the researchers underestimated the ways in which the psychological *and* physical insecurity caused by poverty contributed to the factors they *did* see as being important. In other words, poverty and its associated stresses may have created the conditions wherein love, recognition, spontaneity, and belonging were harder to achieve.

Poverty was also downplayed in a 1965 *Scientific American* article by Alexander Leighton. Leighton acknowledged that there was a "high correlation between the many deprivations suffered by" people in depressed areas and "the extent of psychiatric disorder."[68] He mentioned that, as early as 1950, his team gave a report to county officials detailing how better social integration could be facilitated by more internal community leadership, better education, and enhanced economic opportunities. While the researchers endeavored to foster leadership and education, the development of a nearby public works project created jobs for local people, and, by 1965, the situation in these depressed areas had improved markedly, resulting in better mental health. In analyzing the improvements, however, Leighton implied that community leadership, in particular, was necessary for antipoverty measures to be effective. Referencing Johnson's War on Poverty, he argued that social functioning ("leadership, followership and practice in acting together cooperatively") had to progress in order for people to take advantage of the programs offered to them. In other words, people had to become more deserving recipients of antipoverty measures. Underlying Stirling County (and other social psychiatry studies) was a conservatism that was reflected in how the findings and implications were expressed and how people living in deprived conditions were presented. The social environment might have been the most important epidemiological factor, but it lay alongside a notion held by some researchers that something was simply "wrong with the poor."[69] This helps explain why, despite the evidence that they themselves were building, social psychiatrists were often reluctant to argue that the prevention of mental illness required the elimination of economic, social, and racial inequalities.

PREVENTION IN THE COMMUNITY

If Alexander Leighton was not convinced that antipoverty measures alone could prevent mental illness, he and the other Stirling County researchers were more positive about the preventive potential of CMHCs. BMHC was founded in 1951 with the belief that community approaches to mental health could facilitate preventive psychiatry. The rest of this chapter explores how BMHC and the CMHCs created after the Community Mental Health Act of 1963 attempted to prevent mental illness. Although prevention was meant to be central to the work of CMHCs, its prominence quickly faded. On the one hand, the preventive function of CMHCs was undermined by the pressing need to treat patients, especially in the wake of deinstitutionalization. On the other hand, however, CMHCs could only do so much to address the deep-seated structural issues, including poverty, inequality, social isolation, and social disintegration, that contributed to mental illness. Despite the progressive legislation of the Johnson administration, many of these factors worsened as economic stagnation took hold during the 1970s and the progressive ambitions of the postwar period faded. This was especially true in communities that were already struggling from lack of investment and chronic social problems. As the community psychiatrist Carl C. Bell (1947–2019) reflected in 2004, "Not a great deal of progress has been made in addressing the health needs of the poor and underserved, many of whom are Black Americans."[70] This was chiefly because not enough was done to alleviate poverty and inequality in the United States, including that experienced by Black Americans and other marginalized communities.

During the early years of community mental health, however, there was great optimism about the preventive capacity of

CMHCs. Two of the fundamental principles underlying community mental health were that "psychiatric disorder can be systematically prevented from occurring" and that "the conditions of the social, cultural and economic environments are of at least equal importance to biological endowment and psychological experience in the genesis and maintenance, as well as in the prevention and treatment of mental disorder."[71] As the British-Israeli psychiatrist Gerald Caplan (1917–2008) described, CMHCs could achieve primary, secondary, and tertiary prevention.[72] Primary prevention involved addressing the factors in the community believed to contribute to mental illness, for example, the work of LHMHS's indigenous paraprofessionals in helping community members attain suitable housing or secure welfare benefits.[73] Caplan also put considerable emphasis on pregnancy and mother-child relationships, following the ongoing development and influence of psychoanalytic theory.[74] Secondary prevention concerned early identification of mental health problems and timely intervention to avert chronic illness and hospitalization. Here, liaising with schools, as well as other service providers, was crucial. Finally, tertiary prevention concentrated on reducing the impairment caused by "fully developed disorders," which could include alleviating the social problems contributing to mental illness in the first place.[75]

Alexander Leighton's recollections of BMHC provide an example of how such preventive work was attempted in practice. Overall, BMHC's work, as with all CMHCs, focused mainly on diagnosis and treatment. If potential cases—especially those involving children—were detected and treated early, this contributed to secondary and tertiary prevention. As such, BMHC worked closely with schools, social services, and local clergy to identify those believed to be at risk. But primary prevention was also considered important, not least because it exemplified the belief "that almost every human being had a basic potential for . . . mental health . . . if only given the opportunity." As Leighton described, "The effort in primary prevention was to involve public education regarding mental health and illness so that people might cope better with putative causal factors such as psychological stress and mobilize their personal and social assets effectively. Specific targets were to be parents, teachers, physicians, clergy, people with political influence, and other leaders, opinion setters, and 'gatekeepers' of society." In other words, the idea was not to eliminate these "causal factors" but to help people manage them more effectively. Leighton stated that these efforts were "pursued with vigor for many years" but that success was difficult to determine. Then, in 1970, BMHC's preventive activities intensified and shifted to focus even more squarely on children and, specifically, the education system, in the belief that "the schools of Bristol constituted a psychologically damaging environment for children."[76] Leighton's account of what occurred after this change in tack highlighted how activist CMHCs could find themselves in a difficult position with respect to the broader community. It also demonstrated, yet again, how CMHCs could only do so much to change the structural factors that affected mental health.

BMHC's interest in the school system escalated in 1969 when a young, recently hired teacher wrote a letter to a local newspaper calling for numerous reforms. He was subsequently fired. Although Leighton urged BMHC staff (consisting of a psychiatrist, psychologist, social worker, and a secretary) to stay neutral, they quickly sided with the teacher. In the ensuing furor, BMHC staff openly criticized the School Board and demanded "the ouster of school personnel." As a result, many influential members of the community turned against BMHC and, by extension, the Stirling County Study. These community members included physicians (such as the School Board chair), who were vital to secondary prevention because they provided early identification of mental illness.[77] Some of these physicians already had misgivings about BMHC's approach to patient management, which were intensified by the crisis. The debacle also deepened the suspicions of BMHC's Board of Directors about the effectiveness of its preventive work. Finally, BMHC's opposition to the School Board also reignited the misgivings of many Stirling County residents about participating in the study in the first place.[78] Overall, Leighton concluded that "among the consequences of this crisis for the Centre was a crop of negative opinions and attitudes on the part of the public and a certain amount of isolation from the other subsystems of the area, especially the human service organizations." This negativity especially damaged BMHC's preventive agenda, which relied on community collaboration. Although the insular nature of Bristol exacerbated the situation, Leighton hinted that the problems affecting BMHC were similar to those affecting community mental health more generally. Doubts were emerging about the effectiveness of "programs for prevention and for fostering 'positive mental health.'" Reflecting the higher-than-anticipated rates of mental illness, Leighton added that the "goal of trying to provide services for everyone with a psychological or social need began to seem more and more like trying to drink the ocean."[79]

Leighton's assessment of the situation also sheds light on the political dilemmas facing CMHCs. As Harry Brickman, program chief for Los Angeles County Mental Health Services between 1960 and 1976, explained, "A delicate balance must be set and maintained between the modest, but ultrasafe position that mental health is nothing more than clinical services, and the perhaps over-ambitious, but more daring position that mental health services can and should eventuate in a more humane and emotionally healthy community."[80] Although Leighton wanted to integrate Stirling County's depressed areas, his approach was more conservative than that of his BMHC colleagues. Moreover, it is evident from his description of the issue that he was frustrated by the confrontational and seemingly militant attitude of the BMHC staff, who framed the debate about Bristol's schools as pitting the "establishment against young revolutionaries." They, Leighton believed, were overly influenced by the counterculture and the "behaviors and sentiments characteristic of the sixties." Overall, he thought BMHC staff behavior was marked by "a flavor of contempt, that the local society ought to change its ways and values. These were not well received; they were seen as presumptuous and motivated more by a desire to show off, or by political and economic ideology, than by a desire to cope with mental illnesses in the population."[81]

Such views were reminiscent of how LHMHS administrators interpreted the actions of indigenous paraprofessionals who were impatient for change. They also underlined a disconnect between the research conducted by social psychiatrists—which implied that profound societal changes were required to prevent mental illness—and the willingness of social psychiatrists themselves to admit that such changes were needed, let alone advocate for them. It is worth remembering here that most of the social psychiatrists featured in this book were not particularly radical in either their outlook or action. Some, such as Marvin Opler, had previously been outspoken on political matters but had suffered as a result. Others, such as August Hollingshead, were fundamentally conservative. Moreover, all of them appear to have been primarily motivated by their careers, rather than by a desire to effect societal change. Although social psychiatrists saw themselves as part of a broad movement to transform how mental illness was understood and addressed, they viewed their role as providing the research on which future policy would be based. They were researchers, not revolutionaries.[82]

In turn, mental health professionals working in community mental health were also influenced by career considerations. As discussed in chapter 3's conclusion, community psychiatrists grew disillusioned by what they perceived as their eroding role and dwindling authority within CMHCs. As a result, many left community psychiatry for private practice or academic roles. One example of this was the aforementioned Brickman, who, despite his enthusiasm for community psychiatry, eventually became frustrated by the lack of state support and internal politics and left for private practice in 1976.[83] Psychoanalysis, it should be remembered, remained both culturally popular and professionally lucrative in the United States during the 1970s, though its influence was flagging. Analytic psychiatry was also perceived to be more prestigious than community psychiatry.[84] In addition, there were increasing opportunities for biological psychiatrists in private practice, which could pay even better, since they could treat more patients per day.[85]

Staff retention was also a problem at BMHC. It had always been difficult to recruit and retain qualified staff (especially social workers with master's degrees), as was the case for many CMHCs, but after the community began to turn against the center, staff became frustrated and wanted to leave. There were long periods when one or two out of the four center positions were vacant. Since diagnosis and treatment were thought to be more pressing activities, it was BMHC's preventive work that suffered most from these staff shortages. This, in turn, lowered expectations of what the center could achieve on the part of the general community, the center's Board of Directors, and BMHC staff members themselves. As Leighton concluded, "the Centre was a sand castle, constantly being washed away and rebuilt."[86]

BMHC's difficulties in preventive psychiatry were mirrored in the CMHCs that followed. In California, community mental health was fomented by the Short-Doyle Act of 1957.[87] This legislation allowed cities and counties to claim reimbursement of up to 50 percent from the state for the development of local mental health services.[88] Within five years, three-quarters of Californians were living in participating municipalities.[89] But the services also had to include preventive measures in order to be funded. In the words of the legislation: "Everyone who comes in contact with others at critical times in life—the schools, the courts, law enforcement personnel, the family doctor, the clergy, agencies to whom people in trouble turn—can promote mental health and prevent mental illness."[90] Therefore, much of the preventive activities that emerged in California focused on educating people to facilitate early identification and treatment.

An example of the preventive work California CMHCs undertook can be found in a 1960 article by Ruth J. Levy, a psychologist who worked for the San Jose City Health Department. In 1960, San Jose was a growing, increasingly multicultural city transitioning from an agricultural economy to an industrial one. Its Community Mental Health Service (CMHS) engaged in prevention by providing mental health education to those in human services (including teachers, social workers, ministers, public health nurses, and police officers).[91] Such training was intended "to promote mental health by increasing skills in interpersonal relationships and by effecting attitudinal changes."[92] It was hoped that such workers could then help contribute to early identification of mental disorder and therefore reduce the tensions contributing to such problems. One specific initiative that arose as a result was situated at a "small industrial concern." A psychologist consulted with both staff and management and discussed "feelings evoked by . . . experiences with authority figures; reasons sometimes underlying breakdown in communication; the effects of punitive attitudes; and the evolution of certain biases which impede optimum functioning."[93] Another project focused on educating teachers about how their interactions with students could affect their emotional health. Child health conferences were also established by the Health Department to better assess the mental health dynamics in families. Levy reported that demand for such mental health education and consultation was increasing and was being well received. Yet it was difficult to determine what effect it had in terms of preventing mental illness. Three years later, those involved in the CMHS could claim success with respect to the treatment services they provided, but they could say little about the preventive services apart from the numbers of hours allocated to them.[94]

In a book about their experiences running community mental health programs in Los Angeles, Marvin Karno (b. 1933) and Donald A. Schwartz (1926–2020) noted that difficulties in assessing the effectiveness of preventive services often led to the neglect of such services. If, for example, "resources are spent on prevention at the expense of being applied to serve those known to be ill, as is usually the case, then the expenditure will be seen as even more unwise."[95] Concerns about how resources were being spent escalated "in times of shrinking financial support (such as seem to be upon community mental health programs at present)," resulting in "interprogram competition . . . for scarce funds." For their part, Karno and Schwartz hinted that spending "scarce funds" on treatment was money better spent.

Referencing the work of the Leightons, they questioned whether any "social engineering efforts" at improving social integration had been successful. While much of the beginning of their book discussed historical attempts to prevent mental illness, they spent little time discussing such efforts in California, suggesting that these initiatives had quickly waned. In addition, they did not discuss whether some of the broader, socioeconomically based recommendations that informed California's community mental health legislation (emerging out of the first Governor's Conference on Mental Health in 1949) had been realized. Among these included providing better housing, better schools, secure employment, and increased recreation opportunities, as well as parent and professional mental health education.[96] Similarly, in an earlier article written by Schwartz about community psychiatry, these aspects of prevention were overlooked.[97] California's intentions might have been ambitious with respect to preventing mental illness, but its experience of community mental health proved otherwise.[98]

The California experience of preventing mental illness was replicated in other states after the Community Mental Health Act was passed. As in California, the desire to place prevention at the heart of legislation did not materialize, heaping further pressure on CMHCs to provide treatment:

> With the lack of effective preventive services and the system's inability to respond to indirect needs, people who otherwise might have been diverted from a path of psychiatric disability found themselves requiring more intensive treatment and rehabilitation. This exacerbated the use of hospital-level care and increased the number of patients among those who left inpatient settings to face an uncoordinated, disjointed, and underfunded community system, or nonsystem, of care.[99]

The rhetoric of prevention in community mental health simply did not translate into action. For example, a survey of CMHC directors conducted by NIMH during the early 1970s indicated that prevention remained their first priority. But even by 1967/1968, only 13.4 percent of community mental health funding was allocated to primary prevention.[100] Moreover, a 1970 NIMH report found that only 3–4 percent of CMHC time was spent on preventive activities.[101] A joint APA-NAMH report on CMHCs from the previous year barely mentioned prevention. This was despite what some of its contributors were saying about the role of socioeconomic factors in the triggering of mental illness. In a statement reminiscent of Tom Young's mental breakdown, John Cody, the director of the High Plains Mental Health Center in Kansas, described how "in Western Kansas we have a very serious problem with the small farmer who simply can't make it economically anymore. Generally these are men who have only an eighth-grade education and no skills beyond farming. They develop acute schizophrenic breakdowns under these pressures, and sometimes severe depressions. They usually do very well in the hospital. Their delusions and hallucinations are almost gone after a few days. But we send them right back to the hopeless and isolated situation on the farm."[102] Some CMHCs continued to provide mental health education, ranging from conducting "rap" sessions with adolescents to consulting with community groups and services, but these initiatives were of little use to the individuals Cody described, who were undergoing extensive periods of turmoil.[103]

Overall, by the 1970s, there was thought to be a "dearth of primary prevention activities" in CMHCs.[104] Financial constraints and the pressure to treat current patients attenuated efforts at prevention. By then it was clear that only about a third of the two thousand CMHCs initially planned would ever be built.[105] By 1974, only 591 CMHCs had been built, and only 443 of those were operating.[106] The internal politics of some CMHCs, as well as the difficulty in attaining and retaining staff, also proved problematic. Overarching these barriers were lingering doubts about the preventive mission itself. To those who believed that major social change was required to prevent mental illness, the preventive activities of CMHCs seemed akin to attempting "to fell a giant sequoia with a toy axe."[107] In contrast, other mental health professionals continued to doubt that social action was necessary or even advisable.[108] Still others who were initially enthusiastic about community mental health became disenchanted. Reflecting on his training as a community psychiatrist during the 1980s, Hunter McQuistion (b. 1952) described how "there was a whole cohort of senior colleagues who were disillusioned by the community mental health center movement . . . and they withdrew from the political end of, or broadly speaking, the social advocacy end of our work."[109] Difficulties in proving the effectiveness of preventive activities also added to the growing pessimism.[110] This made it even more difficult to convince both funders and the general public that it was both possible and necessary to prevent mental illness.[111] Finally, there was also the sense among some mental health workers that although the—admittedly often limited—preventive work of CMHCs might help those at risk of minor mental health problems, they did little or nothing to prevent what they saw as serious and persistent mental illness.[112] As discussed in chapter 6, such beliefs became more prevalent after the 1980s, when biological approaches to psychiatry took hold and when genetic, neurological explanations for mental illness began to dominate.

Economic difficulties during the 1970s, ranging from the cost of the Vietnam War to the energy crisis, further exacerbated the problems facing CMHCs.[113] Resources for community mental health were declining at a time when socioeconomic problems were increasing. Still, those advocating for preventive mental health received one final boost when President Jimmy Carter (b. 1924) established the first ever President's Commission on Mental Health (PCMH) in 1977, chaired by First Lady Rosalynn Carter (b. 1927).[114] Among the many task panels created was one assigned to address prevention.[115] Just as the JCMHI formed in the 1950s could reflect on the successes and failures of the mental hygiene and child guidance movements, PCMH could learn from the vicissitudes of community mental health. It recognized that both U.S. society and mental health professionals tended to be "crisis-oriented," rather than "future-oriented," meaning that preventive initiatives were not deemed to be urgent or vital.[116] It also observed that many Americans viewed the principles behind primary prevention—which came out of social psychiatry research—as politically threatening. Finally, it admitted that the preventive efforts made by CMHCs lacked coherence, personnel, administrative support, funding, and sufficient analysis to determine effectiveness.

The panel's recommendations focused squarely on primary prevention and targeted infants and children especially. In addition to a NIMH Center for Primary Prevention and the development of primary prevention programs (including perinatal and parenting initiatives), it recommended that the "national effort to reduce societal stresses produced by racism, poverty, sexism, ageism, and urban blight must be strengthened as an important strategy for primary prevention."[117] This was one of the few times that the social ramifications of social psychiatry research were clearly articulated by such a panel. Although the panel recognized that it had "no magical power to eliminate the above sources of societal stress," this did not "deter us from taking

leadership in pointing clearly to them as factors capable of producing profound emotional distress in individuals." Going
further, it especially emphasized the importance of tackling
racism as part of "a comprehensive national program for primary prevention."

The findings of the task panel on prevention and that of the
other PCMH panels were crucial in developing the Mental
Health Systems Act of 1980, passed during the final months of
Carter's presidency. The act has been described as "a complex and
mysterious statement of conflicting views on community services
for the mentally ill." Nevertheless, it reaffirmed the federal government's commitment to community mental health and sought
to fix some of the problems that emerged since the first Community Mental Health Act in 1963. Chief among these was the
neglect of prevention. The act established the NIMH Center for
Prevention and provided grants to further preventive efforts. It
also prioritized services for the most vulnerable groups, which
contributed to secondary and tertiary prevention.[118] Finally, the
act emphasized patients' rights, thus facilitating increased attention toward patient experiences and understandings of mental
illness, including how they interpreted the role of socioeconomic
factors. It was not perfect legislation, but it was an acknowledg-
ment that, while there were problems with community mental
health, it—and prevention—was worth fighting for.

Within months, however, the legislation had been mostly
scrapped as part of newly elected President Reagan's Omnibus
Budget Reconciliation Act (1981). As contemporary observers
described, "Almost twenty years of federal policy was expunged
within a few days of furious budget activity . . . when the will to
sustain the effort to improve care for the mentally ill was lost
in a powerful political backlash."[119] The federal government

continued to provide block grants for mental health and substance abuse services but cut the amount provided by a quarter. Moreover, the states were left to decide how to spend the funds, effectively removing the influence of the federal government. The NIMH budget was slashed, positions were abolished, and the Center for Prevention was eventually mothballed.[120] CMHCs continued to operate, but the federal impetus behind them and the ambition to prevent mental illness had disappeared.

CONCLUSION: THE INVISIBLE CEILING

Reflecting on how BMHC failed to achieve the aspirations set out for it, Alexander Leighton was reminded of Roy Grinker's article "Psychiatry Rides Madly in All Directions," which, in turn, borrowed from the Canadian humorist Stephen Leacock (1869–1944).[121] Psychiatry, particularly after World War II, was apt to overreach itself, promise too much, and ignore its priorities. All this led to disappointment and disillusionment. Concurrently, Leighton also observed that there had been a history of movements within mental health that had been initially buoyed by high expectations but eventually had been "blocked by a low, invisible ceiling against which it vainly struggled until exhausted." I would argue that then, as now, this invisible ceiling has tended to consist of the structural factors, notably, poverty and inequality, that contribute to and exacerbate mental illness. During the height of the community mental health movement, CMHCs constantly came up against this invisible ceiling.

Historians, such as Grob, have contended that faith in prevention was "illusory" and that "the prevention of mental illness and the promotion of mental health were little more than attractive slogans."[122] Such assessments have often been based on the presumed failure of CMHCs to fulfill the preventive role assigned to them. On the one hand, I would argue that subsequent research into the preventive activities of specific CMHCs (such as LHMHS) might reveal that such efforts were not altogether futile. While the mental health education work of CMHCs was not particularly effective, indigenous paraprofessionals and other CMHC staff did reduce the stress and strife that contributed to mental illness in many communities. But on the other hand—and more importantly—I would also suggest that without broader societal reforms to tackle socioeconomic problems—such as those indicated in the PCMH report—CMHCs could never have lived up to the lofty ambitions set out for them. The fault with community mental health, therefore, was not that prevention was a chimera but that not enough was done outside CMHCs to foster social integration, reduce poverty, and tackle racism and inequality.

Grob and others have also claimed that preventive psychiatry lacked an evidentiary base.[123] Although the flowering of social psychiatry research following World War II would indicate otherwise, social psychiatrists themselves nevertheless were guilty of downplaying the significance of their findings and routinely recommending that more research be done before any firm conclusions could be made. Stirling County provides an excellent example of such reticence. Decades upon decades after the original research was conducted, Murphy and Alexander Leighton were still combing through the original data. While such thoroughness might have demonstrated a certain empirical rigor, it did not help social psychiatric theory translate into practice, where the real test of its mettle would have to occur. As it happened, only a fraction of what social psychiatry research was indicating was ever applied, and even this, the preventive activities of CMHCs, was quickly sidelined by the pressing need to treat patients. Social psychiatry was never truly put to the test, and, when other ways of understanding mental health began to challenge its previous dominance, it was soon forgotten.

6

THE DECLINE OF
SOCIAL PSYCHIATRY

The goal of medicine is peculiarly the goal of making itself unnecessary: of influencing life so that what is medicine today becomes mere commonsense tomorrow.

—Adolf Meyer

On December 27, 1967, John W. Gardner (1912–2002), secretary of health, education, and welfare, spoke to the American Statistical Association about a "crunch between expectations and resources" that was occurring in the United States. Although the Johnson administration had accomplished much in its War on Poverty, Gardner argued that there was a limit to what could be accomplished without fundamental changes to how the nation's income was distributed. "We are in deep trouble as a people. And history is not going to deal kindly with a rich nation that will not tax itself to cure its miseries."[1] A month later, Gardner resigned.

Among the many psychiatrists who would have been struck by Gardner's words was Matthew P. Dumont, then assistant chief of the Center for Studies of Metropolitan Mental Health Problems at NIMH and soon to be assistant commissioner for

Drug Rehabilitation in Massachusetts. In 1968, Dumont published *The Absurd Healer*, which compiled his thoughts about social psychiatry and community mental health.[2] The book was also a call for a more humane and compassionate approach to psychiatry, echoed in its foreword by the NIMH psychiatrist Leonard J. Duhl. Duhl argued that psychiatrists needed to employ an ecological model in order to treat and prevent mental illness. They had to concern themselves with racism and poverty, as well as the inadequacy of the systems meant to address these ills. Psychiatry had to change and, indeed, was "being changed by the events around it."[3]

Dumont went further, arguing that society itself had to transform radically. Unlike most of his peers, Dumont acknowledged the ramifications of social psychiatry research and was willing to articulate them. He likened the link between poverty and mental illness to that of smoking and cancer. Although it was still impossible to establish the correlation absolutely, there was enough evidence to justify action. Just as cancer prevention involved smoking cessation programs, it was "the responsibility of the mental health professions to devote at least some of their attention to these issues [poverty, unemployment, and social discrimination] or the battle against mental illness will be lost."[4] Moreover, Dumont argued that changes required in this battle involved

redistribution of the wealth and resources of this country on a scale that has never been imagined. We should be constructing a society for the urban poor of such beauty and richness, with so many options for behavior, that it becomes nothing less than a privilege to be called poor. The schools and hospitals in the ghettos should be *better* than those in the suburbs. The mechanisms for participating in government should be *more effective* for the poor than for the affluent. The gap between the haves and the have-nots in this country should be closed so quickly that for a while it would seem to be reversed.[5]

Cast against the tentative conclusions made by social psychiatry researchers, Dumont's words appear bold, even brash. But they nevertheless represented a logical application of the epidemiological insights social psychiatry studies were revealing. Dumont might have been channeling the radical and volatile spirit of the 1960s, but his prescription for preventive mental health was rooted in social psychiatry.

Throughout *The Absurd Healer*, Dumont implied that pronounced social change, though difficult to achieve, was possible. By the time he wrote *Treating the Poor* in 1992, his hope had vanished. After sixteen years working in community mental health in Chelsea, Massachusetts, one of the state's most deprived communities (the city would be declared bankrupt in 1991), his career in community psychiatry had been terminated by "a tax-conscious governor," along with those of eight hundred others working in outpatient clinics. This was even though Dumont's time in Chelsea had constantly demonstrated that socioeconomic problems produced mental illness. But the prevention of mental illness in such conditions was "an endless struggle with a hydra-headed beast." Unemployment, homelessness, addiction, racism, pollution (especially from lead), crime, fires, malnutrition, overcrowding, violence, and child sexual abuse were rife in the city, creating a toxic psychological environment. In Chelsea, Dumont explained, "political economy . . . is a mental health issue, not metaphorically but concretely and specifically." Despite increasing socioeconomic problems, however, the shift away from social and community psychiatry continued. By 1991, the community mental health movement had "become a dead leaf blown into a blind alley, its occasional rustle causing the merest sidelong glance from passersby busy with other things." Dumont himself "had to say goodbye to my professional *raison d'être*, community psychiatry. From now on, it would be just a succession of jobs." He eventually found work in a state hospital, representing "the closing of a circle, a return to the place where social psychiatry began."[6]

This chapter explains what happened between *The Absurd Healer* in 1968 and *Treating the Poor* in 1992, when social psychiatry went from being the driving force within mental health policy to being largely forgotten. Just as the "words *poverty* and *racism* disappeared from psychiatric journals and textbooks" by the 1990s, the notion of social psychiatry also vanished.[7] In its place emerged a resurgent biological psychiatry that was more concerned with psychopharmaceutical treatment than prevention. Underlying this transition were numerous factors both internal and external to psychiatry. After touching briefly on some of the external factors that led to a "crunch between expectations and resources" for social psychiatry, the chapter will focus on the factors within psychiatry and mental health that pushed aside the influence social psychiatry once had. On one side were even more radical voices, coming from radical psychiatry, antipsychiatry, and the psychiatric survivors' movement, which often questioned the very notion of mental illness. On the other side, however, was a resurgent biological psychiatry, which emphasized the genetic and neurological aspects of mental illness and emphasized medication. Undermined by both these disparate yet powerful forces within mental health, social psychiatry and its preventive ethos faded into obscurity.

LOST WARS

The demise of social psychiatry was influenced by numerous developments outside of psychiatry, ranging from the election of unsupportive presidents, such as Richard Nixon, and a gradual shift to the political right to the declining U.S. economy during the 1970s and increasing concern about federal spending.[8] Looming over all these factors were two wars: the metaphorical War on Poverty and the very real Vietnam War. Johnson's War on Poverty should have been the ideal policy platform to accompany the community mental health movement and the findings emerging out of social psychiatry. But though it reduced poverty to its lowest level yet by 1973 (especially among children), it focused too much on attacking the so-called culture of poverty, rather than poverty itself.[9] This reinforced the notion of the "undeserving poor," which, in turn, suggested that the poor could not be trusted to help themselves.[10]

As discussed previously, social psychiatrists were typically quiet about the policy implications of their findings regarding socioeconomic deprivation and mental illness. They were reticent partly because they thought that more evidence was required but also because their studies raised awkward questions about what should be done about poverty and inequality. It is worth remembering that, apart from the earlier work of Faris and Dunham, the social psychiatry projects of the postwar period were conducted and largely written up during the 1950s, with much of their activity conducted during the height of McCarthyism. As described in chapter 4, many social scientists were blacklisted, including Marvin Opler and Eleanor Leacock. Other social psychiatrists may have been broadly liberal, but that did not mean that they desired a "redistribution of the wealth and resources of this country on a scale that has never been imagined," as Dumont desired. Reducing poverty might be crucial in the fight against mental illness, but this was not to be accomplished by giving the poor more money. The "culture of poverty" also had to be addressed.

The term "culture of poverty" was coined by the anthropologist Oscar Lewis (1914–1970) in his 1959 book *Five Families: Mexican Case Studies in the Culture of Poverty*.[11] It referred "to the destructive behaviors and values" that "rendered the poor dependent and passive, unable to break out of the cycle of poverty in which they were enmeshed."[12] The poor were imbued with "a sense of resignation or fatalism and an inability to put off the satisfaction of immediate desires in order to plan for the future."[13] Lewis's notion of the culture of poverty was picked up by Michael Harrington (1928–1989), whose book *The Other America* (1962) heavily influenced the antipoverty approaches of both Kennedy and Johnson.[14] As chapters 3 and 5 demonstrate, similar thinking can also be found in the New Haven and Stirling County studies. The descriptions of the homes of the impoverished in both places were marked not by empathy but by aversion and, at times, disgust. The disheveled and unhygienic state of such homes provided evidence that the poor lacked dignity and self-respect. They would squander any resources directed at them. It was the mentality of the poor that needed changing, not their income.

Both the New Haven and Stirling County studies focused primarily on white populations. But, as Mical Raz has shown, the idea of the culture of poverty, as well as the associated notion of cultural deprivation (also described in New Haven and Stirling County), quickly became associated with Black Americans living in impoverished urban environments.[15] Particularly influential was Daniel P. Moynihan's (1927–2003) controversial 1965 report *The Negro Family: The Case for National Action*, written when he was Johnson's assistant secretary of labor. Moynihan began his report by decrying the centuries of racism and prejudice that Black Americans had faced. But the specific problem that needed fixing, Moynihan argued, was the Black family, which was "the fundamental source of the weakness of the Negro community." High rates of marriage breakdown and children born out of wedlock, he continued, meant that a quarter of households were headed by women. This "matriarchal structure" led not only to high levels of welfare dependency but also placed Black males at considerable disadvantage in terms of educational and career achievement.[16] Moynihan's report also fueled ideas about maternal deprivation, which was rooted in part in Freudian theory and had become more prominent during World War II.[17] Concerns about Black families, therefore, did not center on reducing racism and poverty but rather on racialized ideas about cultural and maternal deprivation.[18] Deprivation theory, as Raz has argued, especially influenced the development of Head Start, the most lasting legacy of the War on Poverty. Although the early years of Head Start did address nutritional deprivation, its primary focus was cultural deprivation, stemming from the erroneous beliefs (held, for example, by First Lady Lady Bird Johnson) that Black children had not seen a book, held a flower, or heard one hundred words.[19] Its creation also reinforced the long-standing American idea that education, not income redistribution, was the key to solving social problems.[20]

As many historians have observed, deprivation theory also drew significant criticism, not least from Black Americans.[21] But it nevertheless reinforced the idea of the undeserving poor: that some of the poor effectively brought poverty upon themselves. The racial connotations of such thinking were enhanced further following the race riots of the mid- and late 1960s. These riots may have been about urban poverty and racism, but they paradoxically led some liberal white Americans to question the wisdom of the War on Poverty.[22] As the case of LHMHS demonstrates, white liberals were also threatened and disenchanted by the emergence of the Black Power movement, which felt to some like an attack on them as individuals, rather than the racist and inequitable social structure. White liberals, described Dumont, often had a desire to "save" Black Americans. In turn, this "rescue fantasy" could be interpreted as the white liberal exploiting the Black American "*for the white liberal's own salvation.*"[23] When Black Americans justifiably expressed resentment about the idea that they needed to be saved (a notion that imbued deprivation theory), it further disillusioned white liberals about the War on Poverty. According to Jill Quadagno, "As the furor of the civil rights movement wound down, there was a widespread backlash against spending on social programs that benefited the poor, especially the black poor."[24] When what was needed to end poverty was the socioeconomic empowerment of individuals provided through democratic and bottom-up means, what was provided were top-down programs intended to culturally rehabilitate and control.[25]

The legacy of the War on Poverty's focus on "improving" individuals, rather than progressive structural reforms, has endured.[26] In the immediate term, however, much of the War on Poverty legislation began to be dismantled when Nixon took office. Moreover, by the late 1960s, both economic resources and political energy were being sucked into another conflict, the Vietnam War, which pulled both money and attention away from domestic affairs. As Dumont described, Vietnam also distracted Americans who wanted social change away from issues related to poverty and race and, in turn, away from the prevention of mental illness.[27] This included mental health professionals.

Many psychiatrists, for instance, were drafted or volunteered for service. They would treat combat stress, substance abuse, and other psychiatric problems, as well as attempt to boost morale, control behavioral problems, and reduce alienation. These included John Talbott, later an APA president, who would go on to protest the Vietnam War.[28] At the 1967 American Orthopsychiatric Association conference, for instance, five hundred mental health professionals called for the Vietnam War to end at a White House demonstration, arguing that it was inhumane and that it drew funds away from health, research, and education.[29] The 1969 APA meeting in Miami had even more tumultuous protests. As Lucas Richert describes, the Vietnam War helped galvanize radical psychiatrists, who argued that their more conservative colleagues were complicit in legitimizing it.[30] During the conference, the Radical Caucus of the APA demanded that the draft be ended and that the APA expel members engaged in or researching the war.[31] Although radical psychiatrists were interested in many other issues, including poverty and racism, the all-encompassing and pressing nature of Vietnam and the protests that enveloped it inevitably drew attention from other issues.

The financial burden of the Vietnam War was exacerbated by economic decline during the early 1970s. According to Katz, the 1973 oil crisis and ensuing stagflation precipitated increasing inequality, with poverty concentrating evermore "in inner city districts scarred by chronic joblessness and racial segregation." Child poverty was higher in the United States than anywhere else in the developed world, as were rates of incarceration. As trade union membership fell, "the real value of the minimum wage, welfare benefits, and other social protections . . . erode[d]."[32] Crucially, a wide swathe of observers blamed the Great Society and War on Poverty legislation for these woes, leading both Republicans and Democrats to crack down on welfare dependence and apply market ideology to social policy. Whereas the political and ideological atmosphere of the 1960s had been conducive to social psychiatry, the 1970s and 1980s would prove to be the opposite.[33]

NOT RADICAL ENOUGH

If social psychiatry was undermined by the shifting political terrain of the 1970s, it was also hampered by changes within U.S. psychiatry. Long-dominant psychoanalysis had begun its slow decline from its midcentury heights, and biological psychiatry was in the ascendency.[34] Concurrently, antipsychiatry, radical psychiatry, and the psychiatric survivors' movement were gaining prominence.[35] While biological psychiatry emphasized how mental illness had an objective, organic reality, radical voices often questioned mental illness's very existence, or at least how mainstream psychiatry conceptualized it. Before turning to the rise of radical thought within mental health, it is worth mentioning the waning of psychoanalysis, which paralleled that of social psychiatry.

Although social psychiatry benefited from enormous political influence during the postwar period, within psychiatry itself, psychoanalysis enjoyed significant hegemony. Psychoanalysts dominated academic and administrative posts, psychoanalytical research filled the pages of journals, and psychotherapy remained a lucrative treatment for private practitioners. Psychoanalytical themes and ideas saturated culture in the United States during the 1950s and 1960s, particularly in literature, film, and the visual arts.[36] Many social psychiatrists, such as Rennie and Redlich, were trained in and practiced psychoanalysis, and psychoanalytical thinking heavily influenced their understanding of mental illness and the etiological role of the environment and early childhood experiences. In addition, many of the psychoanalysts who helped psychiatry gain prominence during World War II, including William Menninger and numerous APA presidents, supported social psychiatry after it ended. Psychoanalysis and social psychiatry, therefore, overlapped in the thinking of many psychiatrists during this period, despite the former's focus on treatment and the latter's emphasis on prevention. This meant that community psychiatrists disgruntled by the lack of support for CMHCs could often retreat to private psychoanalytical practice, thus reducing the number of psychiatrists involved in community mental health and often limiting the poor's access to psychotherapy.[37] But while there was some commensurability between psychoanalysis and social psychiatry, this was less the case with either biological psychiatry or the radical approaches that would emerge.

Antipsychiatry, radical psychiatry, and the psychiatric survivors' movement might have been distinctive, and sometimes contradictory, critiques of psychiatry. But what they shared was a willingness to defy conventional understandings of mental illness, how it should be treated, and society's role in relation to it. While these movements had some ideas in common with social psychiatrists, overall, they went much further in demanding fundamental changes in terms of how psychiatry—and society more generally—defined, understood, and dealt with mental illness. In so doing, these movements attracted many adherents, both activists and intellectuals, who could have otherwise pushed social psychiatry to be more bullish in arguing for the sort of progressive social changes needed for preventive mental health.

Alongside the more strident voices of antipsychiatry, radical psychiatry, and the psychiatric survivors' movement, social psychiatry appeared tame, even conservative. Exacerbating the situation was the fact that many medical students interested in social psychiatry were dissuaded from speaking about political issues. Dumont, for instance, recalled how he and a group of his fellow medical students at the University of Chicago were told during the early 1960s that if their discussions about the "'social' aspects of medicine" continued, they would be suspended. As Dumont observed: "A word to the cowardly was sufficient. We were the Silent Generation; our tasks were to do our work, cultivate our careers, and keep our mouths shut."[38] Talbott similarly found himself being reprimanded for protesting the Vietnam War.[39] Social and community psychiatry, though revolutionary in some ways, were still part of mainstream medicine. Embarking upon a career in these medical disciplines still required adherence to the accepted standards of how a physician should think and behave. Antipsychiatry, radical psychiatry, and the psychiatric survivors' movement differed in this respect because many involved in these movements were either not psychiatrists or, if they were, had achieved sufficient standing or notoriety to say what they thought.

Antipsychiatry provided much of the intellectual heft for psychiatry's critics during the 1960s and 1970s. The term "antipsychiatry" was coined in 1967 by the South African psychiatrist David Cooper (1931–1986) and then used retrospectively as an umbrella term to describe the thinking of a range of critics coming from different political, disciplinary, and geographical places, including the psychiatrists Thomas Szasz (1920–2012), Frantz Fanon (1925–1961), and R. D. Laing (1927–1989); the philosopher Michel Foucault (1926–1984); the sociologist Erving Goffman (1922–1982); and even Scientology's founder L. Ron

Hubbard (1911–1986).[40] Although "antipsychiatry" has continued to be a contentious term, underlying it was the idea that mental illness (or madness) was to varying degrees constructed by society to serve different functions, including the control of deviance or to excuse problematic behavior.[41] Moreover, mental illness could not be understood as objectively as other medical conditions; it could only be perceived subjectively as a product of society and social relations. Social psychiatrists would have agreed that mental illness was often produced by society, but in a markedly different way. While they often debated how mental illness should be defined, they nevertheless accepted that most mental illnesses were real, problematic, and justified prevention.[42] Furthermore, social psychiatrists also would have rejected the other core element of antipsychiatry, namely, that psychiatrists were often a force for ill, not good.

Although social psychiatry had significant political influence during the 1950s and 1960s, antipsychiatry had gained much more popular appeal by the 1960s and 1970s. Popular interest in antipsychiatry was fueled partly by the celebrity status of thinkers such as R. D. Laing, but it was also driven by novels such as *The Manchurian Candidate* (1959), *The Caretakers* (1959), and *One Flew Over the Cuckoo's Nest* (1962), all of which were made into films.[43] These works dramatized the abuses occurring in asylums and emphasized the potentially manipulative and coercive power of psychiatrists and other mental health workers. They contributed to what Michael Staub has described as "a moment when a significant portion of the populace . . . believed madness to be a plausible and sane reaction to insane social conditions, and that psychiatrists served principally as agents of repression."[44]

Staub also argues that interest in mental illness generally was often a proxy for "political, emotional, and social" concerns.[45] Antipsychiatry, in particular, was part of a broader "protest against racism, the Vietnam War, professional authority, and hierarchical distinctions common to 'establishment' organizations of all kinds, including state mental hospitals."[46] While this is certainly the case for antipsychiatry, it was not so for social psychiatry, which remained politically coy. The politics connected to antipsychiatry, however, were not homogenous. Whereas most associated with antipsychiatry were left leaning, Thomas Szasz's views were rooted in libertarianism and attracted right-wing adherents.[47] While it may have been a somewhat amorphous concept, antipsychiatry nevertheless occupied a space in the political discourse that could have been taken up by discussions of the implications of social psychiatry research.

Radical psychiatry, which started to coalesce as a movement around 1968, also took attention away from social psychiatry. Radical psychiatry, as with antipsychiatry, is somewhat difficult to define, in part because radical psychiatrists were interested in a range of themes connected to mental health. On the one hand, radical psychiatrists were interested in pushing for radical social change. But, on the other hand, radical psychiatrists were also interested in exploring innovative treatments for mental illness, ranging from LSD to primal scream therapy.[48] Given their willingness to articulate their views vigorously, for example, by protesting at APA conferences and through their publications, radical psychiatrists also drew the ire of establishment psychiatrists. But they also attracted followers. The journal of the Radical Therapist Collective, *Radical Therapist* (which would change its name to *Rough Times* in 1972 and then *State and Mind* in 1976), for example, had a circulation of five thousand.[49] Although radical psychiatry had effectively peaked by the early 1970s, its emergence during the late 1960s stole momentum from social psychiatry and, in so doing, emphasized the case that social psychiatrists were not going far enough.

Political activism was often thought to be central to radical psychiatry. Indeed, the motto of *Radical Therapist* was: "Therapy means social, political, and personal change, not adjustment." But what such change implied was not altogether clear. The psychiatrist John Talbott's analysis of the content of *Radical Therapist* acknowledged that while radical psychiatrists were keen to criticize the psychiatric establishment and, for example, decry community mental health as a front for social control and the status quo, they offered few solutions. Barely any *Radical Therapist* articles, for example, addressed how to approach the mental health needs of poor, nonwhite, and working-class communities. In anticipating the coming revolution, Talbott argued, radical psychiatrists were ignoring current realities embodied in the "chronically ill and severely disabled individuals who inhabit state hospitals, welfare hotels, and skid rows."[50] Nevertheless, they had played an important role in highlighting that many of the theories and assumptions held by more conventional psychiatrists ought to be questioned, if not overturned.

The psychiatric establishment did not always welcome such criticism or how it was articulated. For instance, in his 1970/1971 APA presidential address, entitled "The Proper Business of Psychiatry," Robert S. Garber (1912–2005) lamented that "on the outer fringes of our membership" there was "the disturbing activity of a small group who would convert us into a radical, politically partisan, agitatory, propagandist pressure group. They shout, they disrupt, they insult, they shed heat but not light." Psychiatrists might be frustrated by the current political situation and by the APA's "lack of zeal" in addressing "social problems," but they should not get involved in "partisan politics." Overall, Garber argued that "losing our cool will not help. Building our science may. One hopes that our nuclear center of opinion may yet attract and contain these strange particles that threaten to escape from its outer edges."[51] Garber's criticism of the message and approach of radical psychiatry was made even more scathing by the fact that he had been a leading figure in GAP, serving as its president from 1965 to 1967.[52] As discussed in chapter 1, GAP had been formed in 1946 to show how psychiatry could address issues such as poverty, racism, industrial relations, and international affairs.[53] But, as psychiatrists such as Garber contended, psychiatry could only attain such influence if it maintained its professional propriety. Radicalism was counterproductive. Moreover, the psychiatrists behind the transition to community mental health were dismayed by claims made by radical psychiatrists that community psychiatry was a "weapon of the establishment" and "a means to pacify angry communities and promote harmony rather than work toward social change."[54] CMHCs were not the panacea they were hoped to be. But dismissing them as a kind of establishment psychiatry plot went too far and provided support for Talbott's critique that radical psychiatry was rooted too much in ideology and not enough in reality. It also overlooked the fact that some CMHCs, such as LHMHS, were fulfilling their preventive function and were at least attempting to develop democratic and egalitarian modes of operation. In their desire for revolutionary change, radical psychiatrists rejected the possibility that gradual reform was better than nothing and could contribute something to the prevention of mental illness.

Lucas Richert has emphasized how unconventional treatments also captivated radical psychiatrists. *Radical Therapist* often featured articles that criticized the use of lobotomy, insulin shock treatment, ECT, and even the new psychoactive drugs that had helped facilitate deinstitutionalization.[55] Imbued with the spirit of the counterculture, radical psychiatrists instead experimented with a panoply of novel therapies. These included transactional analysis, ecologically based therapy (for example, Morita therapy), primal scream therapy, meditation, and above all, the use of psychedelic drugs such as LSD.[56] Many of these therapies, including the use of psychedelics, do not seem so radical today.[57] But they were so during the 1960s and 1970s. More importantly, they represented the dissatisfaction of many patients and mental health professionals with conventional psychiatric therapies and their motivation to look elsewhere.[58]

Most of these therapies remained on the fringes of psychiatry, and, therefore, interest in them did not affect social psychiatry directly. They did, however, indicate that a demand for new, effective treatments remained central to both radical and mainstream elements within psychiatry. Prevention was desirable, but the impact of preventive mental health programs, especially the unambitious educative and consultative efforts produced by CMHCs, lacked the immediacy of novel therapies that connected with the contemporary zeitgeist. More importantly, the sheer variety of radical treatments highlighted a shift from a focus on *population* mental health, which had been the lens through which social psychiatrists understood mental health, to *individual* mental health, which would dominate thinking about mental health until very recently. Treatments that could take the form of everything from a psychedelic drug to a psychodrama therapy session may have catered in general to clinicians and patients drawn to the counterculture, but they also provided individuals with considerable choice as consumers of mental health care. These therapies, therefore, were not just part of the counterculture; they were also part of the consumer culture that helped fuel the self-help industry.[59] They were also emblematic of the "me decade," characterized as a period during which

Americans indulged in self-gratification, materialism, and narcissism.[60] The transition from population to individual mental health will be explored further in the final section of the chapter, which focuses on biological psychiatry, but it is worth mentioning here that it was also a facet of radical psychiatry. Radical psychiatrists were concerned about far-reaching social problems, such as poverty and inequality, but their attraction to unconventional therapies also facilitated the shift back to a focus on the mental health of individuals and thus away from the population mental health approach fostered by social psychiatry.

Radical psychiatry may have been an extremist approach to many conventional psychiatrists, but for some patients, its focus was misplaced. The word "psychiatry" in its name implied that medical expertise, however unorthodox, still mattered most. Beginning in the early 1970s, the psychiatric survivors' movement began questioning this axiom, contending that the views of patients also needed consideration and that many long-held ideas about diagnosis, treatment, and the power of psychiatrists should be questioned.[61] This patient-centered approach to understanding mental illness emerged in part out of antipsychiatry (and to a lesser extent radical psychiatry) and partly out of the broader civil rights movement of the 1960s. It was also rooted in earlier crusades in support of patient rights and freedoms, including those spearheaded by Elizabeth Packard (1816–1897) and Clifford Beers. In the United States, the movement began with the founding of advocacy groups on the east and west coasts (for example, the Insane Liberation Front, founded in Portland in 1970, and the Mental Patients' Liberation Front, founded in Boston in 1971).[62] Canadian groups, such as Vancouver's Mental Patient Association, emerged concurrently.[63] The demands of these groups varied, ranging from an end to invasive therapies and involuntary hospitalization to dismantling the psychiatric profession altogether.[64] Above all, however, such groups championed the rights of psychiatric patients, questioned the medical model of mental illness and the hegemony of psychiatry, and validated and celebrated the experiences and insights of survivors.[65]

In some ways, the aims of the psychiatric survivors' movement coalesced with those of social psychiatrists. Social psychiatrists did not see patients merely as patients but rather as unique individuals who existed in complex social environments that were shaped by politics, culture, and economics. Part of the motivation behind the CMHCs was to provide treatment and preventive initiatives in ways that reflected such understanding. Equally, most psychiatric survivors would have concurred with the findings of social psychiatrists that poverty, inequality, and social disintegration were significant drivers and exacerbators of mental illness. But, as with antipsychiatry and radical psychiatry, the psychiatric survivors' movement nevertheless provided an alternative way of conceptualizing and dealing with mental illness that distracted from social psychiatry and its preventive focus. As the term "psychiatric survivor" suggested, those involved in psychiatric survivor groups concentrated on the rights, needs, and perspectives of those already coping with a system of mental health care that they deemed to be harmful. To them, preventing mental illness was more about changing the way it was defined and treated than psychiatric epidemiology. Moreover, while social psychiatry and its primary application, community mental health, could be interpreted as progressive attempts to make psychiatry more democratic, they were still bound up in a system of mental health care that privileged the knowledge held by educated elites, not patients.[66] Social psychiatry was not nearly radical enough.

BACK TO BIOLOGY

Antipsychiatry, radical psychiatry, and the psychiatric survivors' movement had all eroded the influence of social psychiatry by the early 1970s, particularly among those seeking to challenge the current political and psychiatric systems. For mental health professionals, patients, intellectuals, and anyone else interested in unorthodox approaches to mental health, it was these novel, exciting, and innovative perspectives that captivated, not those of social psychiatry. But while debates about radical therapies and patient rights were fomenting on psychiatry's fringes, a much more significant development was occurring in the mainstream: the resurgence of biological approaches to psychiatry that privileged genetic and neurological explanations for mental illness and relied heavily on pharmaceutical treatments. It was this momentous shift to seeing mental illness as predominantly a brain disease that was most damaging to social psychiatry. Most obviously, the focus on the brain meant that psychiatrists were less interested in the social determinants of mental health. But the emphasis on psychopharmacology and the genetic aspects of mental illness also meant that prevention was considered less important. Why worry about preventing mental illness if you thought it was genetic (and could not be prevented, barring eugenics) and believed it could be treated easily (and profitably) with a pill? Finally, the rebirth of biological psychiatry was also accompanied by new ways of diagnosing patients. In *DSM-III*, the APA's bible, mental disorders were presented as discrete categories of pathology that often had precise biological markers and could be treated with specific psychiatric medications. While *DSM* has often (and rightly) been implicated in pathologizing "normal" behavior, it also contributed to removing psychiatric disorder from the social contexts in which it emerged and through which it was experienced.[67] It was no longer society that was flawed and needed fixing, only individuals.

Biological approaches to psychiatry were certainly influential before its period of dominance at the end of the twentieth century. But they existed alongside the other ways of understanding and treating mental illness, namely, social psychiatry and psychoanalysis. Lobotomy, ECT, and insulin shock therapy, for example, became common in the United States during the 1940s and 1950s, roughly the same time as the zenith of psychoanalysis and the emergence of social psychiatry.[68] Whereas lower-class patients tended to receive more somatic therapies and upper-class patients were treated more often with psychoanalysis, this was not always the case, as the botched lobotomy of Rosemary Kennedy (1918–2005) demonstrates. As the psychiatrist Melvin Sabshin (1925–2011) observed, psychiatrists during the postwar period tended to gravitate toward psychotherapeutic, somatotherapeutic, and sociotherapeutic ideologies.[69] Psychiatrists negotiated their position with regards to these different camps in various ways. Jonathan Metzl has argued that Freudian ideas, particularly about gender, continued to inform the thinking of biological psychiatrists, influencing how and why they prescribed medications.[70] Most psychiatrists who became interested in social and community psychiatry were analytically trained initially, and some continued to identify as psychoanalysts. Other psychoanalysts, as Sabshin described, were more "purist" and resisted community mental health.[71] Still others, such as the child psychiatrist Leon Eisenberg (1922–2009), despised psychoanalysis but were sympathetic toward both biological and social psychiatry.[72] As the psychiatrist Wes Sowers (b. 1953) recalled of his training at AECM, "There were definite sort of tribes . . . among the faculty members . . . many of those who were interested in community psychiatry also had an interest in . . . psychodynamic theory . . . and there were also . . . people who had . . . a biologic focus, but . . . for many who were community psychiatrists, taking elements of those . . . was fairly common."[73] Overall, however, it was biological psychiatry's turn at the helm.

As with the rise of social psychiatry, biological psychiatry's ascendency rested on both scientific and political changes. Specifically, it benefited from and, in turn, spurred new research in neurology, psychopharmacology, and genetics, as well as the way in which advancements in these fields mapped neatly onto those in Western biomedicine more generally. These developments began during the 1940s and 1950s (and, like social psychiatry, would be accelerated by World War II), culminating in the 1990s, the "decade of the brain," of the human genome project, and of mass-marketed psychiatric drugs such as Prozac. All of this helped biological psychiatrists make the case that their approach, and not social psychiatry or psychoanalysis, was the most "scientific," modern, and technologically sophisticated way to understand and treat mental illness. Unlike social psychiatry, which suffered from the erosion of the Great Society policies of the 1970s and the rise of neoliberalism during the 1980s, biological psychiatry took advantage of the shift to the political right. Interest in the mental health of populations and prevention, briefly reaffirmed by Carter's commission, was soon replaced by a focus on individual patients and the drugs needed to treat their *DSM*-determined diagnoses.

Arguably, the most important of these developments for biological psychiatry was the emergence of psychopharmacology. The proliferation of psychiatric drugs aligned psychiatry closer to the rest of medicine. As Charles Rosenberg has described, psychiatry had long struggled for respectability, especially during the asylum era.[74] Biological treatments during midcentury, such as lobotomy and insulin shock therapy, may have been perceived as technologically sophisticated, but they were also controversial. Psychoanalysis and social psychiatry may have captivated many, but to others they could appear (perhaps unfairly) not particularly scientific. Psychopharmacology, in contrast, made psychiatry seem legitimate and authoritative.

Before the 1950s, drugs, especially sedatives such as opiates, barbiturates, bromides, and choral hydrate, were used by psychiatrists, but they were not thought to be very effective in treating symptoms.[75] These drugs, even more than the ones that followed, also had undesirable side effects, including toxicity and dependency.[76] The modern era of psychopharmacology really emerged with the first antipsychotic: chlorpromazine (trademarked in the United States as Thorazine), which was discovered by the French pharmaceutical firm Laboratoires Rhône-Poulenc in 1950, just as social psychiatry was gaining influence.[77] It was soon followed by the first tranquilizers, or antianxiety drugs, such as Miltown and Valium, and antidepressants, such as Tofranil, as well as more controversial psychedelics, such as LSD, and amphetamines, such as Ritalin.[78] A second generation of antidepressants, the selective serotonin reuptake inhibitors (SSRIs), such as Prozac, became even more popular and profitable during the 1980s and 1990s.

In addition to boosting the respectability of psychiatry and facilitating lucrative ties with the pharmaceutical industry, psychopharmacology provided hope to both psychiatrists and patients. During the postwar period, many endemic infectious diseases, ranging from tuberculosis to syphilis, could finally be treated effectively using antibiotics. Other dreaded diseases, such as polio, were being tackled through vaccination. Drugs were also being developed to treat cancer effectively, transforming diagnoses such as childhood leukemia from being "hopeless" to having high survival rates.[79] Many psychiatrists were confident that psychiatric patients would also be the beneficiaries of similar magic bullets. While the thalidomide tragedy (which was prevented in the United States) may have raised questions about drug safety and pharmaceutical company ethics, psychiatric drugs such as Thorazine seemed clearly preferable to lobotomy or prolonged institutionalization, despite their side effects. As opposed to a lengthy course of psychoanalysis, drugs were also a speedy treatment, which also boosted optimism. As the child psychiatrist Maurice Laufer declared in 1970 with respect to the hyperactivity drug Ritalin, they created "one of the few situations in which you can do something quickly for people."[80] As with many other facets of medicine, drugs appeared to be the future for psychiatry, making the need to prevent mental illness appear less urgent.

The promise of psychiatric drugs was mirrored by an increasing emphasis on the neurological aspects of mental disorder beginning in the 1970s. Neurology had been closely associated with psychiatry as early as the nineteenth century, but the discipline was still relatively new at the turn of the century, with only a few neurological centers existing in central Europe.[81] In the United States, the first neurologists, including William A. Hammond (1828–1900) and Silas Weir Mitchell (1829–1914), were stimulated by the experience of treating soldiers during the Civil War. The American Neurological Association was founded in 1875, and neurologists used electrotherapy and other measures to treat neurasthenia, one of the neurological (and psychiatric) diseases of the day.[82] U.S. developments in neurology advanced further during and after World War I, as physicians were once again faced with the challenge of treating and understanding soldiers' neurological injuries. One early center was the Yale Neurology Study Unit, founded in 1924, just as the Yale Mental Hygiene Center (see chapter 1) was getting established.[83] Another was the Montreal Neurological Institute, founded by the pioneering neurosurgeon Wilder Penfield (1891–1976) in 1934. As Yvan Prkachin's recent article about Penfield's flirtation with psychosurgery experiments during the 1940s explains, psychiatric interest in neurology (and vice versa) was stimulated in part by a desire to treat patients.[84]

Although the dominance of psychoanalysis in American psychiatry during the postwar period meant that neurology and psychiatry became somewhat "estranged," this soon began to change. One reason for this was the "integrative" approach of neurologists in seeking to inform knowledge about other medical specialties rather than focusing on specialization. Stephen Casper has described how the neurologist was a "cooperative labourer . . . at the centre of medicine's and sciences' many divisions."[85] Biological psychiatry was ideally placed to capitalize on neurology's integrative tendencies, most notably when it began to capitalize on rapidly improving brain-imaging technology. Beginning in the 1960s, for example, neurophysiological studies of dreams and sleep that utilized rapid eye movement (REM) and the measurement of brainwaves would contradict influential Freudian ideas about what dreams were and what they represented.[86] A decade later, neuroscientists were able to use MRIs to apparently "map" the brains of people with mental disorders, including Alzheimer's disease, depression, bipolar disorder, and schizophrenia.[87] Although the clinical use of such scans was typically only to rule out the existence of organic brain diseases, these images, typically juxtaposed against the scan of a "normal" brain, provided convincing evidence for many that mental disorder was purely biological.[88] By the late 1990s, neuroscience was being used to explain (and explain away) everything from art appreciation to religion.[89] We were, as it were, our brains. This trend to understand everything through the lens of neurology

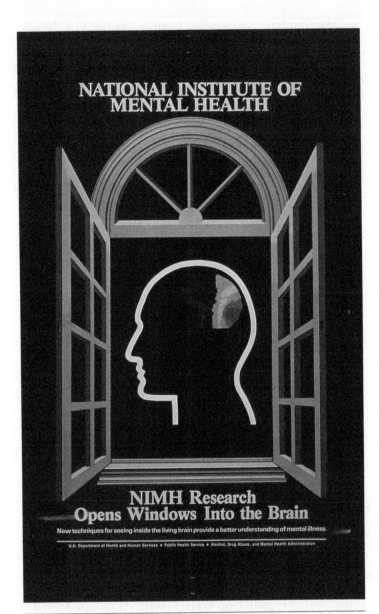

FIGURE 6.1 NIMH brain.

Source: National Library of Medicine. Creative Commons.

extended naturally to mental illness, thus entrenching biological psychiatry's growing hegemony.

Along with neuroscience, the other explanation for understanding health, medicine, and human nature that became dominant toward the end of the twentieth century was genetics. Theodore Porter has recently demonstrated how statistical analysis by asylum doctors during the early nineteenth century began to establish the link between insanity and heredity.[90] These physicians would be instrumental in pushing eugenic strategies to prevent the reproduction of the insane, feebleminded, and other undesirables. While these ideas remained prominent during the early twentieth century, they were sidelined somewhat by mid-century by explanations from psychoanalysis and social psychiatry, which emphasized nurture, rather than nature.[91] The discovery of the structure of DNA in 1953, coming at the height of psychoanalytical and social psychiatry influence, did not immediately shift the focus of psychiatrists back onto genetics, but gradually—and as interest in psychopharmacology and neurology grew—genetic explanations became more common. Articles discussing the genetic origins of diagnoses ranging from ADHD to schizophrenia flooded psychiatric journals. By 2001, APA President Daniel B. Borenstein could confidently state that "now the human genome has been mapped, additional research will disclose how specific genetic expressions lead to psychiatric illnesses."[92]

Genetic explanations were attractive to psychiatrists in part because they aligned with a growing tendency to stress the hereditary nature of other chronic diseases, such as diabetes, cancer, and heart disease. These were often at the expense of explanations related to the environment and lifestyle, factors frequently linked to socioeconomic circumstance. They also, however, provided patients and their families with a more acceptable cause for mental disorder at a time when both psychoanalysts and social psychiatrists were likely to highlight the role of early childhood experiences and, in particular, parenting practices. Mothers were especially implicated.[93] One example of such "mother blame" can be found in the case of autism and the so-called refrigerator mother; another can be found in the case of ADHD, before its reimagination as a neurological disorder.[94] Parents, as well as schools and society more generally, embraced genetic explanations in part because they expunged them of such blame. Many parents of children diagnosed with either ADHD or autism would get diagnosed themselves after their children were, further reinforcing the supposedly genetic nature of the disorder. Assuming that such disorders were genetic, however, was easier than identifying the genes responsible for them. As Jennifer Singh has argued with respect to autism, billions of dollars have been spent searching for the elusive autism gene, to no avail. Much of this money, Singh suggests, would have been better spent supporting people with such diagnoses who increasingly self-identify as being "neurodiverse," as opposed to being disordered.[95] Ultimately, the history of these disorders (and many others) demonstrates a wide range of contributing factors, not least the increasing willingness of clinicians, teachers, and parents to label children as disordered.[96] But establishing the supposedly genetic nature of such disorders proved to be pivotal.

By 1980, biological psychiatry had succeeded both psychoanalysis and social psychiatry as the preeminent psychiatric approach. One significant indicator of its dominance was the publication of *DSM-III* in that year, which marked a fundamental change from its more analytically oriented predecessors.[97] On the surface, *DSM-III* was merely a manual that helped clinicians define and diagnose mental disorders, promising more clarity, accuracy, and objectivity in the process. But it also served other functions. As the *DSM* historian Hannah Decker has explained, *DSM* became the psychiatric shorthand for everyone from mental health professionals and medical students to judicial officials and teachers. A *DSM* diagnosis could pave the way for more support for children struggling at school and for people in the workplace. If a mental health researcher wanted to win funding, they had to frame their project in *DSM* terms. Finally, psychiatrists needed to submit *DSM* codes in order to get reimbursed by health insurance companies.[98] *DSM-III* also entrenched biological psychiatry as the default model for understanding mental health.

One of the chief critiques of *DSM-III* and its successors has been how it greatly expanded the numbers of disorders that could be diagnosed and, subsequently, treated. In so doing, critics argued it "made us crazy" by pathologizing many behaviors that could otherwise be interpreted as normal.[99] To a degree, doing so was not so different from social psychiatrists after World War II, who warned how mental illness was much more prominent in U.S. society than previously thought. But while social psychiatrists argued that the mental health of all would suffer from adverse socioeconomic circumstances, *DSM-III* disorders were depicted instead as flaws in the neurological makeup of specific individuals, likely from genetic factors. If people blighted with such defects desired to succeed in the increasingly competitive and cutthroat atmosphere of the 1980s, they had to embrace the diagnosis provided by the psychiatric bible and the treatments that would follow.

The proliferation of mental disorder in *DSM-III* and subsequent editions implied that mental disorders were discrete categories that had the qualities of timelessness and universality.[100] In other words, these disorders existed in the same precise form regardless of where they were found in the world or, indeed, when. They were real, objective, and unalterable entities.[101] Categorizing mental disorders in this way helped make such conditions appear more similar to somatic diseases, while deemphasizing the role of the social environment in shaping how they were understood or experienced. This was particularly the case when combined with the increasingly common notion that mental illness was fundamentally neurological and genetic in nature. There was no difference, therefore, between the depression experienced by someone in an impoverished slum in Detroit than that experienced by an individual living in a wealthy suburb of Los Angeles.

In addition to reinforcing the biological nature of mental illness, *DSM-III* also facilitated the pharmaceutical treatment of mental disorder. Pharmaceutical companies developed drugs to treat specific *DSM* diagnoses, which were "relentlessly marketed to psychiatrists and the lay public."[102] Since health insurance companies were more likely to cover the cost of such drugs, as opposed to, for example, psychotherapy, the pathway from the initial presentation of symptoms to the prescription of a drug was simplified. A social worker familiar with *DSM-III* diagnoses might complete the manual's checklist for a particular diagnosis and then refer their client to a physician (not necessarily a psychiatrist) for an official diagnosis and the recommended prescription of drugs, which would be covered by health insurance.[103] The simplicity of this process distracted from the need to consider either the precise circumstances of the patient or the environmental context in which they, and their mental health, existed. In the rush to pin *DSM* diagnoses on patients and prescribe them drugs, even less attention, therefore, was devoted to prevention.

CONCLUSION: BIO-PSYCHO-SOCIAL

In many ways, *DSM-III* helped commoditize mental illness, transmuting it from a costly drag on postwar U.S. society (as Kennedy had described) to a driver of enormous wealth and influence for pharmaceutical companies, health insurers, mental health researchers, and, indeed, psychiatrists. It is not surprising that this transformation began during the 1980s, when the welfare state was being dismantled, when neoliberalism was on the rise, and when one of its spokespersons, Ronald Reagan's top ally Prime Minister Margaret Thatcher (1925–2013), was declaring that "there is no such thing as society." With its focus on individual, rather than population, mental health and its ties to the medical-industrial complex, biological psychiatry capitalized on this shift to the right, just as social psychiatry suffered from it. As Matthew Dumont declared, "Right-wing politics and conventional psychiatry always go hand in hand."[104] By conventional, Dumont meant an approach to psychiatry that emphasized the provision of marketized treatments to individuals (which could apply to psychoanalysis), as opposed to approaches that focused on population mental health and prevention.

It is also unsurprising that social psychiatry failed to thrive under these altered political circumstances. Any assessment of social psychiatry, its legacy, or what insights it might offer today, therefore, should take this broader political context into consideration. Social psychiatry did not fail to reach its potential because its ideas about preventing mental illness were inherently flawed. Instead, a variety of factors combined to undermine it. These ranged from social psychiatrists not going far enough in articulating the implications of their research to changes in the political landscape that rendered biological psychiatry more palatable. Any analysis of the longue durée of the history of psychiatry in the United States will demonstrate how similar vicissitudes have affected the rise and fall of other approaches.

And times continue to change. Even before the COVID-19 pandemic concentrated attention once again on the social determinants of mental illness, there were signs that biological psychiatry's supremacy was fading, if only somewhat. Leading up to the publication of *DSM-5*, there were heated debates about how "normal" human behaviors, such as sadness and naughtiness, were being pathologized and drugged away. Concurrently, advocates for neurodiversity (as opposed to neuroenhancement through drugs) argued that many of the world's existential problems, not least climate change, required the input of those who were "wired" differently, such as Greta Thunberg. Moreover, while some antistigma campaigns have concentrated on the idea that mental illness is a disease just like any other, others have emphasized that mental health problems can affect anyone at some point, thus undermining the idea that some people are innately disordered and require "fixing" with drugs.[105] Finally, an increasing number of pharmaceutical industry scandals, most notably the OxyContin tragedy involving Purdue Pharma (which was recently told in the Disney+ miniseries *Dopesick*), have raised questions about how drugs are approved, regulated, and marketed.[106] At the same time, cognitive behavior therapy and other "talk" therapies have emerged once again as alternatives. Biological psychiatry remains dominant, but not as much as before.

One lesson we could learn from psychiatry's proclivity for rise-and-decline narratives is that of the desirability of plurality, interdisciplinarity, and open-mindedness with respect to how mental illness is conceptualized and addressed. Throughout this book I have been arguing that social psychiatry and its emphasis on prevention should be rehabilitated. The mental health side-plot of the COVID-19 pandemic is only the latest piece of evidence to convince us that social factors contribute to mental illness and that prevention should and must be at the heart of mental health policy and practice. But that does not mean that other approaches to mental health should be sidelined. As my previous work on the history of ADHD has highlighted, the best way to understand the behavioral problems of children is to take a flexible and holistic view that situates the child in their cultural, socioeconomic, ecological, and biomedical context and, most importantly, takes their own perspectives on board. This requires insights from all psychiatric disciplines, as well as those of the humanities and social sciences. The same applies for mental health more generally. Instead of lurching from one paradigm to another, psychiatry should reaffirm the need for a biopsychosocial approach where there is mutual respect for the insights different models can offer. History can explain why paradigm shifts in psychiatry have occurred. But it can also make the case for more integration, collaboration, and nuance in future.

EPILOGUE

Social Psychiatry and Universal Basic Income

Standing in the supermarket
Hiding my calculator from view
Hoping no one can feel my despair
As I get closer to the queue
An empty wallet, what a mess
Are we all standing here, feeling the same distress?
Drowning in the damage, full of shame and self-doubt
It's hard to stay sane and find your voice when all you want
    to do is shout

—Rachel Meach

This book has argued that it is time to revisit social psychiatry. From a historiographical perspective, the history of social psychiatry has largely been ignored, dismissed, or demonized, leaving us with an inaccurate picture of twentieth-century psychiatry in the United States. I have instead attempted to reinsert social psychiatry and its preventive ethos back into this broader history. I have contended that social psychiatrists did not fail to achieve their aims because their ideas were incorrect, overly idealistic, or naïve but rather because they did not go far enough in articulating what their findings implied about how to prevent mental illness. Equally, it is vital to consider the broader political context in which social psychiatry initially thrived and latterly declined. Social psychiatry built on the achievements and ambitions of the mental hygiene and child guidance movements, both of which put preventing mental illness at the heart of their activities. It benefited from the blossoming of social science in places like the Chicago School and the willingness of both psychiatrists and social scientists to engage energetically in genuine interdisciplinarity, the likes of which have rarely been seen since. And it capitalized on the deep concerns about mental illness that developed during World War II, as well as the faith placed in psychiatry to deal with this perceived crisis in mental health. Finally, the findings of social psychiatrists began to be digested just as presidents Kennedy and Johnson were embarking on momentous changes in terms of how the federal government tackled both poverty and mental illness. While the Community Mental Health Act that emerged did not meet the aspirations set out for it, this was more to do with lack of resources and changing priorities, rather than with the ideas that spurred it. Just as social psychiatry was a product of a particular time and place, its declining relevance during the 1980s and 1990s was attributable in large part to seismic changes in the political landscape and within psychiatry. Neither the biological psychiatrists nor the small-government, neoliberal politicians that came to prominence had much time for social psychiatry or preventive mental health. Social psychiatry was relegated to the margins of psychiatry, its story forgotten.

As important as it is to challenge and extend the rich historiography of U.S. psychiatry, however, this book has also had another purpose, namely, to inform, invigorate, and inspire current attempts to develop preventive approaches to mental health.

The term "social psychiatry" might not be very familiar to many mental health professionals today, but the idea that socioeconomic circumstances have a profound effect on mental health is becoming popular again.[1] Research on psychiatric epidemiology beginning in the late 1990s, for instance, began to emphasize the role of Adverse Childhood Experiences (ACEs), such as experiencing neglect, witnessing violence, or exposure to substance abuse, in poor health outcomes, including mental illness.[2] In 2009, Robert Wilkinson and Kate Pickett published *The Spirit Level*, followed by *The Inner Level* in 2018, both of which stressed how societal inequalities led to poor mental health outcomes.[3] WHO's 2014 report *Social Determinants of Mental Health* also indicated that researchers were returning to how poverty, inequality, and social isolation contributed to mental disorder.[4] Finally, even biomedically oriented scientists are turning to socioeconomic factors, linking poverty, for example, to impaired brain development and cognitive problems.[5]

It would be a tremendous shame, however, for today's enthusiasm about preventive mental health to share the same fate as social psychiatry and to be swept to the sidelines as the political and intellectual sands shift. As with social psychiatry during the 1950s and 1960s, too much time continues to be spent on cementing the links between socioeconomic problems and mental illness at the expense of determining how to apply such insights. As the sixtieth anniversary of Kennedy's "Special Message on Mental Illness" looms, this must change. Rather than endlessly confirming what social psychiatrists were concluding decades ago, the focus must shift toward transforming society in ways that promote mental health and prevent mental illness. One way to do this could be by introducing a universal basic income, or UBI.

UBI is a guaranteed, unconditional income that is set at a level that would lift every individual out of poverty. During the past decade, UBI has become increasingly attractive to both those on the left and right, given the global financial crisis of 2007–2008, concerns about workplace automation eliminating millions of jobs, and increasing frustration about the welfare systems in many countries. Andrew Yang recently raised the profile of UBI in his 2020 presidential bid, and in the 2021 Scottish Holyrood elections, four of the five major parties included in their manifestos a plan to introduce it. The COVID-19 pandemic has accelerated interest in UBI even further, as many countries introduced schemes to provide income to people made unemployed by lockdown measures. Despite its recent popularity, the idea of guaranteed income is not new. Similar concepts can be found in the writing of Thomas More (1478–1535), Thomas Paine (1737–1809), and especially Thomas Spence (1750–1815).[6] UBI also emerged briefly during the zenith of social psychiatry in 1969 in a sadly overlooked report completed by JCMHC with the provocative title *Crisis in Child Mental Health: Challenge for the 1970s*.[7]

JCMHC was founded in 1966 as an extension of the work of JCMIH, which had culminated in the publication of *Action for Mental Health* in 1961. Just like its predecessor, JCMHC was expected to produce bold recommendations. Upon the announcement of the commission, its chair, the child psychiatrist Reginald Lourie (1908–1988), declared that JCMHC would use its "zeal, courage, and determination" to "be ready to recommend a radical reconstruction of the present system" of mental health care for children.[8] The American Orthopsychiatric Association went further, arguing that the primary barriers to child mental health were social and economic. To address this problem, it argued that a minimum income of $10,000 should be guaranteed for every family of four.[9] JCMHC did not disappoint. Among its many recommendations to improve child mental health, including the provision of a child advocacy system, employment for all willing to work, and a national health service, was a guaranteed minimum income for all Americans.[10] Unfortunately, this recommendation, along with most of the others, was not heeded. While both Nixon and Carter attempted to pass guaranteed income legislation, their efforts faltered, and the idea of a basic income drifted to the political margins.[11]

The members of JCMHC clearly saw how a guaranteed income could result in better mental health outcomes, especially for children. But, just as mental health advocates have been slow to consider how UBI could improve mental health, UBI's proponents have typically failed to articulate how the financial benefits of better mental health could help justify the cost of such a system.[12] Mental health has not typically been formally assessed in the small number of UBI pilots that have been undertaken, though anecdotal reports from and analyses of pilots have indicated improvements in mental health.[13] One fascinating example comes from Dauphin, Manitoba, where a UBI experiment was held between 1974 and 1979. The health economist Evelyn Forget analyzed health data from the experiment and found that during that time psychiatric hospitalizations dropped, indicating improvements in mental health.[14] The Great Smoky Mountain Study, though not studying UBI per se, also demonstrated how family income supplements (from a casino) was associated with fewer mental health and substance abuse problems in Cherokee adolescents as they became adults.[15] Finally, the mental distress caused by the cancellation of an already underway UBI pilot in Ontario in 2019 unintentionally showed how quickly the mental health benefits of a secure income could accrue—and then vanish.[16]

Overall, more research is required to make the case to politicians, mental health workers, and the public that UBI could be a powerful tool in preventive mental health strategies.[17] But the history of social psychiatry can provide additional evidence. Social psychiatrists found that high levels of poverty, inequality, and social disintegration led to more mental illness, whether you were in Manhattan or rural Nova Scotia. A guaranteed income, just as JCMHC's members suspected in 1969, is ideally suited to alleviate each one of these social ills.

The most immediate impact of UBI would be to eliminate poverty, which social psychiatrists argued was particularly pathological for mental health. If set sufficiently, UBI would provide individuals with the means to meet their basic needs. This would include parents and carers, whose unpaid work contributes enormously to society yet comes at great financial cost to them as individuals. Progressive anti-inflationary measures such as rent control, free public transportation, and local food schemes

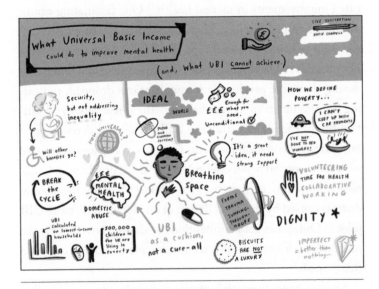

FIGURE E.1 Peace of mind.

Source: Illustration created by live-event illustrator and graphic recorder Katie Chappell, http://www.katiechappell.com. Permission granted by Katie Chappell.

could ensure that costs were kept under control and that the income provided would continue to keep people above the poverty line. Crucially, since UBI is a universal, guaranteed source of income with no strings attached, the stress associated with navigating the welfare system would be eliminated. Recent films, including *I, Daniel Blake* (2016), *Rocks* (2019), and *Nomadland* (2019) illustrate just how easy it is for individuals to run afoul of the system and suffer the consequences.[18] In turn, welfare workers, who currently exist primarily as gatekeepers, preventing the "undeserving poor" from accessing benefits, could then be reassigned to help individuals deal with other pressing and overlooked problems. These may include addictions, ongoing or historical abuse, physical health, domestic discord, or even career-related issues, all of which may *also* affect mental health. By guaranteeing an income—a relatively simple process—the welfare system could reorient itself toward dealing with these thornier problems. An example of this could be providing more comprehensive support to a mother who, now in receipt of a guaranteed income, has the means to escape domestic abuse. The same could be said for the mental health system. With the burden of mental illness caused by socioeconomic problems eased, mental health workers could focus more on the intractable causes, ranging from genetic and organic factors to sexual abuse and other forms of trauma.[19]

UBI could also help improve mental health by reducing the entrenched inequalities that social psychiatrists linked to mental illness. Although Hollingshead and Redlich associated inequality primarily with class, others have shown that discrimination on the basis of race, gender, disability, sexuality, ethnicity, and religion also contributes to poor mental health.[20] UBI could reduce the hopelessness associated with inequality and the so-called diseases of despair (for example, substance abuse and suicidal behaviors) by improving social mobility.[21] With a guaranteed income, individuals would have the means to pursue higher education, start their own business, engage in artistic endeavors, or leave unrewarding jobs for something better. It could provide individuals with the time and space to determine what they really want to do with their lives and with the means to pursue those dreams. Empowered in this way, employees would also be in a much stronger position to bargain with employers for better pay, working conditions, and training opportunities. Although more research on employment is needed, many UBI trials have seen increases in employment levels, possibly because people are able to seek out more desirable jobs.[22] Finally, since UBI is a universal payment, paid to all regardless of wealth or status, the stigma and shame attached to receiving welfare would be greatly reduced.

Finally, social psychiatrists linked mental illness with social or community disintegration and social isolation. The Stirling County Study focused specifically on this theme, but it featured implicitly in other social psychiatry research, as well as contemporary studies, such as Herbert Gans's influential work on Boston's West End and its demolition, *The Urban Villagers*.[23] UBI could help reintegrate communities in profound ways. As we have all experienced during the pandemic, social connection is vital for mental health. What the pandemic also did, however, was convince many people that their lives were not structured in ways that were conducive to their mental health. Yes, the pandemic was stressful, but before the pandemic, so too was managing work, parenting or caring responsibilities, commuting, and fitting in time for exercise or leisure activities. Millions of people unable to work during the pandemic (and often surviving on government furlough schemes) turned to baking, art, physical activity, engaging with nature, language learning, or countless other valuable "distractions." UBI could permit such people to rebalance their time in ways that provide more opportunities to conduct such activities, many of which are beneficial for mental health or could lead to employment opportunities. Even more importantly, however, it could allow people more time to engage with their communities in ways they find meaningful. Such activities could range from teaching painting or music in an after-school program to vital ecological work that could help protect vulnerable communities from the ravages of climate change.[24] This sort of community building is currently done on a volunteer basis, which works for those with the financial means and time but is simply not possible for those who lack such security. UBI could liberate people to reintegrate with their communities in meaningful ways that improved their mental health *and* the viability, safety, beauty, cohesiveness, and environmental sustainability of their neighborhoods. It could help societies shift away from focusing endlessly on economic growth, which does not benefit everyone, to social and emotional growth, which does.

Last, but certainly not least, UBI could help improve the mental health of those already dealing with mental illness, along with their family members, community support workers, and clinicians. This would include the millions of American homeless who are believed to suffer from mental illness.[25] Financial insecurity poses enormous challenges to those facing mental illness, especially when governments change welfare policies or change criteria for benefits. As a recent series of workshops on financial insecurity and mental health illustrated, even filling out the forms required by different income-granting bodies can be a source of considerable stress, contributing to feelings of despair. UBI would provide people coping with mental illness, as well as those trying to support them, a much more stable platform for their recovery. This includes individuals who feel pressured into returning to paid employment before they have recovered, thereby running the risk of relapsing.

UBI would not be a magic bullet. Mental illness has many causes, many of which need to be addressed in precise, specific ways. But by preventing or mitigating mental disorders caused or exacerbated by socioeconomic factors, UBI could ease the gigantic burden currently faced by both formal and informal mental health services. In so doing, it could allow researchers, clinicians, and health policy makers more time to address how to treat and prevent other, more intractable forms of mental illness, such as those triggered by childhood sexual abuse or other traumatic experiences. It could also provide a robust foundation onto which more social programs geared toward preventing mental illness could be built. Such programs could include those related to career development, community building, or intergenerational mentoring. Above all, a UBI is a clear message to everyone in society, no matter their race, ethnicity, religion, sexuality, class, or gender, that they are worthy of an income and they have an inalienable right to an income—no matter what. UBI will not solve our ongoing mental health crisis. But it is a good start.

ACKNOWLEDGMENTS

This spark for this project came in 2004, when I bumped into my former MA co-supervisor Patricia Prestwich outside Athabasca Books in Edmonton's Old Strathcona. I mentioned how social psychiatry had popped up unexpectedly during my research on the history of ADHD, and she encouraged me to explore it further. It took a while before I did, but I'm grateful to Patricia for lighting the kindling and to the Arts and Humanities Research Council for providing the fuel to keep the fire going. Thanks also to Columbia University Press for their support and, in particular, the hard work of Stephen Wesley, Jennifer Crewe, and Meredith Howard.

Since 2004, I've had the support of many kind and generous historians. Above all, I'd like to pay tribute to Ed Ramsden, whose knowledge, insight, and support was always invaluable; Cathy Coleborne, whose energy and passion has always been inspiring; and Despo Kritsotaki and Vicky Long, who have been wonderful coeditors and friends. Allan Beveridge, Gayle Davis, Erika Dyck, Rob Ellis, Sarah Marks, Mikko Myllykangas, Luc Richert, Mat Savelli, Helen Spandler, Martin Summers, Jesper Vaczy Kragh, and many other mental health historians have also provided encouragement and motivation. All my work has been built on the foundations of my postgraduate studies, so I am forever indebted to Lesley Cormack, Mark Jackson, and Rima Apple.

This book is a product of the University of Strathclyde's Centre for the Social History of Health and Healthcare, where I am grateful to work. I thank all my Strathclyde pals for their support, especially Patricia Barton, Richard Finlay, Emma Newlands, Laura Kelly, Arthur McIvor, and Jim Mills. Thanks in particular to Linsey Robb, who did many of the oral histories. Douglas Brodie ensured that I had ample time to research and write while I was vice dean of research and has been a wonderful mentor. Lizann Bonner, Mark Ellis, Mark Irvine, and Michelle Stewart in the Faculty Office have also been great colleagues. I am forever thankful to Strathclyde for giving me a career in academia. I hope this book counts as "useful learning."

I first heard about universal basic income during a lecture by the late sociologist Erik Olin Wright. I thank Jamie Cooke, Mike Danson, and the Scottish Universities Insight Institute for helping me explore UBI further. Thanks also to everyone who participated in our "Peace of Mind" project. I am also grateful to all of my oral history interviewees for taking the time to talk to me about their experiences and to all the knowledgeable archivists who helped me out, particularly those at the Rockefeller Archive Center, who also funded my visit.

I owe a great debt to close friends and family. Tindy Agaba, Mark Doidge, Matt Eisler, Bryce Evans, Peter Jackson, Ross MacFarlane, and Cory Segin have been there to listen to my rants and reflections and to share their wisdom with me. Thanks also to Mom, Dad, the Herberts, and the Burkes for their encouragement and support. Most importantly, I want to express my gratitude to Michelle, Dashiell, and Solveigh for their patience and support, especially when we were all crammed into the house during lockdown. Finally, Star has been my lovely writing companion for the last year. It's time for a walk, pup.

NOTES

INTRODUCTION: THE MAGIC YEARS

1. Lucy Ozarin, "Daniel Blain: Founder of This Journal," *Psychiatric Services* 50 (1999): 1563.

2. Starr's ancestor James Logan (1674–1751) had been the secretary to William Penn (1644–1718), served as the fourteenth mayor of Philadelphia, and was the founding trustee of the College of Pennsylvania, the predecessor of the University of Pennsylvania.

3. "Daniel Blain: History in Personal Introduction, Drafted 10/30/72 and 12/1/72," in Melvin Sabshin Library and Archives, American Psychiatric Association: Daniel Blain (1898–1982) Papers, Box 100662, Folder 219.

4. Albert Deutsch, *The Shame of the States* (1948; New York: Arno, 1973).

5. Daniel Blain, "Twenty-Five Years of Hospital and Community Psychiatry," *Hospital and Community Psychiatry* 26 (1975): 605.

6. Blain, "Twenty-Five Years."

7. William C. Menninger, *Psychiatry in a Troubled World: Yesterday's War and Today's Challenge* (New York: Macmillan, 1948).

8. "Daniel Blain: History in Personal Introduction, Drafted 10/30/72 and 12/1/72," in Melvin Sabshin Library and Archives, American Psychiatric Association: Daniel Blain (1898–1982) Papers, Box 100662, Folder 221.

9. In the United Kingdom and elsewhere, social psychiatry also involved therapy, specifically, therapeutic communities. It has also been

associated with transcultural psychiatry. See Maxwell Jones, *Social Psychiatry: In the Community, in Hospitals, and in Prisons* (Springfield, IL: Charles C. Thomas, 1962); Marvin K. Opler, *Culture, Psychiatry, and Human Values: The Methods and Value of a Social Psychiatry* (Springfield, IL: Charles C. Thomas, 1956).

10. See Theresa R. Richardson, *The Century of the Child: The Mental Hygiene Movement and Social Policy in the United States and Canada* (Albany: State University of New York Press, 1989); Kathleen W. Jones, *Taming the Troublesome Child: American Families, Child Guidance, and the Limits of Psychiatric Authority* (Cambridge, MA: Harvard University Press, 1999).

11. Hans Pols and Stephanie Oak, "War and Mental Health: The US Psychiatric Response in the 20th Century," *American Journal of Public Health* 97 (2007): 2132–42; Andrew Scull, "The Mental Health Sector and the Social Sciences in Post–World War II USA. Part 1: Total War and Its Aftermath," *History of Psychiatry* 22 (2010): 3–19.

12. Thomas A. C. Rennie, "Social Psychiatry: A Definition," *International Journal of Social Psychiatry* 1 (1955): 5–13.

13. Charles E. Rosenberg, *Explaining Epidemics and Other Studies in the History of Medicine* (Cambridge: Cambridge University Press, 1992), chap. 11.

14. Blain received roughly $20,000 per year for three years from the National Library of Medicine to complete his project. "Daniel Blain: History in Personal Introduction, Drafted 10/30/72 and 12/1/72," in Melvin Sabshin Library and Archives, American Psychiatric Association: Daniel Blain (1898–1982) Papers, Box 100662, Folder 260.

15. Oral history interview with Michael Barton, July 22, 2015.

16. Blain, "Twenty-Five Years," 605–9. Blain was also assisted by Robert L. Robinson (1915–1980), who served as the APA's director of public affairs for thirty-one years and edited the APA newspaper, *Psychiatric News*.

17. See David Healy, *The Antidepressant Era* (Cambridge, MA: Harvard University Press, 1997); Andrea Tone, *Age of Anxiety: A History of America's Turbulent Affair with Tranquilizers* (New York: Basic Books, 2009); David Herzberg, *Happy Pills in America: From Miltown to Prozac* (Baltimore, MD: Johns Hopkins University Press, 2010).

18. Andrew Scull, *Decarceration: Community and the Deviant—a Radical View* (Englewood Cliffs, NJ: Prentice Hall, 1977); John A. Talbott, *The*

Death of the Asylum: A Critical Study of State Hospital Management, Services, and Care (New York: Grune and Stratton, 1978); Despo Kritsotaki, Vicky Long, and Matthew Smith, eds., *Deinstitutionalisation and After: Post-War Psychiatry in the Western World* (Basingstoke: Palgrave Macmillan, 2016).

19. E. Fuller Torrey, *American Psychosis: How the Federal Government Destroyed the Mental Illness Treatment System* (Oxford: Oxford University Press, 2013), ix–x, 43–44, 58, 115, 165.

20. Gerald N. Grob, *From Asylum to Community: Mental Health Policy in Modern America* (Princeton, NJ: Princeton University Press, 1991), 303.

21. U.S. Department of Housing and Urban Development, *The Applicability of Housing First Models to Homeless Persons with Serious Mental Illness* (Rockville, MD: U.S. Department of Housing and Urban Development, 2007), https://www.huduser.gov/portal/publications/hsgfirst.pdf.

22. Gerald N. Grob, "Presidential Address: Psychiatry's Holy Grail: The Search for the Mechanisms of Mental Diseases," *Bulletin of the History of Medicine* 72 (1998): 212.

23. Dennis Doyle, *Psychiatry and Racial Liberalism in Harlem, 1936–1968* (Rochester, NY: University of Rochester Press, 2016); Gabriel N. Mendes, *Under the Strain of Color: Harlem's Lafargue Clinic and the Promise of an Antiracist Psychiatry* (Ithaca, NY: Cornell University Press, 2015); Mical Raz, *What's Wrong with the Poor? Psychiatry, Race, and the War on Poverty* (Chapel Hill: University of North Carolina Press, 2013); Jonathan M. Metzl, *The Protest Psychosis: How Schizophrenia Became a Black Disease* (Boston: Beacon, 2009). For an account of the racist origins of American psychiatry, see Mab Segrest, *Administrations of Lunacy: Racism and the Haunting of American Psychiatry at the Milledgeville Asylum* (New York: New Press, 2020).

24. Martin Summers, *Madness in the City of Magnificent Intentions: A History of Race and Mental Illness in the Nation's Capital* (Oxford: Oxford University Press, 2019).

25. Michael Neve, "Commentary on the History of Social Psychiatry and Psychotherapy in Twentieth-Century Germany, Holland, and Great Britain," *Medical History* 48 (2004): 407–12.

26. Heinz-Peter Schmiedebach and Stefan Priebe. "Social Psychiatry in Germany in the Twentieth Century: Ideas and Models," *Medical History* 48 (2004): 449–72.

27. Christof Beyer, "'Islands of Reform': Early Transformation of the Mental Health Service in Lower Saxony, Germany in the 1960s," in *Deinstitutionalisation and After: Post-War Psychiatry in the Western World*, ed. Despo Kritsotaki, Vicky Long, and Matthew Smith (Basingstoke: Palgrave, 2016), 99–114. This was similar to how the term was used in Holland. Harry Oosterhuis, "Between Institutional Psychiatry and Mental Health Care: Social Psychiatry in the Netherlands, 1916–2000," *Medical History* 48 (2004): 413–28.

28. Despo Kritsotaki, "From 'Social Aid' to "Social Psychiatry': Mental Health and Social Welfare in Post-War Greece (1950s–1960s)," *Humanities and Social Sciences Communications* 4 (2018), https://www.nature.com/articles/s41599-018-0064-1.

29. Harry Yi-Jiu Wu, "World Citizenship and the Emergence of the Social Psychiatry Project of the World Health Organization, 1948–c.1965," *History of Psychiatry* 26 (2015): 166–81.

30. Edward Shorter, *A Historical Dictionary of Psychiatry* (Oxford: Oxford University Press, 2005). Neither does Shorter pay much attention to social psychiatry in *A History of Psychiatry*. Edward Shorter, *A History of Psychiatry: From the Era of the Asylum to the Age of Prozac* (New York: Wiley, 1997).

31. Hans Pols, "Anomie in the Metropolis: The City in American Sociology and Psychiatry," *Osiris* 18 (2003): 194–211; Dan Blazer, *Age of Melancholy: Major Depression and Its Social Origins* (New York: Routledge, 2005); Michael Staub, *Madness Is Civilization: When the Diagnosis Was Social, 1948–1980* (Chicago: University of Chicago Press, 2011); Dana March and Gerald M. Oppenheimer, "Social Disorder and Diagnostic Order: The U.S. Mental Hygiene Movement, the Midtown Manhattan Study, and the Study of Psychiatric Epidemiology in the 20th Century," *International Journal of Epidemiology* 43 Supplement (2014): 129–142; Matthew Smith, "A Fine Balance: Individualism, Society, and the Prevention of Mental Illness in the United States, 1945–1968," *Humanities and Social Sciences Communications* 2 (2016): 1–11; David G. Satin, *Community Mental Health, Erich Lindemann, and Social Conscience in American Psychiatry*, 3 vols. (New York: Routledge, 2020).

32. See Despo Kritsotaki, Vicky Long, and Matthew Smith, eds., *Preventing Mental Illness: Past, Present, and Future* (Basingstoke: Palgrave, 2018).

33. World Health Organization, *Mental Disorders* (Geneva: World Health Organization, 2019), https://www.who.int/news-room/fact-sheets/deta il/mental-disorders.

34. Substance Abuse and Mental Health Services Administration, *Behavioral Health Spending and Use Accounts, 1986–2014* (Rockville, MD: Department of Health and Human Services, 2016), https://store.sa mhsa.gov/product/Behavioral-Health-Spending-and-Use-Accounts -1986-2014/SMA16-4975.

35. World Health Organization, *Mental Health in the Workplace* (Geneva: World Health Organization, 2019), https://www.who.int/mental_hea lth/in_the_workplace/en/.

36. Holly Hedegaard, Sally C. Curtin, and Margaret Warner, "Suicide Rates in the United States Continue to Increase," *NCHS Data Brief* 309 (2018), https://www.cdc.gov/nchs/data/databriefs/db309.pdf.

37. Joel Paris, *Overdiagnosis in Psychiatry: How Modern Psychiatry Lost Its Way While Creating a Diagnosis for Almost All of Life's Misfortunes,* 2nd ed. (Oxford: Oxford University Press, 2020); Steven K. Kapp, ed., *Autistic Community and the Neurodiversity Movement: Stories from the Frontline* (Basingstoke: Palgrave, 2020).

38. Diana Frasquilho, Margarida Gaspar Matos, Ferdinand Salonna, Diogo Guerreiro, Cláudia C. Storti, Tânia Gaspar, and José M. Caldas-de-Almeida, "Mental Health Outcomes in Times of Economic Recession: A Systematic Literature Review," *BMC Public Health* 16 (2016), doi:10.1186/s12889-016-2720-y.

39. Mike Baker, Jennifer Valentio-DeVries, Manny Fernandez, and Michael LaForgia, "Three Words. 70 Cases. The Tragic History of 'I Can't Breathe,'" *New York Times,* June 29, 2020.

40. Lola Jaye, "Why Race Matters When It Comes to Mental Health," BBC, August 12, 2020, https://www.bbc.com/future/article/20200804 -black-lives-matter-protests-race-mental-health-therapy. See also Lillian Comez-Días, Gordon Nagayama Hall, and Helen A. Neville, "Racial Trauma: Theory, Research, and Healing: Introduction to the Special Issue," *American Psychologist* 74 (2019): 1–5.

41. Office of the Surgeon General, *Mental Health: Culture, Race, and Ethnicity: A Supplement to Mental Health: A Report of the Surgeon General* (Rockville, MD: Substance Abuse and Mental Health Services Administration, 2001), https://www.ncbi.nlm.nih.gov/books/NBK44246/.

42. Robert E. L. Faris and H. Warren Dunham, *Mental Disorders in Urban Areas: An Ecological Study of Schizophrenia and Other Psychoses* (Chicago: University of Chicago Press, 1939).

43. August B. Hollingshead and Frederick C. Redlich, *Social Class and Mental Illness* (New York: John Wiley and Sons, 1958).

44. Leo Srole, Thomas S. Langner, Stanley T. Michael, Marvin K. Opler, and Thomas A. C. Rennie, *Mental Health in the Metropolis: The Midtown Manhattan Study* (New York: McGraw Hill, 1962).

45. Stirling County is a pseudonym for a real county in Nova Scotia.

46. Alexander H. Leighton, *My Name Is Legion: Foundations for a Theory of Man in Relation to Culture* (New York: Basic Books, 1959); Charles C. Hughes, Marc-Adelard Tremblay, Robert N. Rapoport, and Alexander H. Leighton, *People of Cove and Woodlot* (New York: Basic Books, 1960); Dorothy C. Leighton, John S. Harding, David B. Macklin, Allister M. MacMillan, and Alexander H. Leighton, *The Character of Danger: Psychiatric Symptoms in Selected Communities* (New York: Basic Books, 1963).

I. THE ORIGINS OF SOCIAL PSYCHIATRY

1. Thomas A. C. Rennie, "Social Psychiatry—a Definition," *International Journal of Social Psychiatry* 1 (1955): 5–13.

2. E. E. Southard, "Alienists and Psychiatrists: Notes on Divisions and Nomenclature of Mental Hygiene," *Mental Hygiene* 1 (1917): 567–71.

3. Joseph M. Gabriel, "Mass Producing the Individual: Mary C. Jarret, Elmer E. Southard, and the Industrial Origin of Psychiatric Social Work," *Bulletin of the History of Medicine* 79 (2005): 430–58. Social psychiatry was also the topic of a 1925 article by the psychiatrist Clinton P. McCord (1881–1953), but he, too, emphasized the connection between psychiatry and social services. Clinton P. McCord, "Social Psychiatry—Its Significance as a Specialty," *AJP* 82 (1925): 233–40.

4. Rennie, "Social Psychiatry," 6, 10, 9.

5. Rennie, "Social Psychiatry," 12.

6. For more on preventing mental illness, see Despo Kritsotaki, Vicky Long, and Matthew Smith, eds., *Preventing Mental Illness: Past, Present and Future* (Basingstoke: Palgrave, 2018).

7. Gerald N. Grob, *The Mad Among Us: A History of the Care of America's Mentally Ill* (New York: Free Press, 1994), 60, 151.

8. Albert Deutsch, *The Mentally Ill in America: A History of Their Care and Treatment from Colonial Times* (Garden City, NY: Doubleday, Doran and Company, 1937), 489.

9. Deutsch, *Mentally Ill in America*, 490. The original can be found in Henry C. Schumacher, "The Depression and Its Effect on the Mental Health of the Child," *American Journal of Public Health* 24 (1934): 367–71.

10. Deutsch, *Mentally Ill in America*, 491, 490.

11. The social psychologist Marie Jahoda (1907–2001) also argued that there was already enough evidence linking deprivation to mental illness and that, rather than attempting "to prove what is already known," "all available social energy is needed to eliminate these conditions." Marie Jahoda, "Toward a Social Psychology of Mental Health," in *Symposium on the Healthy Personality*, ed. Milton J. E. Senn (New York: Josiah Macy, Jr. Foundation, 1950), 211–30.

12. Rennie, "Social Psychiatry," 8–9, 10. The historian Gerald Grob would have concurred with Rennie, stating that "the modern psychiatric concept of prevention had little meaning; it was largely a myth that offered assurance to a wide public and provided the specialty with a measure of legitimacy." He added that even if the link between environmental factors and mental illness could be ascertained, there was no guarantee "that individuals would consent to environmental modifications which limited their freedom and autonomy." Gerald N. Grob, *From Asylum to Community: Mental Health Policy in Modern America* (Princeton, NJ: Princeton University Press, 1991), 14.

13. Émile Durkheim, *Le suicide. Étude de sociologie* (Paris: Ancienne Librairie Germer Bailière et Cte., 1897); Georg Simmel, "The Metropolis and Mental Life," in *The Urban Sociology Reader*, ed. Jan Lin and Christopher Mele (London: Routledge, 2012), 23–31.

14. Roy R. Grinker and John P. Spiegel, *Men Under Stress* (Philadelphia: Blakiston, 1945).

15. William C. Menninger, *Psychiatry in a Troubled World: Yesterday's War and Tomorrow's Challenge* (New York: Macmillan, 1948), viii.

16. Milton J. Rosenau, *Preventive Medicine and Hygiene* (New York: D. Appleton and Co., 1913), vii.

17. Thomas W. Salmon, "Mental Hygiene," in *Preventive Medicine and Hygiene*, ed. Milton Joseph Rosenau (New York: D. Appleton and Co., 1913), 298–303.

18. Salmon, "Mental Hygiene," 307. Immigrants, Salmon continued, were particularly vulnerable to such causes. See also Thomas W. Salmon, "The Relation of Immigration to the Prevalence of Insanity," *American Journal of Insanity* 64 (1907): 53–71.

19. Gerald N. Grob, *Mental Illness in American Society, 1875–1940* (Princeton, NJ: Princeton University Press, 1983), 145.

20. William Sweetser, *Mental Hygiene or an Examination of the Intellect and Passions Designed to Illustrate Their Influence on Health and the Duration of Life* (New York: J & H. G. Langley, 1843); Isaac Ray, *Mental Hygiene* (Boston: Ticknor and Fields, 1863). The term "mental hygiene" is still used today, for example in the name of the New York City Department of Health and Mental Hygiene.

21. Clifford Whittingham Beers, *A Mind That Found Itself: An Autobiography* (New York: Longmans, Green, 1908).

22. Norman Dain, *Clifford W. Beers: Advocate for the Insane* (Pittsburgh, PA: University of Pittsburgh Press, 1980), 89.

23. Dain, *Clifford W. Beers*, 150–51.

24. Salmon, "Mental Hygiene," in *Preventive Medicine and Hygiene*, ed. Milton Joseph Rosenau (New York: D. Appleton and Co., 1916), 331.

25. Another contemporaneous example of the trend toward exploring the social context of mental illness was the foundation of the American Orthopsychiatric Association in 1924.

26. Grob, *Mental Illness*, 159–61.

27. Meyer and Brush obtained $53,000 over five years from the Commonwealth Fund to pay for the following salaries: $3,000 for the psychiatrist, $1,050 for the psychologist ("for intelligence tests"), $1,500 for the chief social worker, $1,200 for the social worker, and $750 for a clinical secretary. Commonwealth Fund Records, Series 18, Box 199, Folder 1870, Rockefeller Archive Center.

28. Commonwealth Fund Records, Series 18, Box 199, Folder 1870. NCMH published numerous "Parent-Teacher Packets," as well as a series of primers for "advanced readers." These titles were authored both by well-known psychiatrists, such as William A. White (1870–1937), and social workers, such as Jessie Taft (1882–1960).

29. Theodore Porter has demonstrated how the record keeping of asylum superintendents led to the association of insanity and heredity and, subsequently, eugenic solutions. Theodore M. Porter, *Genetics in the Madhouse: The Unknown History of Human Heredity* (Princeton, NJ: Princeton University Press, 2018). See also Ian Dowbiggin, *Keeping America Sane: Psychiatry and Eugenics in the United States and Canada, 1880–1940* (Ithaca, NY: Cornell University Press, 1997); Erika Dyck, *Facing Eugenics: Reproduction, Sterilization, and the Politics of Choice* (Toronto: University of Toronto Press, 2013).

30. Grob, *Mental Illness*, 166–67.

31. Dowbiggin contends that, given the widespread support of eugenics during this period, the "mystery is not why some U.S. psychiatrists endorsed eugenics but why all of them were not seduced by it." Dowbiggin, *Keeping America Sane*, 128–29, 132.

32. Grob, *Mentally Ill*, 173–74. In addition, 17,000 mostly "feebleminded" individuals were sterilized. In Britain, the Mental Deficiency Act (1913) rejected sterilization but mandated the segregation of the feebleminded, not least for eugenic purposes. See Mark Jackson, *The Borderland of Imbecility: Medicine, Society, and the Fabrication of the Feeble Mind in Victorian and Edwardian Britain* (Manchester: Manchester University Press, 2000).

33. Theresa R. Richardson, *The Century of the Child: The Mental Hygiene Movement and Social Policy in the United States and Canada* (Albany: State University of New York Press, 1989), 2.

34. Kathleen W. Jones, *Taming the Troublesome Child: American Families, Child Guidance, and the Limits of Psychiatric Authority* (Cambridge, MA: Harvard University Press, 1999), 2.

35. Richardson, *Century of the Child*, 77, 82–86, describes how two conferences in New Jersey in 1920 involving mental hygienists, the Rockefeller Foundation, and the Commonwealth Fund helped emphasize the role of childhood in preventive psychiatry. The Laura Spelman Rockefeller Memorial Fund (established in 1918) would come to focus considerably on child development.

36. Alice Smuts, *Science in the Service of Children, 1893–1935* (New Haven, CT: Yale University Press, 2006), 107–12.

37. Richardson, *Century of the Child*, 11.

38. Jones, *Taming the Troublesome Child*, 3; Julia Grant, *Raising Baby by the Book: The Education of American Mothers* (New Haven, CT: Yale

University Press, 1998); Heather Munro Prescott, *A Doctor of Their Own: The History of Adolescent Medicine* (Cambridge, MA: Harvard University Press, 1998); Rima Apple, *Perfect Motherhood: Science and Childrearing in America* (New Brunswick, NJ: Rutgers University Press, 2006).

39. Jones, *Taming the Troublesome Child*, 2–3.

40. Grob, *Mental Illness*, 121.

41. Jones, *Taming the Troublesome Child*, 62–90. An exception to this was the pioneering Judge Baker Foundation in Boston, the direction of which was shared by the psychiatrist William Healy and the psychologist Augusta Bronner (1881–1966). Jones, *Taming the Troublesome Child*, 70.

42. Jones, *Taming the Troublesome Child*, 73.

43. For example, see Elnora E. Thomson, "Case Work in the Field of Mental Hygiene," *Annals of the American Academy of Political and Social Science* 77 (1918): 71–78.

44. Jones, *Taming the Troublesome Child*, 82.

45. Jones, *Taming the Troublesome Child*, 82–83.

46. Jones, *Taming the Troublesome Child*, 66.

47. William Healy estimated that 13 percent of repeat delinquents in Chicago had "encountered some early sexual experience sufficiently serious to be accounted . . . [as] a causative factor of delinquency." Jones, *Taming the Troublesome Child*, 75–76.

48. Jones, *Taming the Troublesome Child*, 75.

49. Jones states that "psychiatric interviewers did not frame questions to elicit stories of incest, although they did seek evidence of 'sex play' (the clinic's term) between siblings." During the 1920s and 1930s, incest was not always considered particularly harmful. While psychoanalysts saw children as inherently sexual beings who would not necessarily be damaged by sex with adults, racialist child guiders believed that Black children matured earlier than their white counterparts and were, therefore, not vulnerable to such abuse. Elizabeth Pleck, *Domestic Tyranny: The Making of Social Policy Against Family Violence from Colonial Times to the Present* (New York: Oxford University Press, 1987); Stephen Robertson, *Crimes Against Children: Sexual Violence and Legal Culture in New York City, 1880–1960* (Chapel Hill: University of North Carolina

Press, 2005); Lynn Sacco, *Unspeakable: Father-Daughter Incest in American History* (Baltimore, MD: Johns Hopkins University Press 2009); Dennis Doyle, *Psychiatry and Racial Liberalism in Harlem, 1936–1968* (Rochester, NY: University of Rochester Press, 2016), 48–51.

50. Ernest W. Burgess Papers, Box 11, Folder 4, Special Collections Research Center, University of Chicago Library. I have deliberately not used the name of the girl and her family.

51. The case notes suggested, however, that the mother's equivocation may have been caused by intimidation from her older daughter (the rapist's wife). A few weeks later, when this older daughter was not present in the interview, she "expressed herself freely" and berated her son-in-law, stating that his prison sentence was not sufficient.

52. Burgess Papers, Box 11, Folder 4.

53. Burgess Papers, Box 11, Folder 4.

54. Given some inconsistencies and apparent inaccuracies in the file, the numbers of residents in the flat vary, but this also appears to be attributable to the chaotic circumstances of the family.

55. Burgess Papers, Box 11, Folder 4.

56. Burgess Papers, Box 11, Folder 4. In the case notes, the wording was initially "the biggest flirt [the teacher] ever had in her room," but the typed words "the biggest" are scored out and replaced in pen with the word "a." It is not clear who corrected the report, but the revised version also added some quotation marks in pen, which suggest that the teacher (whose words were being quoted) might have been given the initial draft and felt obliged to edit or correct what the social worker wrote down. This was one of only a handful of handwritten corrections to an eight-page report (plus added letters and other documentation), suggesting that such characteristics had to be expressed precisely.

57. Burgess Papers, Box 11, Folder 4.

58. Burgess Papers, Box 11, Folder 4.

59. Burgess Papers, Box 11, Folder 4.

60. Burgess Papers, Box 11, Folder 4.

61. The factors identified in this case mirror those highlighted by the Maryland Mental Hygiene Clinic at roughly the same time. In order of frequency: "training and discipline; broken home; low standards—early

home life; poor physical condition; domestic friction (b/w child and parents); neurotic parents; inferior intellect—parents; poor placement—foster or institutional; psychopathic parents; domestic friction (adults); financial stress; organic disease; psychosis in parents; physically ill parents; 'Old World Standards in home'; change in family life; stress of involutional period; childbirth—puerperal infection." Commonwealth Fund records, Series 18, Box 199, Folder 1870.

62. "Troubled Students Seek and Get Aid," *Welfare Magazine*, April 1927, in Commonwealth Fund Records, Series 18, Box 387, Folder 3718. For more on the origins of psychiatry at Yale, see Jonathan W. Engel, "Early Psychiatry at Yale: Milton C. Winternitz and the Founding of the Department of Psychiatry and Mental Hygiene," *Yale Journal of Biology and Medicine* 67 (1994): 33–47. Mental hygiene clinics were also being established at high schools: Marian McBee, "A Mental Hygiene Clinic in a High School: An Evaluation of Problems, Methods, and Results in the Cases of 328 Students," *Mental Hygiene* 19 (1935): 238–80.

63. Commonwealth Fund Records, Series 18, Box 387, Folder 3718.

64. Commonwealth Fund Records, Series 18, Box 387, Folder 3718.

65. James Rowland Angell, quoted in "Mental Hygiene at Yale," *New York Times*, June 23, 1926, 9.

66. For more on Scoville's views, see Mildred C. Scoville, "An Inquiry Into the Status of Psychiatric Social Work," *American Journal of Orthopsychiatry* 1 (1931): 145–51.

67. For more on the origins of psychiatric social work in the United States, see Gabriel, "Mass Producing the Individual," 430–58.

68. Commonwealth Fund Records, Series 18, Box 387, Folder 3718.

69. Emphasis in original. Commonwealth Fund Records, Series 18, Box 387, Folder 3719.

70. Commonwealth Fund Records, Series 18, Box 387, Folder 3719.

71. Commonwealth Fund Records, Series 18, Box 387, Folder 3720.

72. Commonwealth Fund Records, Series 18, Box 387, Folder 3720.

73. Commonwealth Fund Records, Series 18, Box 388, Folder 3721.

74. Commonwealth Fund Records, Series 18, Box 387, Folder 3719.

75. Commonwealth Fund Records, Series 18, Box 387, Folder 3719.

76. Commonwealth Fund Records, Series 18, Box 387, Folder 3720.

77. Commonwealth Fund Records, Series 18, Box 387, Folder 3720.

78. Commonwealth Fund Records, Series 18, Box 387, Folder 3720.

79. Commonwealth Fund Records, Series 18, Box 388, Folder 3721.

80. For more on IHR, see J. G. Morawski, "Organizing Knowledge and Behavior at Yale's Institute of Human Relations," *Isis* 77 (1986): 219–42.

81. Engel, "Early Psychiatry at Yale," 44.

82. Robert M. Hutchins, "An Institute of Human Relations," *AJS* 35 (1929): 191–92.

83. Rosenau, *Preventive Medicine*, ix.

84. Gustavo Tosti, "Suicide in the Light of Recent Studies," *AJS* 3 (1898): 464–78. Tosti's article did generate a lengthy clarification from Durkheim in a subsequent issue of *AJS*.

85. Howard B. Woolston, "The Urban Habit of Mind," *AJS* 17 (1912): 602–14. Robert E. Park, one of the driving forces behind the Chicago School, studied under Simmel in Germany. Robert E. L. Faris, *Chicago Sociology: 1920–1932* (Chicago: University of Chicago Press, 1967), 108. For more on urban mental health, see chapter 4 in this volume.

86. Guillaume de Greef, "Introduction to Sociology: IV," trans. Eben Mumford, *AJS* 9 (1903): 69–104.

87. "Notes and Abstracts," *AJS* 6 (1901): 575–76.

88. For instance, H. C. Stevens, "Review of *The Mental Health of the Schoolchild*," *AJS* 21 (1915): 272–74.

89. The "Recent Literature" in a 1925 issue of *AJS* included summaries of *AJP* articles on the emotional problems of "superior children" and on "Immigration and the Problem of the Alien Insane." See "Recent Literature," *AJS* 25 (1931): 123–44.

90. Jules Morel, "Prevention of Mental Diseases," trans. C. R. Henderson, *AJS* 5 (1899): 72–97.

91. Morel, "Prevention of Mental Diseases, 74.

92. Seba Eldridge, *Problems of Community Life: An Outline of Applied Sociology* (New York: Thomas Y. Crowell, 1915), 122–23.

93. Most of Park's review, in fact, simply copied from the book to illustrate its "rough analysis and classification of the problems of modern city life." The section copied was "Care and Prevention of Insanity and Feeblemindedness." Robert E. Park, "Review of *Problems of Community Life: An Outline of Applied Sociology*," *AJS* 21 (1915): 121.

94. Ernest R. Groves, "Sociology and Psycho-Analytic Psychology: An Interpretation of the Freudian Hypothesis," *AJS* 23 (1917): 107–16.

95. H. Warren Dunham, "The Field of Social Psychiatry," in *Mental Health and Mental Disorder: A Sociological Approach*, ed. Arnold M. Rose (London: Routledge and Kegan Paul, 1956), 61.

96. Georg Schweinfurth, *The Heart of Africa*, vol. 2, trans. Ellen E. Frewer (New York: Harper and Brothers, 1874); Henri A. Junod, *The Life of a South African Tribe*, vol. 2: *The Psychic Life* (Neuchatel: Attinger-Frêres, 1913); John H. Weeks, *Among the Primitive Bakongo* (London: Seeley, Service and Co., 1914); Margaret Mead, *Coming of Age in Samoa* (New York: William Morrow, 1928). Mead would become quite involved in the World Federation of Mental Health after World War II. Harry Yi-Jiu Wu, *Mad by the Millions: Mental Disorders and the Early Years of the World Health Organization* (Cambridge, MA: MIT Press, 2021), 43.

97. For an early discussion of this, see Ellen Winston, "The Alleged Lack of Mental Diseases Among Primitive Groups," *American Anthropologist* 36 (1934): 234–38.

98. A. L. Kroeber, "Anthropology of Hawaii," *American Anthropologist* 23 (1921): 129–37. Kroeber had previously written a critique of Freud's *Totem and Taboo*. A. L. Kroeber, "Totem and Taboo: An Ethnic Psychoanalysis," *American Anthropologist* 22 (1920): 48–55.

99. Kroeber, "Anthropology of Hawaii, 134–35.

100. Kroeber, "Anthropology of Hawaii, 136.

101. Ellen Winston, "The Assumed Increase in Mental Disease," *AJS* 40 (1935): 427–39; A. J. Jaffe and Ethel Shanas, "Economic Differentials in the Probability of Insanity," *AJS* 39 (1944): 534–39.

102. Maurice H. Kraut, "The Province of Social Psychiatry," *Journal of Abnormal and Social Psychology* 28 (1933): 155–59.

103. L. Guy Brown, "The Field and Problems of Social Psychiatry," in *Fields and Methods of Sociology*, ed. L. L. Bernard (New York: Ray Long and Richard R. Smith Publishers, 1934), 129.

104. Lawrence K. Frank, "Society as Patient," *AJS* 42 (1936): 335–44. Frank's influence was highlighted by Burgess twenty years later. Ernest W. Burgess, "Problems of Social Psychiatry and Theoretical Overview," in *Mental Health in Modern Society*, ed. Arnold M. Rose (London: Routledge and Kegan Paul, 1956), 3–17. For more on Frank, see Matthew Smith, "A Fine Balance: Individualism, Society, and the Prevention of Mental Illness in the United States, 1945–1968," *Humanities and Social Sciences Communications* 2 (2016): 1–11.

105. Ernest W. Burgess, "The Influence of Sigmund Freud Upon Sociology in the United States," *AJS* 45 (1939): 356–74.

106. For more on the history of the Chicago School, see Ruth Shonle Cavan, "The Chicago School of Sociology, 1918–1933," *Urban Life* 11 (1983): 407–20; Martin Bulmer, *The Chicago School of Sociology* (Chicago: University of Chicago Press, 1984); Anthony J. Cortese, "The Rise, Hegemony, and Decline of the Chicago School of Sociology, 1892–1945," *Social Science Journal* 32 (1995): 235–54.

107. Robert E. Park, *The Principles of Human Behavior* (Chicago: Zalaz Corporation, 1915); Nels Anderson, *The Hobo: The Sociology of the Homeless Man* (1923; Chicago: University of Chicago Press, 1965); Louis Wirth, *The Ghetto* (Chicago: University of Chicago Press, 1925); Frederick Thrasher, *The Gang: A Study of 1,313 Gangs in Chicago* (Chicago: University of Chicago Press, 1927); Harvey W. Zorbaugh, *The Gold Coast and the Slum* (Chicago: University of Chicago Press, 1927); Ruth Shonle Cavan, *Suicide* (Chicago: University of Chicago Press, 1928); E. Franklin Frazier, *The Negro Family in Chicago* (Chicago: University of Chicago Press, 1931).

108. Robert E. Park and Ernest W. Burgess, *The City* (Chicago: University of Chicago Press, 1925).

109. Louis Wirth, "Clinical Sociology," *AJS* 37 (1931): 49–66. For more on the history of clinical sociology, see Jan M. Fritz, "The History of Clinical Sociology," *Sociological Practice* 7 (1989): 72–95.

110. Some sociologists did work at mental hygiene and child guidance clinics, including Leonard Cottrell (1899–1985), who—arranged by Burgess—worked at IJR, investigating the social networks of juvenile delinquents. James T. Carey, *Sociology and Public Affairs: The Chicago School* (London: Sage, 1975), 88–89.

111. There were certainly exceptions, most notably Karen Horney (1885–1952), Alfred Adler (1870–1937), Franz Alexander (1891–1964), and Gregory Zilboorg (1890–1959), the last also being a pioneering historian of psychiatry. Thomas D. Eliot, "Interactions of Psychiatric and Social Theory Prior to 1940," in *Mental Health and Mental Disorder: A Sociological Approach*, ed. Arnold M. Rose (London: Routledge and Kegan Paul, 1956), 18–41.

112. J. T. Searcy, "The Sociology of Insanity," *Southern Bench and Bar Review* 1 (1913): 286, 287, 289.

113. J. T. Searcy, "An Epidemic of Acute Pellagra," *Transactions of the Medical Association of the State of Alabama* (April 1907): 387–97. For more on the history of pellagra in the United States, including the unwillingness to accept that the disease was caused by vitamin deficiency, see Elizabeth W. Etheridge, *The Butterfly Caste: A Social History of Pellagra in the South* (Westport, CT: Greenwood, 1972); and Mary Katherine Crabb, "An Epidemic of Pride: Pellagra and the Culture of the American South," *Anthropologica* 34 (1992): 89–103.

114. Susan Lamb, "Social Skills: Adolf Meyer's Revision of Clinical Skill for the New Psychiatry of the Twentieth Century," *Medical History* 59 (2015): 443–64.

115. Grob, *Mad Among Us*, chap. 6.

116. Herman M. Adler, "The Relation Between Psychiatry and the Social Sciences," *AJP* 83 (1927): 661–69.

117. Dunham, "Field of Social Psychiatry," 61; Naoko Wake, *Private Practices: Harry Stack Sullivan, the Science of Homosexuality, and American Liberalism* (New Brunswick, NJ: Rutgers University Press, 2011), 92.

118. American Psychiatric Association, *Proceedings of the First Colloquium on Personality Investigation* (New York: APA, 1928).

119. Wake, *Private Practices*, 94–99.

120. Eliot, "Psychiatric and Social Theory," 32–33.

121. Dunham, "Field of Social Psychiatry," 62.

122. Adolf Meyer, "Presidential Address," *AJP* 85 (1928): 1–31.

123. Edward Sapir, "The Contribution of Psychiatry to an Understanding of Behavior in Society," *AJS* 42 (1937): 862.

124. Physicians were first offered training in the social sciences in the 1930s, with Sullivan's Washington School of Psychiatry among the first to offer such courses. Wake, *Private Practices*, 96, 114–15.

125. The participation of social scientists during World War II was also extensive, which meant that they enjoyed an enhanced profile after the war, too. Andrew Scull, "The Mental Health Sector and the Social Sciences in Post–World War II USA. Part I: Total War and Its Aftermath," *History of Psychiatry* 22 (2010): 3–19.

126. United States Army Medical Department, *Neuropsychiatry in World War II* (Washington, DC: Office of the Surgeon General, 1966), 1:xix.

127. Scull, "Mental Health Sector," 6.

128. United States Army Medical Department, *Neuropsychiatry in World War II*, 1:xiii, 159–63.

129. Grob, *From Asylum to Community*, 10.

130. Naoko Wake, "The Military, Psychiatry, and 'Unfit' Soldiers, 1939–1942," *Journal of the History of Medicine and Allied Sciences* 62 (2007): 461–94.

131. Ellen Dwyer, "Psychiatry and Race During World War II," *Journal of the History of Medicine and Allied Sciences* 61 (2006): 124, 127.

132. Grob, *From Asylum to Community*, 11–13, 16–17.

133. William C. Menninger, "Presidential Address," *AJP* 106 (1949): 2–3.

134. Grob, *From Asylum to Community*, 16.

135. John C. Whitehorn, quoted in Grob, *From Asylum to Community*, 16.

136. Grob, *From Asylum to Community*, 14–15, 16.

137. Albert Deutsch, *The Shame of the States* (New York: Harcourt, Brace, 1948).

138. Grinker and Spiegel, *Men Under Stress*, vii. See also Mark Jackson, *The Age of Stress: Science and the Search for Stability* (Oxford: Oxford University Press, 2013), chap. 4.

139. William Menninger, quoted in Group for the Advancement of Psychiatry, "History," https://ourgap.org/History.

140. Menninger, "Presidential Address," 4. For more on GAP and its attempts to reorganize the APA, see Grob, *From Asylum to Community*, 28–43.

141. GAP, *The Social Responsibility of Psychiatry: A Statement of Orientation* (New York: GAP, 1950).

142. Grob, *From Asylum to Community*, 54.

143. Menninger, "Presidential Address," 5.

144. Michael Staub, *Madness Is Civilization: When the Diagnosis Was Social* (Chicago: University of Chicago Press, 2011), 13.

145. Menninger, "Presidential Address," 12.

146. William C. Menninger, quoted in Marvin Karno and Donald A. Schwartz, *Community Mental Health: Reflections and Explorations* (New York: John Wiley and Sons, 1974), 10–11.

2. FROM HOBOHEMIA TO THE GOLD COAST

1. See Richard Noll, *American Madness: The Rise and Fall of Dementia Praecox* (Cambridge, MA: Harvard University Press, 2011).

2. Ernest W. Burgess Papers, Box 97, Folder 6, Special Collections Research Center, University of Chicago Library.

3. The phenomenon of "jack-rolling" and of the "jack-roller" was explored in Clifford R. Shaw, *The Jack-Roller* (Chicago: University of Chicago Press, 1930).

4. Burgess Papers, Box 97, Folder 6.

5. Robert E. L. Faris and H. Warren Dunham, *Mental Disorders in Urban Areas: An Ecological Study of Schizophrenia and Other Psychoses* (Chicago: University of Chicago Press, 1939).

6. Faris and Dunham, *Mental Disorders*, chap. 9.

7. H. Douglas Singer, in Faris and Dunham, *Mental Disorders*, vii.

8. Ernest W. Burgess, "Introduction," in Faris and Dunham, *Mental Disorders*, ix.

9. Robert E. Park and Ernest W. Burgess, *Introduction to the Science of Sociology* (Chicago: University of Chicago Press, 1921); Robert E. L. Faris, *Chicago Sociology: 1920–1932* (Chicago: University of Chicago Press, 1967); Ruth Shonle Cavan, "The Chicago School of Sociology, 1918–1933," *Urban Life* 11 (1983): 407–20.

10. Robert E. Park, Ernest W. Burgess, and Roderick D. McKenzie, *The City* (Chicago: University of Chicago Press, 1925), chap. 2. Burgess's theory—and Chicago's place as a model American city—was challenged in the 1980s by those who argued that the sprawl of Los Angeles now exemplified urban development in the United States. Andrew J. Diamond, *Chicago on the Make: Power and Inequality in a Modern City* (Berkeley: University of California Press, 2017), 4.

11. Faris and Dunham, *Mental Disorders*, 1.

12. Dennis Doyle, *Psychiatry and Racial Liberalism in Harlem, 1936–1968* (Rochester, NY: University of Rochester Press, 2016), 20–30. As Doyle explains, the psychiatric statistician Benjamin Malzberg's (1893–1975) research also questioned the racist assumptions made about the nature of mental disorder in Black Americans. Benjamin Malzberg, "Migration and Mental Disease Among Negroes in New York State," *American Journal of Physical Anthropology* 21 (1936): 107–13.

13. There have been debates about whether the Chicago School was a "monolithic, homogeneous tradition" of sociology or, instead, a more heterogeneous collection of ideas and approaches. I present it here as a highly influential and often dominant player in shaping how sociology would be conducted and utilized in shaping social policy. See James T. Carey, *Sociology and Public Affairs: The Chicago School*

(London: Sage, 1975); Lester R. Kutz, *Evaluating Chicago Sociology* (Chicago: University of Chicago Press, 1984), 99; Lee Harvey, *Myths of the Chicago School of Sociology* (Aldershot: Avebury, 1986); Jonathan H. Turner, "The Mixed Legacy of the Chicago School of Sociology," *Sociological Perspectives* 31 (1988): 325–38.

14. See William I. Thomas and Florian Znaiecki, *The Polish Peasant in Europe and America* (New York: Knopf, 1927). See also Carey, *Sociology and Public Affairs*, chap. 4.

15. Ernest W. Burgess and Donald J. Bogue, eds., *Contributions to Urban Sociology* (Chicago: University of Chicago Press, 1964), 488.

16. Nels Anderson, *The Hobo: The Sociology of the Homeless Man* (1923; Chicago: University of Chicago Press, 1965); Louis Wirth, *The Ghetto* (Chicago: University of Chicago Press, 1925); Frederick Thrasher, *The Gang: A Study of 1,313 Gangs in Chicago* (Chicago: University of Chicago Press, 1927); Harvey W. Zorbaugh, *The Gold Coast and the Slum* (Chicago: University of Chicago Press, 1927); Ruth Shonle Cavan, *Suicide* (Chicago: University of Chicago Press, 1928); Walter Reckless and Mapheus Smith, *Juvenile Delinquency* (New York: McGraw-Hill, 1932); Walter Reckless, *Vice in Chicago* (Chicago: University of Chicago Press, 1933). Jack Faris, "Robert E. Lee Faris, ASA Past President, 1907–1998," *Footnotes* 26 (1998): 8.

17. Robert G. Spinney, *City of Big Shoulders: A History of Chicago* (Dekalb: Northern Illinois Press, 2000), 100–104, 47–66.

18. Spinney, *City of Big Shoulders*, 123–45, 167–69; Anderson, *The Hobo*, 3.

19. William T. Stead, *If Christ Came to Chicago!* (Chicago: Laird and Lee, 1894).

20. Stead, *If Christ Came*, 157–59; Kathleen W. Jones, *Taming the Troublesome Child: American Families, Child Guidance, and the Limits of Psychiatric Authority* (Cambridge, MA: Harvard University Press, 1999), 31–34; Jane Addams, *Twenty Years at Hull House* (New York: Macmillan, 1911).

21. Anderson, *The Hobo*, v–xiv; Noel Iverson, "Nels Anderson: A Profile," *Labour/Le Travail* 63 (2009): 181–205.

22. Iverson, "Nels Anderson," xi.

23. Iveson, "Nels Anderson," xi–xii; Cavan, "Chicago School," 417.

24. It was also a question posed in Alice Solenberger, *One Thousand Homeless Men: A Study of Original Records* (Philadelphia: Wm. F. Fell Co., 1911), 89.

25. Robert E. Park, "Editor's Preface," in Anderson, *The Hobo*, xxiii.

26. Park, in Anderson, *The Hobo*, xxv. See also Park and Burgess, *Science of Sociology*, chaps. 3–4.

27. Hobohemia was nearly "womanless and childless." Anderson, *The Hobo*, 5.

28. Solenberger, *One Thousand Homeless Men*, 89–90. For more on the impact of Solenberger's work, see Kenneth L. Kusmer, *Down and Out, On the Road: The Homeless in American History* (Oxford: Oxford University Press, 2002), 93–94. For a more positive view on the life on the tramp, which interpreted tramping as a chosen occupation, see Stephen Graham, *The Gentle Art of Tramping* (New York: Appleton, 1926).

29. Solenberger, *One Thousand Homeless Men*, 91.

30. Anderson, *The Hobo*, 61.

31. Zorbaugh, *The Gold Coast and the Slum*.

32. Wirth, *The Ghetto*.

33. Faris and Dunham, *Mental Disorders*, 8.

34. Faris and Dunham, *Mental Disorders*; Louis Wirth, "The Ghetto," *AJS* 33 (1927): 68–71.

35. Wirth, "The Ghetto," 71.

36. Wirth, "The Ghetto," 70. As discussed in chapter 4, however, such insights did not prevent mass slum removal projects in the decades that followed.

37. Faris and Dunham, *Mental Disorders*, 177.

38. E. Franklin Frazier, *The Negro Family in Chicago* (Chicago: University of Chicago Press, 1931); Clifford Shaw and Frederick Zorbaugh, *Delinquency Areas: A Study of the Geographic Distribution of School Truants, Juvenile Delinquents, and Adult Offenders in Chicago* (Chicago: University of Chicago Press, 1929).

39. Shaw conducted similar studies of Cleveland, Philadelphia, Birmingham, Richmond, Denver, and Seattle. He also recorded numerous life histories of delinquents, which resulted in three monographs. Shaw, *The Jack-Roller*; Clifford Shaw, *The Natural History of a Delinquent Career* (Chicago: University of Chicago Press, 1931); Clifford Shaw, *Brothers in Crime* (Chicago: University of Chicago Press, 1938).

40. E. H. Sutherland, "Review of *Delinquency Areas: A Study of the Geographic Distribution of School Truants, Juvenile Delinquents, and Adult Offenders in Chicago*," *AJS* 36 (1930): 139–40.

41. Park and Burgess, *The City*, 50–58.

42. Faris and Dunham, *Mental Disorders*, 2.

43. Faris and Dunham, *Mental Disorders*, 9–10.

44. The supervisors of Chicago School doctoral projects often wrote the introductions of their students' monographs.

45. Ernest W. Burgess Papers, Box 11, Folder 5. For more on debates about sociologists and social policy, see Carey, *Sociology and Public Affairs*.

46. Faris, *Chicago Sociology*, 84.

47. The American Society of Criminology established an award for young scholars in Cavan's honor in 1997. Imogene L. Moyer, "Ruth Shonle Cavan (1896–1993): A Tribute," *Women and Criminal Justice* 7 (1996): 3–22.

48. Cavan, *Suicide*, 77–78.

49. In contrast, many regions reported no suicides at all. Cavan, *Suicide*, 81.

50. Cavan also employed maps effectively to illustrate the distribution of suicide.

51. Cavan, *Suicide*, 100, 103, 104.

52. The term was used by Kathryn McGonigal and John F. Galliher, who accused Faris of plagiarizing Mabel Agnes Elliott (1898–1990) in his sociology textbook *Social Disorganization* (1948). Putting this issue to one side (though the evidence is convincing), the Faris family continued in the sociology tradition. Faris's son Jack earned a PhD in sociology, and his grandson Robert is also a sociologist. Another grandchild is the actor Anna Faris. Kathryn McGonigal and John F. Galliher, *Mabel Agnes Elliott: Pioneering Feminist, Pacifist Sociologist* (Lanham, MD: Lexington, 2009), 97–101.

53. Faris, *Chicago Sociology*.

54. Faris, "Robert E. Lee Faris," 8.

55. It is noted in *Mental Disorders in Urban Areas*, xxi, that the sociologist (and professional football player) Herbert Blumer (1900–1987) also suggested to Faris that he study the distribution of mental disorders for his doctoral dissertation.

56. Faris, "Robert E. Lee Faris," 8.

57. H. Warren Dunham, "Mental Disorders in Urban Areas: A Retrospective View," in *Community Surveys of Psychiatric Disorders*, ed. Myrna M. Weissman, Jerome K. Myers, and Catherine E. Ross (New Brunswick, NJ: Rutgers University Press, 1986), 66.

58. Dunham, "Mental Disorders," 66, 65, 70.

59. Robert E. L. Faris, "Reflections on the Ability Dimension in Human Society," *American Sociological Review* 26 (1961): 835–43.

60. Robert Faris, much like Daniel Blain, also attempted to write the history of American sociology in his retirement. As with Blain, this history was sadly not completed. Faris interview.

61. Gerald N. Grob, *From Asylum to Community: Mental Health Policy in Modern America* (Princeton, NJ: Princeton University Press, 1991), 243.

62. R. A. Schermerhorn, "Review of *Sociological Theory and Mental Disorder*," *Social Forces* 39 (1961): 364–65; H. Warren Dunham, *Sociological Theory and Mental Disorder* (Detroit, MI: Wayne State University Press, 1959).

63. "Dr H. Warren Dunham Dead; Studied Urban Schizophrenia," *New York Times*, December 31, 1985, B10.

64. Faris and Dunham, *Mental Disorders*, 21–22. See also H. Warren Dunham, "The Ecology of Functional Psychoses in Chicago," *American Sociological Review* 2 (1937): 467–79.

65. J. F. Sutherland, "Geographical Distribution of Lunacy in Scotland," *British Association for Advancement of Science* (1901): 742–43; William A. White, "Geographical Distribution of Insanity in the United States," *Journal of Nervous and Mental Disease* 30 (1903): 257–79. For more on White, see Suzanne Hollman, "White's Restraint and Progressive American Psychiatry at St. Elizabeth's Hospital: 1903–1937," University College London, 2020. Sutherland's son, Halliday Sutherland, was also a physician and produced the first British public health film, *The Story of John M'Neil* (1911).

66. Sutherland, "Geographical Distribution," 742–43.

67. White, "Geographical Distribution," 263.

68. David Schuster, *Neurasthenic Nation: America's Search for Health, Happiness, and Comfort, 1869–1920* (New Brunswick, NJ: Rutgers University Press, 2011).

69. White, "Geographical Distribution," 257–58, 279.

70. Before dismissing weather altogether, it should be noted that "airs, waters, and places" were central to humoral understandings of madness since the time of Hippocrates, as White noted. Researchers still explore

the link between weather and mental health, with particular emphasis on suicide, which is found to increase with certain weather conditions. In addition, researchers also suspect that extreme weather as a result of climate change will result in poorer mental health. Apocryphally, in my home province of Alberta, it was said that suicide rates were high in the southern city of Lethbridge because it was so windy. See Selvi Kayipmaz, Ishak San, Eren Usul, and Semih Korkut, "The Effect of Meteorological Variables on Suicide," *International Journal of Biometeorology* 64 (2020): 1593–98.

71. Faris and Dunham, *Mental Disorders*, 188–93.

72. Other maps were broken down further into 120 "subcommunities."

73. Faris and Dunham, *Mental Disorders*, 24–25. Kenwood has gained attention recently for being the home of President Barack Obama.

74. Faris and Dunham, *Mental Disorders*, 24. The Lake Calumet region has also been long afflicted by environmental degradation.

75. Faris and Dunham, *Mental Disorders*, chap. 9.

76. Faris and Dunham, *Mental Disorders*, 143–44, 145–46, 147.

77. Patients in private hospitals also had much shorter stays.

78. Faris and Dunham, *Mental Disorders*, 30–31, 31–32.

79. Faris and Dunham, *Mental Disorders*, 38.

80. Faris and Dunham, *Mental Disorders*, 40, 194.

81. Faris and Dunham, *Mental Disorders*, 40.

82. Although the rates for males were somewhat higher than that for females, the overall geographical pattern of distribution held. The only exceptions to this were in Hobohemia, which had an almost exclusively male population, and two other regions in the west of the city, where no explanation for the discrepancy was provided. Faris and Dunham, *Mental Disorders*, 42–44.

83. Martin Summers, *Madness in the City of Magnificent Intentions: A History of Race and Mental Illness in the Nation's Capital* (Oxford: Oxford University Press, 2019), 3–9.

84. For more on the history of schizophrenia, see Kiernan McNally, *A Critical History of Schizophrenia* (Basingstoke: Palgrave, 2016).

85. Faris and Dunham, *Mental Disorders*, 85.

86. Faris and Dunham, *Mental Disorders*, 88–89, 84, 98–99, 83, 92.

87. Faris and Dunham, *Mental Disorders*, 104–5.

88. Racist attitudes were certainly present then in U.S. sociology. However, Robert Park's influence likely kept them in check within the Chicago School. In addition to studying race relations, he worked for seven years as a secretary and press agent for the educator and author Booker T. Washington (1856–1915) before joining the University of Chicago. There he offered the course "The Negro in America," the first class on Black Americans offered at a predominantly white university. Winifred Raushenbush, *Robert E. Park: Biography of a Sociologist* (Durham, NC: Duke University Press, 1979); Robert Washington, "Robert E. Park Reconsidered," *International Journal of Politics, Culture, and Society* 7 (1993): 97–107.

89. Faris and Dunham, *Mental Disorders*, 134–39, 69, 206–7.

90. Faris and Dunham, *Mental Disorders*, 63, 78, 79–80.

91. Faris and Dunham, *Mental Disorders*, 160.

92. Burgess, "Introduction," ix.

93. Dunham stated elsewhere that psychiatrists at the time indicated a diagnostic error rate of 30–40 percent for the functional psychoses. Dunham, "Ecology of Functional Psychoses," 478.

94. Faris and Dunham, *Mental Disorders*, 172–173.

95. Faris and Dunham, *Mental Disorders*, 173.

96. Robert E. L. Faris, "Cultural Isolation and the Schizophrenic Personality," *AJS* 40 (1934): 163.

97. According to his son Jack, Faris meant to have conducted one hundred interviews to simplify the statistical calculations. When he went back and counted them, however, he found that he had one extra. Faris interview.

98. Faris, "Cultural Isolation," 162.

99. Echoing this downplaying of the role of poverty and unemployment, in his introduction Burgess noted that the "financial depression beginning in 1929 was accompanied by little or no increase in mental disorders." Burgess, "Introduction," xii.

100. Robert E. L. Faris, "Insanity Distribution by Local Areas," *Journal of the American Statistical Association* 27 (1932): 57.

101. Faris and Dunham, *Mental Disorders*, 159.

102. Dunham, "Mental Disorders," 71.

103. Faris, *Chicago Sociology*, 35.

104. Carey, *Sociology and Public Affairs*, 87–89.

105. Burgess, "Introduction," xvii.

106. Faris, "Robert E. Lee Faris," 8.

107. Jack Faris interview.

108. "Staying Healthy to Age 85," *US News and World Report*, June 22, 1964, 66–67.

109. Robert E. L. Faris, "Sociological Factors in the Development of Talent and Genius," *Journal of Educational Sociology* 9 (1936): 538–44.

110. H. Warren Dunham, "Social Psychiatry," *American Sociological Review* 13 (1948): 183–97.

111. Robert M. Frumkin, "Occupation and Major Mental Disorder," in *Mental Health and Mental Disorder: A Sociological Approach*, ed. Arnold M. Rose (London: Kegan Paul, 1956), 136–60.

112. H. Warren Dunham, "Social Structures and Mental Disorders: Competing Hypotheses of Explanation," *Milbank Memorial Fund Quarterly* 39 (1961): 263.

113. S. M. Miller and Elliott G. Mishler, "Social Class, Mental Illness, and American Society: An Expository Review," *Milbank Memorial Fund Quarterly* 37 (1959): 174.

114. Dunham, "Social Structures," 280, 290.

115. Dunham, *Sociological Theory*, 62.

116. Faris and Dunham, *Mental Disorders*, 160–69.

117. H. Warren Dunham, "Some Persistent Problems in the Epidemiology of Mental Orders," *AJP* 109 (1953): 568.

118. John H. Mueller, "Review of *Mental Disorders in Urban Areas*," *Journal of Abnormal and Social Psychology* 35 (1940): 593.

119. Abraham Myerson, "Review of *Mental Disorders in Urban Areas*," *AJP* 96 (1940): 997.

120. Myerson, "Review of *Mental Disorders in Urban Areas*," 996, 997.

121. James S. Plant, "Review of *Mental Disorders in Urban Areas*," *AJS* 44 (1939): 1000–1001.

122. Faris, "Reflections on Social Disorganization."

123. James D. Page, "Review of *Mental Disorder in Urban Areas*," *Journal of Educational Psychology* 30 (1939): 707.

124. Emphasis in original. Georges Devereux, "Review of *Mental Disorders in Urban Areas*," *Psychoanalytic Review* 27 (1940): 251–52.

125. A. W. Stearns, "Review of *Mental Disorders in Urban Areas*," *Annals of the American Academy of Political and Social Science* 204 (1939): 223–24;

Walter A. Adams, "Review of *Mental Disorders in Urban Areas*," *Social Service Review* 13 (1939): 545–46.

126. J. D. M. Griffin, S. R. Laycock, and W. Line, *Mental Hygiene: A Manual for Teachers* (New York: American Book Company, 1940).

127. Stuart A. Queen, "The Ecological Study of Mental Disorders," *American Sociological Review* 5 (1940): 201–9; Clarence W. Schroeder, "Mental Disorder in Cities," *AJS* 48 (1942): 40–47.

128. Dunham, *Sociological Theory*, 146–48.

129. See Matthew Smith, "A Fine Balance: Individualism, Society, and the Prevention of Mental Illness in the United States, 1945–1968," *Humanities and Social Sciences Communications* 2 (2016): 1–11.

130. Melvin L. Kohn, "Social Class and Schizophrenia: A Critical Review," in *Social Psychology and Mental Illness*, ed. Henry Weschler, Leonard Solomon, and Bernard M. Kramer (New York: Holt, Rinehart, and Winston, 1970), 113–28; John J. Schwab and Mary E. Schwab, *Sociocultural Roots of Mental Illness: An Epidemiological Survey* (New York: Plenum, 1978), 172–78; R. Neugebauer, B. P. Dohrenwend, and B. S. Dohrenwend, "Formulation of Hypotheses About the True Prevalence of Functional Psychiatric Disorders Among Adults in the United States," in *Mental Illness in the United States*, ed. ed. B. P. Dohrenwend (New York: Praeger, 1980), 45–94.

131. H. Warren Dunham, "Community Psychiatry: The Newest Therapeutic Bandwagon," *Archives of General Psychiatry* 12 (1965): 303–13; Grob, *From Asylum to Community*, 243.

132. D. L. Gerard and L. G. Houston, "Family Setting and the Social Ecology of Schizophrenia," *Psychiatric Quarterly* 27 (1953): 90–101; E. M. Goldberg and S. L. Morrison, "Schizophrenia and Social Class," *British Journal of Psychiatry* 109 (1963): 785–802.

133. Rema Lapouse, Mary A. Monk, and Milton Terrace, "The Drift Hypothesis and Socioeconomic Differentials in Schizophrenia," *American Journal of Public Health* 46 (1956): 984.

134. Melissa J. Perry, "The Relationship Between Social Class and Mental Disorder," *Journal of Primary Prevention* 17 (1996): 18–30.

135. Dunham, "Social Psychiatry," 183.

136. In a 1944 article, Faris foreshadowed Laing in one of his last publications on mental illness. He provided an in-depth analysis of a single

patient diagnosed with schizophrenia, described as "the most violent patient in the 'violent ward'" and, according to patients, "the craziest one here." Faris argued that the patient's abnormal behavior should not be considered "mental disorder" but "an elaborate and orderly system of thought, privately worked out as a solution to a number of severe life-problems." Robert E. L. Faris, "Reflections of Social Disorganization in the Behavior of a Schizophrenic Patient," *AJS* 50 (1944): 134.

137. "Conference on Physical Environment as Determinant of Mental Health," John B. Calhoun Papers, 1909–1996, National Library of Medicine, Box 56, Folder 7.

138. Faris interview.

139. See Matthew Smith, "Mixing with Medics," *Social History of Medicine* 24 (2011): 142–50.

140. Diamond, *Chicago on the Make*, 3.

3. SWAMP YANKEES AND PROPER NEW HAVENERS

1. One reason for the Kennedy family's interest in mental illness was the botched lobotomy suffered by the president's sister Rosemary Kennedy (1918–2005) at the hands of Walter J. Freeman Jr. (1895–1972), the foremost American psychosurgeon. The 1941 procedure left her permanently incapacitated and unable to speak. Edward Shorter, *The Kennedy Family and the Story of Mental Retardation* (Philadelphia: Temple University Press, 2000).

2. John F. Kennedy, "Special Message to the Congress on Mental Illness and Mental Retardation," February 5, 1963, https://www.presidency.ucsb.edu/documents/special-message-the-congress-mental-illness-and-mental-retardation.

3. Leopold Bellack, *Handbook of Community Psychiatry and Community Mental Health* (New York: Grune and Stratton, 1964).

4. Deinstitutionalization was also triggered by growing concerns about the perilous state of many psychiatric institutions. Albert Deutsch, *The Shame of the States* (1948; New York: Arno, 1973); Gerald N. Grob, *From Asylum to Community: Mental Health Policy in Modern America* (Princeton, NJ: Princeton University Press, 1991); Despo Kritosotaki, Vicky

Long, and Matthew Smith, *Deinstitutionalization and After: Post-War Psychiatry in the Western World* (Basingstoke: Palgrave, 2016), chap. 1.

5. Grob, *From Asylum to Community*, chap. 8; JCMIH, *Action for Mental Health: Final Report of the Joint Commission on Mental Health and Illness* (New York: Basic Books, 1961).

6. This would have resulted in 3,500 CMHCs. The actual size of catchment areas eventually grew to approximately 250,000 people, but the staffing pressures remained.

7. Fourteen states had introduced community mental health legislation before the federal act, starting with New York in 1954. Lucy D. Ozarin, "Recent Community Mental Health Legislation: A Brief Review," *American Journal of Public Health* 52 (1962): 436–42.

8. R. H. Felix and R. V. Bowers, "Mental Hygiene and Socio-Environmental Factors," *Milbank Memorial Fund Quarterly* 26 (1948): 144.

9. Felix and Bowers, "Mental Hygiene," 125.

10. Felix and Bowers, "Mental Hygiene," 139.

11. Felix and Bowers, "Mental Hygiene," 140. The social psychiatry projects explored in this and the next two chapters would be socioclinical studies of individuals and cross-cultural studies. In terms of the other types of studies recommended by Felix and Bowers, Erich Lindemann had already undertaken research on trauma and grief, focusing on Boston's deadly Cocoanut Grove nightclub fire in 1942, where 492 people were killed. With respect to laboratory studies, Felix and Bowers might have had Hans Selye's stress research in mind. Stanley Cobb and Erich Lindemann, "Symposium on the Management of the Cocoanut Grove Burns at the Massachusetts General Hospital: Neuropsychiatric Observations," *Annals of Surgery* 117 (1943): 814–24; Hans Selye, "The General Adaptation Syndrome and the Diseases of Adaptation," *Journal of Clinical Endocrinology* 6 (1946): 117–230; David G. Satin, "Erich Lindemann as Humanist, Scientist, and Change Agent," *American Journal of Community Psychology* 12 (1984): 519–27; Mark Jackson, *Age of Stress: Science and the Search for Stability* (Oxford: Oxford University Press), 2013.

12. With NIMH's support, Erving Goffman (1922–1982) would set the benchmark for sociological research on mental hospitals with *Asylums:*

Essays on the Social Situation of Mental Patients and other Patients (New York: Anchor, 1961).

13. Felix and Bowers, "Mental Hygiene," 142.

14. Martin Summers, "Inner City Blues: African Americans, Psychiatry, and the Post-War 'Urban Crisis,'" Seminar Paper given to the University of Strathclyde, March 16, 2021.

15. Felix and Bowers, "Mental Hygiene," 144.

16. Another early NIMH-funded project was the sociologist Joseph W. Eaton (1919–2012) and the psychiatrist Robert J. Weil's study of Hutterite communities. Joseph W. Eaton and Robert J. Weil, *Culture and Mental Disorders: A Comparative Study of the Hutterites and Other Populations* (Glencoe, IL: Free Press, 1955).

17. August B. Hollingshead and Frederick C. Redlich, *Social Class and Mental Illness* (New York: John Wiley, 1958); Jerome K. Myers and Bertram H. Roberts, *Family and Class Dynamics in Mental Illness* (New York: John Riley and Sons, 1959).

18. Edward Said, *Orientalism* (New York: Pantheon, 1978); Michal Krumer-Nevo and Orly Benjamin, "Critical Poverty Knowledge: Contesting Othering and Social Distancing," *Current Sociology* 58 (2010): 693–714.

19. For another example of activism relating to community mental health in New York City, see Gerald Markovitz and David Rosner, *Children, Race, and Power: Kenneth and Mamie Clark's Northside Center* (Charlottesville: University of Virginia Press, 1996); and Zoe M. Adams and Naomi Rogers, "'Services Not Mausoleums': Race, Politics, and the Concept of Community in American Medicine (1963–1970)," *Journal of Medical Humanities* 41 (2020): 515–29.

20. Hollingshead and Redlich, *Social Class and Mental Illness*, 3.

21. Hollingshead and Redlich, *Social Class and Mental Illness*, 4–5.

22. Hollingshead and Redlich, *Social Class and Mental Illness*, 3.

23. See Samuel L. Bloom, *Word as Scalpel: A History of Medical Sociology* (Oxford: Oxford University Press, 2002), chap. 7.

24. Mark A. May, "A Retrospective View of the Institute of Human Relations at Yale," *Behavior Science Notes* 6 (1971): 142.

25. Bloom, who served on the Committee on Medical Sociology that was founded by Hollingshead and Robert Straus (1923–2020), distinguished

the terms "medical sociology" and "social psychiatry" as representing sociologists and psychiatrists respectively. Although this shorthand is somewhat accurate, it is also misleading. While some sociologists, including Hollingshead, identified with medical sociology, others, such as Dunham, were identified as representing social psychiatry. Moreover, the academic appointment of other social scientists, such as the anthropologist Marvin Opler (see chapter 4), was that of professor of social psychiatry. Medical sociology also went beyond just psychiatry. Equally significant is that while medical sociology, as described by Bloom, aspired toward objectivity, rather than advocacy, social psychiatry, as defined by Rennie and others, was intended to inform mental health policy, especially regarding prevention. Bloom, *Word as Scalpel*, chap. 7.

26. Julia Adams and David L. Weakliem, "August B. Hollingshead's 'Four Factor Index of Social Status': From Unpublished Paper to Citation Classic," *Yale Journal of Sociology* 8 (2011): 11–19.

27. Jerome K. Myers and Robert Straus, "A Sociological Profile of August B. Hollingshead," *Sociological Inquiry* 59 (1989): 1–6.

28. August B. Hollingshead, *Elmtown's Youth: The Impact of Social Class on Adolescents* (New York: John Wiley and Sons, 1949); Lloyd H. Rogler and August B. Hollingshead, *Trapped: Families and Schizophrenia* (New York: John Wiley and Sons, 1965); Raymond S. Duff and August B. Hollingshead, *Sickness and Society* (New York: Harper and Row, 1968).

29. Bloom, *Word as Scalpel*, 150.

30. August B. Hollingshead, "Commentary on 'The Indiscriminate State of Social Class Measurement,'" *Social Forces* 49 (1971): 563–67.

31. Bloom, *Word as Scalpel*, 149.

32. Calvin J. Frederick, Peter Loewenberg, and Robert O. Pasnau, "In Memoriam: Frederick C. Redlich," University of California, https:// senate.universityofcalifornia.edu/_files/inmemoriam/html /FrederickC.Redlich.htm.

33. In addition to *Psychotherapy with Schizophrenics* and *The Initial Interview in Psychiatric Practice*, Redlich wrote a "pathography" of Adolf Hitler in which he concluded that, while the dictator had numerous physical health problems, he was not likely mentally ill. Eugene B. Brody and Frederick C. Redlich, *Psychotherapy with Schizophrenics* (New York: International Universities Press, 1952); Merton Max Gill,

Frederick C. Redlich, and Richard Newman, *The Initial Interview in Psychiatric Practice* (New York: International Universities Press, 1954); Frederick C. Redlich, *Hitler: Diagnosis of a Destructive Prophet* (New York: Oxford University Press, 1999).

34. Lazarsfeld was originally Redlich's mathematics teacher and then later taught him psychology. Redlich acknowledged Lazarsfeld for encouraging him to shift from psychology to medicine and, ultimately, psychiatry. Bloom, *Word as Scalpel*, 151.

35. Bloom, *Word as Scalpel*, 151.

36. Adams and Weakliem, "August B. Hollingshead," 16.

37. Frederick C. Redlich, quoted in Bloom, *Word as Scalpel*, 152.

38. Eugene Brody, quoted in Bloom, *Word as Scalpel*, 152.

39. William Caudill and Bertram H. Roberts, "Pitfalls in the Organization of Interdisciplinary Research," *Human Organization* 10 (1951): 12–15. After his death, Roberts's family and friends established the Bertram H. Roberts Memorial Fund to host a lecture series in social psychiatry and to support medical students interested in the subject. Shane Seger, "Memorial Fund Continues to Support Training in Social Psychiatry," February 14, 2013, https://medicine.yale.edu/news-article/4783/.

40. Jerome K. Myers and L. L. Bean, *A Decade Later: A Follow-up of Social Class and Mental Illness* (New York: John Wiley and Sons, 1968).

41. Hollingshead and Redlich, *Social Class and Mental Illness*, chap. 2.

42. Hollingshead and Redlich, *Social Class and Mental Illness*, 388.

43. Hollingshead distilled the factors contributing to social stratification into a series of influential indices of social status that were widely used by sociologists. While the two-factor index Hollingshead eventually adopted for the New Haven Study consisted of education and occupation, he later developed a four-factor index that also included sex and marital status in response to criticisms that too much of the family's status depended on data pertaining to the male "head of the household." Hollingshead never published this index during his lifetime (in 2011 it was published in the *Yale Journal of Sociology*, an undergraduate journal), but it nevertheless became widely used, with Yale's sociology department inundated with requests to copy his original typescript. August B. Hollingshead, "Four Factor Index of Social Status," *Yale Journal of Sociology* 8 (2011): 21–52; Adams and Weakliem, "August B. Hollingshead."

44. Hollingshead and Redlich relied on a recently published history of New Haven for their historical chapter. Rollin G. Osterweis, *Three Centuries of New Haven* (New Haven, CT: Yale University Press, 1953).

45. Hollingshead and Redlich, *Social Class and Mental Illness*, 47.

46. Hollingshead and Redlich, *Social Class and Mental Illness*, 49, 53–55.

47. Hollingshead and Redlich, *Social Class and Mental Illness*, 61.

48. In terms of race, it is important to recognize that the New Haven of 1950–1951 that Hollingshead and Redlich researched had changed considerably by 1960. Black Americans, who made up 4 percent of New Haven's population in 1950, made up 16 percent by 1960 and rose to one-third of the population by 1975. White flight of middle-class workers to suburbia contributed to this shift in racial composition. In 1954, Mayor Richard C. Lee (1916–2003), sometimes called "Mr. Urban America," embarked upon an ambitious urban renewal program, but this failed to halt the economic and population decline that afflicted central New Haven and contributed to social problems. Class may have remained as an important factor in understanding mental health in New Haven in 1975, but it likely would have fallen behind race and community disintegration in importance. Michael Sletcher, *New Haven: From Puritanism to the Age of Terrorism* (Charleston, SC: Arcadia, 2004).

49. Hollingshead and Redlich, *Social Class and Mental Illness*, 62.

50. John W. McConnell, *The Evolution of Social Classes* (Washington, DC: American Council on Public Affairs, 1942).

51. Hollingshead and Redlich, *Social Class and Mental Illness*, 122.

52. Hollingshead and Redlich, *Social Class and Mental Illness*, 69–85, 162–63.

53. Hollingshead and Redlich, *Social Class and Mental Illness*, 85–95.

54. Hollingshead and Redlich, *Social Class and Mental Illness*, 95–104.

55. Hollingshead and Redlich, *Social Class and Mental Illness*, 104–14.

56. Hollingshead and Redlich, *Social Class and Mental Illness*, 118, 114–35.

57. Frustratingly, Hollingshead and Redlich often lumped together classes I and II in their statistics, possibly because of the small proportion of the overall population concentrated in these classes. This was despite the fact that Hollingshead and Redlich noted that people in class II were the most "status sensitive" and could "slip into depression" if their

attempts at upward mobility were unsuccessful. Hollingshead and Redlich, *Social Class and Mental Illness*, 85, 94.

58. Hollingshead and Redlich, *Social Class and Mental Illness*, 199, 175.

59. Hollingshead and Redlich's findings countered the downward drift criticisms leveled at Faris and Dunham. Most class V residents had lived in slums all of their lives. Hollingshead and Redlich, *Social Class and Mental Illness*, 246.

60. Hollingshead and Redlich, *Social Class and Mental Illness*, 184, 192.

61. Hollingshead and Redlich, *Social Class and Mental Illness*, 265, 156.

62. Joanna Ryan has recently explored the relationship between psychoanalysis and class in depth. Although she argues that there has been a "silence" about psychoanalysis and class (at least within the United Kingdom), Hollingshead and Redlich's observations indicate that psychiatrists have been aware of such tensions for decades. The Columbia psychiatrist Viola Bernard (1907–1998) was also writing about psychoanalysis and minority groups as early as the 1950s. As Dennis Doyle has written, many white psychoanalysts during this time were simply unwilling to take Black patients. In contrast, Elizabeth Danto's work on ambulatory psychoanalytic clinics demonstrates that Freud and his early followers did want to provide psychoanalysis to those in lower social classes. Viola W. Bernard, "Psychoanalysis and Members of Minority Groups," *Journal of the American Psychoanalytic Association* 1 (1953): 256–67; Elizabeth Ann Danto, *Freud's Free Clinics: Psychoanalysis and Social Justice, 1918–1938* (New York: Columbia University Press, 2005); Dennis Doyle, *Psychiatry and Racial Liberalism in Harlem, 1936–1968* (Rochester: University of Rochester Press, 2016), 19; Joanna Ryan, *Class and Psychoanalysis: Landscapes of Inequality* (London: Routledge, 2017).

63. Hollingshead and Redlich, *Social Class and Mental Illness*, 301.

64. Andrew Scull, "The Mental Health Sector and the Social Sciences in Post–World War II USA. Part 2: The Impact of Federal Research Funding and the Drugs Revolution," *History of Psychiatry* 22 (2011): 274–75.

65. In their follow-up study, Myers and Bean also suspected that class V psychiatric patients were also more impaired or "sicker" than patients from other classes upon admission to hospital and, thus, less likely to be discharged. Myers and Bean, *A Decade Later*, 208.

66. Hollingshead and Redlich, *Social Class and Mental Illness*, 358, 360–61, 363, 364.

67. Hollingshead and Redlich, *Social Class and Mental Illness*, 372.

68. Some still thought that Hollingshead and Redlich went too far. In the preface to *Mental Health of the Poor* (1964), the authors began by questioning that there was "a one-to-one relationship between class position and mental illness." One of these authors was Frank Riessman, who would also write about indigenous paraprofessionals. Frank Riessman, Jerome Cohen, and Arthur Pearl, *Mental Health of the Poor* (New York: Free Press of Glencoe, 1964), vii.

69. Hollingshead and Redlich, *Social Class and Mental Illness*, 119.

70. Hollingshead and Redlich, *Social Class and Mental Illness*, 119–20.

71. Hollingshead and Redlich, *Social Class and Mental Illness*, 120.

72. "Number of TV Households in America 1950–1978," *American Century*, https://americancentury.omeka.wlu.edu/items/show/136.

73. Hollingshead and Redlich, *Social Class and Mental Illness*, 128.

74. Hollingshead and Redlich, *Social Class and Mental Illness*, 134, 132.

75. Hollingshead and Redlich, *Social Class and Mental Illness*, 134.

76. I have used the term "indigenous paraprofessional," but the terms "indigenous nonprofessional" and mental health aide were also used. There were also "indigenous professionals" (trained mental health workers from the local area) and nonindigenous paraprofessionals (for instance, college students who might volunteer at a mental health facility). Robert Reiff and Frank Riessman, *The Indigenous Nonprofessional* (New York: Behavioral Publications, 1965).

77. Werner I. Halpern, "The Community Mental Health Aide," *Mental Hygiene* 53 (1969): 82.

78. Halpern, "Community Mental Health Aide," 82.

79. JCMIH, *Action for Mental Health*, 271.

80. Robert Shaw and Carol J. Eagle, "Programmed Failure: The Lincoln Hospital Story," *Community Mental Health Journal* 7 (1971): 255–63.

81. The Office of Economic Security was created as part of the Economic Opportunity Act of 1964, the centerpiece legislation of the War on Poverty. Martha J. Bailey and Nicholas J. Duquette, "How Johnson Fought the War on Poverty: The Economics and Politics of Funding at the Office of Economic Opportunity," *Journal of Economic History* 74 (2014): 351–88.

82. Emanuel Hallowitz, "The Role of a Neighborhood Service Center in Community Mental Health," *American Journal of Orthopsychiatry* 28 (1968): 705–14.

83. Frank Riessman, "Strategies and Suggestions for Training Nonprofessionals," *Community Mental Health Journal* 3 (1967): 103–10.

84. This quotation comes from an article written by Shaw and Eagle that supported the actions of LHMHS's indigenous paraprofessionals and was highly critical of its management. Shaw and Eagle, "Programmed Failure," 256.

85. Third World Newsreel, *Lincoln Hospital* (New York: Third World Newsreel, 1970), https://www.twn.org/catalog/pages/responsive/cpage .aspx.

86. Emanuel Hallowitz and Frank Riessman, "The Role of the Indigenous Nonprofessional in a Community Mental Health Neighborhood Service Center Program," *American Journal of Orthopsychiatry* 37 (1967): 766–78.

87. By 2000, the population consisted almost entirely of Black Americans and/or Latinos, but some revitalization was occurring. Evelyn Gonzalez, *The Bronx* (New York: Columbia University Press, 2004), 1.

88. Hallowitz and Riessman, "Indigenous Nonprofessional," 769.

89. Hallowitz's coauthor in one article, Frank Riessman, was co-director of LHMHS during its first year.

90. Hallowitz and Riessman, "Indigenous Nonprofessional," 767–68; emphasis in original.

91. Hallowitz and Riessman, "Indigenous Nonprofessional," 771.

92. Hallowitz and Riessman, "Indigenous Nonprofessional," 771.

93. Hallowitz, "Neighborhood Service Center," 707.

94. Hallowitz and Riessman, "Indigenous Nonprofessional," 769.

95. Hallowitz and Riessman, "Indigenous Nonprofessional," 775.

96. Hallowitz and Riessman, "Indigenous Nonprofessional," 775, 776.

97. Seymour R. Kaplan and Melv Roman, *The Organization and Delivery of Mental Health Services in the Ghetto* (New York: Praeger, 1973).

98. Emanuel Hallowitz, "Issues and Strategies in the Use of Nonprofessionals," paper presented at the National Association of Social Workers' National Conference of Social Welfare, San Francisco, May 25, 1968, University of Chicago School of Social Service Administration, Office of the Dean, Harold Richman. Records, 1969–1978, Box 105,

Folder 11, Hanna Holborn Gray Special Collections Research Center, University of Chicago Library.

99. Hallowitz, "Issues and Strategies."

100. Hallowitz, "Issues and Strategies."

101. Hallowitz, "Issues and Strategies." This paternalistic attitude may not have been in place so much in CMHCs run by women. Annelle Primm (b. 1956), a Black psychiatrist, described how she tried to employ an "inclusive" approach to leadership and to instill a "strong camaraderie" in the CMHCs she directed in the 1990s. She admitted, however, that disagreements about roles (for example, between nurses and social workers) still existed. Beverly Hicks (b. 1938), a psychiatric nurse, also recollected similar disputes in Montreal during the 1970s. Oral history interview with Annelle Primm, June 5, 2015; oral history interview with Beverly Hicks, March 10, 2015.

102. Hallowitz, "Issues and Strategies."

103. Kaplan and Roman, *Mental Health Services in the Ghetto*, 25–27.

104. Emphasis in original. Hallowitz, "Issues and Strategies."

105. John Talbott, Anita M. Ross, Alan F. Skerrett, Marion D. Curry, Stuart I. Marcus, Helen Theodorou, and Barbara J. Smith, "The Paraprofessional Teaches the Professional," *AJP* 130 (1973): 805–8.

106. Kaplan and Roman, *Mental Health Services in the Ghetto*, 56.

107. Oral history interview with Diana Ralph, July 12, 2016.

108. C. Gerald Fraser, "Community Takes Over Control of Bronx Mental Health Service," *New York Times*, March 6, 1969, 35.

109. Shaw and Eagle, "Programmed Failure," 256–57.

110. Bertram S. Brown and Harold Goldstein, "The Lightning Rod of Human Service Delivery," in *Controversy in Psychiatry*, ed. John Paul Brady and H. Keith H. Brodie (Philadelphia: W. B. Saunders, 1978), 1041–54.

111. "Cleo Silvers Interview 2," March 12, 2007, Interview with Bronx African American History Project, BAAHP Digital Archive at Fordham, https://research.library.fordham.edu/baahp_oralhist/232/.

112. Third World Newsreel, *Lincoln Hospital*.

113. Third World Newsreel, *Lincoln Hospital*.

114. Emphasis in original. Quoted in Kaplan and Roman, *Mental Health Services in the Ghetto*, 36.

115. Cleo Silvers, Leon Fink, and Brian Greenberg, *Upheaval in the Quiet Zone: A History of Hospital Workers' Union 1199* (Urbana: University of Illinois Press, 1989); Alondra Nelson, "'Genuine Struggle and Care: An Interview with Cleo Silvers," *American Journal of Public Health* 106 (2016): 1744–48.

116. Untitled article by Health Revolutionary Unity Movement in *For the People's Health*, reprinted in *Berkeley Tribe*, February 18–March 2, 1972, 14–15; Shaw and Eagle, "Programmed Failure," 257.

117. Ellen Herman, *Romance of American Psychology: Political Culture in the Age of Experts* (Berkeley: University of California Press, 1995), 256.

118. Joseph T. English, foreword to Kaplan and Roman, *Mental Health Services in the Ghetto*, ix.

119. English, foreword, x.

120. Kaplan and Roman *Mental Health Services in the Ghetto*, 27.

121. In a series of case studies included in their book's appendix, the contributions of the paraprofessionals were made obvious, even though they were underemphasized. Other psychiatrists, however, viewed the events at LHMHS more positively. Robert Marin, who trained at AECM, "identified" with what was going on: "What I was conscious of was this was an impoverished black community that was there in the downstream of slavery and racism. And that in some way, which I couldn't articulate at that point, were caught in some system and some way of life that was incapacitating." Oral history interview with Robert Marin, August 8, 2016.

122. Fitzhugh Mullan, *White Coat, Clenched Fist: The Political Education of an American Physician* (1976; Ann Arbor: University of Michigan Press, 2006), 106.

123. Sessi Kuwabara Blanchard, "How the Young Lords Took Lincoln Hospital, Left a Health Activism Legacy," *Filter*, October 30, 2018, https://filtermag.org/how-the-young-lords-took-lincoln-hospital -and-left-a-health-activism-legacy.

124. Additional efforts were also made to train LHMHS paraprofessionals during the 1970s, with mixed results. Although fifty-six of the ninety-one eligible LHMHS paraprofessionals enrolled in the program, twenty-three dropped out. Three, however, received a master's degree, and twenty-four were pursuing degree qualifications. It

was acknowledged, however, that the structure of the programs did not support the time pressures faced by many paraprofessionals, especially women. According to Diana Ralph, a social worker, paraprofessionals were also not given sufficient support to adapt to postsecondary education and also faced racist attitudes from faculty. Pedro Ruiz, "A Seven-Year Evaluation of a Career-Escalation Training Program for Indigenous Nonprofessionals," *Hospital and Community Psychiatry* 27 (1976): 253–57; Ralph interview.

125. Gill Scott-Heron, "Whitey on the Moon," *Small Talk at 125th and Lenox* (Flying Dutchman Records, 1970).

126. Daniel X. Freedman, "Community Mental Health: Slogan and a History of the Mission," *Controversy in Psychiatry*, ed. John Paul Brady and H. Keith H. Brodie (Philadelphia: W. B. Saunders, 1978), 1060–70.

127. Oral history interview with Gordon H. Clark Jr., May 20, 2015.

128. Gordon H. Clark Jr., *Community Psychiatry: Problems and Possibilities* (Spring House, PA: McNeil Pharmaceutical, 1987), 7. See also Paul J. Fink and Stephen P. Weinstein, "Whatever Happened to Psychiatry? The Deprofessionalization of Community Mental Health Centers," *AJP* 136 (1979): 406–9.

129. Clark, *Community Psychiatry*, 8.

130. J. S. Eaton and L. S. Goldstein, "Psychiatry in Crisis," *AJP* 134 (1977): 642–45.

131. Torrey argues that the "chilling" strike at LHMHS was a pivotal moment in discrediting the preventive potential of CMHCs, but this interpretation seems to be very much from the psychiatric, rather than the community, perspective. E. Fuller Torrey, *American Psychosis: How the Federal Government Destroyed the Mental Illness Treatment System* (Oxford: Oxford University Press, 2013), 69–71.

132. Pedro Ruiz, "The Fiscal Crisis in New York City: Effects on the Mental Health Care of Minority Populations," *AJP* 136 (1979): 93–96.

133. Richard Wilkinson and Kate Pickett, *The Spirit Level: Why Equal Societies Almost Always Do Better* (London: Allen Lane, 2009); Richard Wilkinson and Kate Picket, *The Inner Level: How More Equal Societies Reduce Stress, Restore Sanity, and Improve Everyone's Well-being* (London: Allen Lane, 2018). Pickett has recently, however, launched a

project to explore the relationship between basic income and adolescent mental health. "New Research Will Assess the Impact of Universal Basic Income on Young People's Health," University of York Health Sciences, https://www.york.ac.uk/healthsciences/news-and -events/news/2021/universal-benefit-mental-health/.

134. Although the use of indigenous paraprofessionals waned by the 1980s, a similar model was adopted in recruiting people with lived experience of mental illness as peer support workers. This was a positive development, but it should not have replaced the use of indigenous paraprofessionals. Oral history interview with Jules Ranz, September 9, 2016.

4. MADNESS IN THE METROPOLIS

1. "Materials Relating to *Mental Health in the Metropolis* (articles, pamphlets, etc)," Box 1, Folder 20a, Leo Srole Papers, 1933–1993, SC-54, Hobart and William Smith Colleges Archives and Special Collections; John Dollard, "Scratch a New Yorker, and What Do You Find?," *New York Times*, April 22, 1962, 2.

2. Ironically, Thomas Szasz had published *The Myth of Mental Illness* in the previous year, in which he argued the opposite. Thomas Szasz, *The Myth of Mental Illness: Foundations of a Theory of Personal Conduct* (New York: Hoeber-Harper, 1961).

3. Leo Srole, Thomas S. Langner, Stanley T. Michael, Marvin K. Opler, and Thomas A. C. Rennie, *Mental Health in the Metropolis: The Midtown Manhattan Study*, vol. 1 (New York: McGraw-Hill, 1962).

4. Thomas S. Langner and Stanley T. Michael, *Life Stress and Mental Health: The Midtown Manhattan Study* (New York: Free Press of Glencoe, 1963); Leo Srole and Anita K. Fischer, *Mental Health in the Metropolis: The Midtown Manhattan Study*, rev. and enlarged ed. (New York: New York University Press, 1978); Srole and Millman, *Personality and Mental Health*.

5. Srole et al., *Mental Health in the Metropolis*, 376–77.

6. For more on Midtown, see Hans Pols, "Anomie in the Metropolis: The City in American Sociology and Psychiatry," *Osiris* 18 (2003): 194–211; Dan Blazer, *Age of Melancholy: Major Depression and Its Social Origins*

(New York: Routledge, 2005); Dana March and Gerald M. Oppenheimer, "Social Disorder and Diagnostic Order: The US Mental Hygiene Movement, the Midtown Manhattan Study and the Study of Psychiatric Epidemiology in the 20th Century," *International Journal of Epidemiology* 43 suppl 1 (2014): 129–142.

7. American Sociological Association, "Manhattan Study: A Classic," *Footnotes* 16 (1988): 10.

8. As discussed in the previous chapter, Hollingshead and Redlich relied largely on hospital admissions data but also conducted interviews with a sample of New Haven residents.

9. See Pols, "Anomie in the Metropolis," 194–211; Edmund Ramsden and Matthew Smith, "Remembering the West End: Social Science, Mental Health, and the American Urban Environment, 1939–1968," *Urban History* 45 (2018): 128–49.

10. Michael Harrington, *The Other America: Poverty in the United States* (New York: Simon and Schuster, 1962).

11. The key archival sources are the Marvin Opler Papers at Columbia University Health Sciences Library and the Leo Srole Papers at the Hobart and William Smith Colleges Archives and Special Collections. A substantial portion of the Srole papers remains embargoed and will provide subsequent historians important material to study in future.

12. Edward Shorter, "History of Urban Mental Illness," in *Mental Health and Illness in the City*, ed. N. Okkels, C. Kristiansen, and P. Munk-Jorgensen (Singapore: Springer, 2017), 23.

13. Shorter, "Urban Mental Illness," 23.

14. For a new take on the sociology of cities, see Nikolas Rose and Des Fitzgerald, *The Urban Brain: Mental Health in the Vital City* (Princeton, NJ: Princeton University Press, 2022).

15. Pols, "Anomie in the Metropolis," 194–95.

16. It would continue to be diagnosed in China and Japan. Yu-Chuan Wu, "A Disorder of Qi: Breathing Exercise as a Cure for Neurasthenia in Japan, 1900–1945," *Journal of the History of Medicine and the Allied Sciences* 71 (2016): 322–44; Wen-Ji Wang, "Neurasthenia, Psy Sciences, and the 'Great Leap Forward' in Maoist China," *History of Psychiatry* 30 (2019): 443–56.

17. David Schuster, *Neurasthenic Nation: America's Search for Health, Happiness, and Comfort, 1869–1920* (New Brunswick, NJ: Rutgers University Press, 2011). For more on "pathologies of progress," see Charles E. Rosenberg, "Pathologies of Progress: The Idea of Civilization at Risk," *Bulletin of the History of Medicine* 72 (1998): 714–30.

18. George M. Beard, *American Nervousness, Its Causes and Consequences: A Supplement to Neurasthenia (Nervous Exhaustion)* (New York: G. P. Putnam's Sons, 1881).

19. Georg Simmel, "The Metropolis and Mental Life," in *The Urban Sociology Reader*, ed. Jan Lin and Christopher Mele (London: Routledge, 2012), 23–31.

20. Simmel, "Metropolis and Mental Health," 25. Dietmar Jazbinsek has argued that Simmel based his influential ideas primarily on his own experiences of living in Berlin. Dietmar Jazbinsek, "The Metropolis and the Mental Life of Georg Simmel: On the History of an Antipathy," *Journal of Urban History* 30 (2003): 102–25.

21. Pols, "Anomie in the Metropolis," 198.

22. Simmel, "Metropolis and Mental Life," 25.

23. Ferdinand Tönnies, "Community and Society," in *The Urban Sociology Reader*, ed. Jan Lin and Christopher Mele (London: Routledge, 2012), 16–22; Pols, "Anomie in the Metropolis," 198.

24. Simmel, "Metropolis and Mental Life," 27.

25. Pols, "Anomie in the Metropolis," 198.

26. Simmel, "Metropolis and Mental Life," 31.

27. Moritz Föllmer, "The Sociology of Individuality and the History of Urban Society," *Urban History* 47 (2020): 311–26.

28. Pols, "Anomie in the Metropolis," 201. Cities, according to Park, "lay bare all the human characteristics and traits which are ordinarily obscured and suppressed in small communities." Robert E. Park, Ernest W. Burgess, Roderick Duncan Mackenzie, and Louis Wirth, *The City* (Chicago: University of Chicago Press, 1925), 45–46.

29. Pols, "Anomie in the Metropolis," 201; Louis Wirth, "Urbanism as a Way of Life," *AJS* 44 (1938): 1–24.

30. Wirth, "Urbanism as a Way of Life," 23.

31. Pols, "Anomie in the Metropolis."

32. Pols, "Anomie in the Metropolis."

33. Kenneth T. Jackson, *Crabgrass Frontier: The Suburbanization of the United States* (New York: Oxford University Press, 1985).

34. Ramsden and Smith, "Remembering the West End," 135–37.

35. Edmund Ramsden, "Rats, Stress, and the Built Environment," *History of the Human Sciences* 25 (2012): 123–47. Jon Adams and Edmund Ramsden show how, while rats became "a symbol of all that was wrong with the city—dirt, corruption, degeneracy," the beehive was seen, in contrast, as the model of how to develop a dense, urban environment that did not lead to social problems and decay. Jon Adams and Edmund Ramsden, "Rat Cities and Beehive Worlds: Density and Design in the Modern City," *Comparative Studies in Society and History* 53 (2011): 724.

36. Calhoun's research was the inspiration for the Robert C. O'Brien's Newberry Medal–winning novel *Mrs. Frisby and the Rats of NIMH*. But, unlike the rats in Calhoun's experiments, O'Brien's rats are given various treatments to increase their strength and intelligence. Robert C. O'Brien, *Mrs. Frisby and the Rats of NIMH* (New York: Athenaeum, 1971).

37. Homosexuality was only removed from the *Diagnostic and Statistical Manual of Mental Disorders* (*DSM*) in 1973. Jack Drescher, "Out of *DSM*: Depathologizing Homosexuality," *Behavioral Sciences* 5 (2015): 565–75.

38. Edmund Ramsden, "The Urban Animal: Population Density and Social Pathology in Rodents and Humans," *Bulletin of the World Health Organization* 87 (2009): 82.

39. John B. Calhoun, "Population Density and Social Pathology," *Scientific American* 206 (1962): 139–48.

40. John B. Calhoun, "Space and the Strategy of Life," in *Behavior and Environment*, ed. A. H. Esser (New York: Plenum, 1971), 329–86.

41. John B. Calhoun Papers 1909–1996, Box 56, Folder 7, National Library of Medicine. Sincere thanks to Edmund Ramsden for generously sharing his notes on the Space Cadets.

42. Daniel M. Wilner, Roseabelle Price Walkley, Thomas C. Pinkerton, and Matthew Tayback, *The Housing Environment and Family Life: A Longitudinal Study of the Effects of Housing on Morbidity and Mental Health* (Baltimore, MD: Johns Hopkins University Press, 1962).

43. Jane Jacobs, *The Death and Life of Great American Cities* (New York: Random House, 1961).

44. See Ramsden and Smith, "Remembering the West End." Stephen Spielberg's recent remake of *West Side Story* emphasized the impact of slum removal in New York City in its storyline.

45. For more on Lindemann, see David G. Satin, *Community Mental Health, Erich Lindemann, and Social Conscience in American Psychiatry*, vols. 1–3 (New York: Routledge, 2020).

46. Herbert J. Gans, *The Urban Villagers: Group and Class in the Life of Italian-Americans* (New York: Free Press of Glencoe, 1962). Although Gans was initially a critic of urban renewal, his later work on Levittown, New Jersey, one of the infamous, segregated, and lower-middle-class suburbs built for returning veterans during the late 1940s, countered arguments that suburbia was always sterile and—as many were beginning to argue—pathological. Herbert J. Gans, *The Levittowners: Ways of Life and Politics in a New Suburban Community* (1966; New York: Columbia University Press, 2017). For how American suburbia was represented in literature, see Jo Gill, *The Poetics of the American Suburbs* (Basingstoke: Palgrave, 2013).

47. Marc Fried, "Grieving for a Lost Home: The Psychological Costs of Relocation," in *Urban Renewal: The Record and the Controversy*, ed. James Q. Wilson (Cambridge, MA; MIT Press, 1966), 360, 370–78.

48. Srole et al., *Mental Health in the Metropolis*, 8.

49. Srole et al., *Mental Health in the Metropolis*, 31.

50. S. D. Lamb, *Pathologist of the Mind: Adolf Meyer and the Origins of American Psychiatry* (Baltimore. MD: Johns Hopkins University Press, 2014), 98.

51. For more on psychobiology, see Lamb, *Pathologist of the Mind*, chap. 2. Rennie would write one of Meyer's many obituaries. Thomas A. C. Rennie, "Adolf Meyer (1866–1950)," *Psychosomatic Medicine* 12 (1950): 71–72.

52. Gladys C. Terry and Thomas A. C. Rennie, *Analysis of Parergasia* (New York: Nervous and Mental Disease Monographs, 1938); Luther E. Woodward and Thomas A. C. Rennie, *Jobs and the Man* (Springfield, IL: Charles C. Thomas, 1945); Thomas A. C. Rennie, "Psychiatric Social Work," *AJP* 102 (1946): 542–44; Thomas A. C. Rennie, "National Planning for Psychiatric Education," *Mental Hygiene* 30 (1946): 186–98; Thomas A. C. Rennie and Luther E. Woodward, *Mental Health in Modern Society* (New York: Commonwealth Fund, 1948); Michael

N. Healey, "Assembling Adjustment: Parergasia, Paper Technologies, and the Revision of Recovery," *Culture, Medicine, and Psychiatry* 45 (2021): 405–28.

53. Jacob S. Kasanin, "Review of *Analysis of Parergasia*," *American Journal of Orthopsychiatry* 9 (1939): 817–18.

54. Srole et al., *Mental Health in the Metropolis*, 12.

55. "Letter from Thomas Rennie to Adolf Meyer, undated," Unit 1/3237, Folder 1, Adolf Meyer Collection, Alan Mason Chesney Medical Archives of the Johns Hopkins Medical Institutions. Sincere thanks to Michael N. Healey for sending me these correspondences.

56. "Letter from Hilbert F. Day to Adolf Meyer, March 20, 1931," Unit 1/3237, Folder 1, Adolf Meyer Collection.

57. "Letter from Henry A. Christian, Physician-in-Chief at Peter Bent Brigham Hospital, to Adolf Meyer, March 31, 1931," Unit 1/3237, Folder 1, Adolf Meyer Collection.

58. "Letter from Thomas Rennie to Adolf Meyer, April 6, 1931," Unit 1/3237, Folder 1, Adolf Meyer Collection; "Letter from Adolf Meyer to Thomas Rennie, April 7, 1931," Unit 1/3237, Folder 1, Adolf Meyer Collection.

59. "Letter from Thomas Rennie to Adolf Meyer, April 19, 1940," Unit 1/3237, Folder 4, Adolf Meyer Collection.

60. "Letter from Thomas Rennie to Adolf Meyer, August 20, 1942," Unit 1/3237, Folder 5, Adolf Meyer Collection.

61. Srole et al., *Mental Health in the Metropolis*, vii–viii.

62. Ernest Gruenberg, "Review of *Mental Health in the Metropolis*," *Millbank Memorial Fund Quarterly* 41 (1963): 79.

63. Srole et al., *Mental Health in the Metropolis*, 5, 6.

64. Srole et al., *Mental Health in the Metropolis*, 6, 411–13.

65. Srole et al., *Mental Health in the Metropolis*, 8.

66. Srole et al., *Mental Health in the Metropolis*, 28.

67. Srole et al., *Mental Health in the Metropolis*, 31.

68. Yorkville was described by Srole as 99 percent white, whereas Manhattan as a whole was stated to be 20 percent nonwhite, largely from the racial makeup of Harlem (Puerto Ricans were considered white and consisted of 1.2 percent of Midtown's population, as opposed to 7 percent of Manhattan as a whole). A third of the white population

of Midtown, however, was foreign born. Midtown was criticized for not including Black Americans, but the authors did encourage subsequent studies to address them and the role of race. Srole later claimed that including these groups, as well as children and the elderly, would have exceeded both the budget and the capabilities of the investigators. Leo Srole and Ernest Joel Millman, *Personal History and Health: The Midtown Longitudinal Study, 1954–1974* (New Brunswick, NJ: Transaction, 1997).

69. Srole et al., *Mental Health in the Metropolis*, 32.

70. "Rennie, Thomas A. C., General, 1953–1954," Box 13, Folder 17, Marvin Kaufmann Opler Papers, 1915–1979, Archives and Special Collections, Columbia University Health Sciences Library.

71. Opler Papers; emphasis in original.

72. Srole et al., *Mental Health in the Metropolis*, 60.

73. Srole et al., *Mental Health in the Metropolis*, 62.

74. Srole et al., *Mental Health in the Metropolis*, 62.

75. Srole et al., *Mental Health in the Metropolis*, 38.

76. Srole et al., *Mental Health in the Metropolis*, 60; "Questionnaires: Memoranda Re: Questionnaire, 1953–55," Box 15, Folder 5, Opler Papers.

77. "Numerical Srole Printouts," Box 56, Srole Papers.

78. Srole et al., *Mental Health in the Metropolis*, 40, 398.

79. Srole et al., *Mental Health in the Metropolis*, 390, 40–41.

80. "Numerical Srole Printouts," Srole Papers, Box 56.

81. Examples of how the psychiatrists arrived at their ratings of four respondents were provided in appendix F.

82. Srole et al., *Mental Health in the Metropolis*, 64–65; emphasis in original.

83. "Minutes and Memoranda, 1952–54," Box 14, Folder 8, Opler Papers.

84. "Minutes and Memoranda, 1952–54."

85. "Lectures for Cornell Staff, 1952–58," Box 14, Folder 6, Opler Papers.

86. Srole et al., *Mental Health in the Metropolis*, 29, 69, 80.

87. Harvey Warren Zorbaugh, *The Gold Coast and the Slum: A Study of Chicago's Near North Side* (Chicago: University of Chicago Press, 1929).

88. Srole et al., *Mental Health in the Metropolis*, 80, 81. The relatively small number of children was important since shaping childhood experiences was thought to be central to preventive psychiatry.

89. "Letter from Opler to Rennie, September 30, 1954," Box 13, Folder 17, Opler Papers. Before this letter, there is little hint of tension in the surviving archival records.

90. Leacock's papers are being catalogued at the University of Michigan.

91. Rubin and Leacock's correspondences concerning this dispute are not included in the record, leaving only Opler's take on the matter. However, my analysis of the situation is not to assess who was right or wrong but rather to explore the impact of these tensions on the legacy of Midtown.

92. "Memo from Opler to Midtown Anthropologists, September 24, 1954," Box 14, Folder 8, Opler Papers.

93. Another example of Opler's short temper can be found in a series of correspondences with the psychiatrist Joshua Bierer (1901–1984) pertaining to their joint organization of the First International Congress of Social Psychiatry, held in London in 1964. "First Int'l Conf of Social Psych, Correspondence, Bierer, Joshua, Dec 1963–Dec 1964," Box 22, Folder 4, Opler Papers.

94. "Opler to Rennie, September 30, 1954," Box 13, Folder 17, Opler Papers; emphasis in original.

95. "Rennie to Opler, October 4, 1954," Box 13, Folder 17, Opler Papers.

96. "Opler to Rennie, October 29, 1954," Box 13, Folder 17, Opler Papers.

97. The tensions between Opler and Srole are also highlighted in a handwritten note to Rennie describing how Opler was "thoroughly disgusted" by the proposals of Srole, Rubin, and Leacock to split up the anthropology studies. "Opler to Rennie, March 11, 1955," Box 13, Folder 18, Opler Papers.

98. "Opler to Rennie, January 26, 1955," Box 13, Folder 17, Opler Papers.

99. "Opler to Rennie, February 18, 1955."

100. "Opler to Rennie, February 19, 1955," Box 13, Folder 17, Opler Papers.

101. "Leacock to Rennie, February 28, 1955," Box 13, Folder 18, Opler Papers.

102. "Individuals, Rennie, Thomas A. C., General, Undated, ca. 1953–56," Box 13, Folder 19, Opler Papers; emphasis in original.

103. "Rennie to Opler, September 30, 1954," Box 13, Folder 17, Opler Papers.

104. Ruth Benedict, *Patterns of Culture* (Boston: Houghton Mifflin, 1934), 46; Ruth Benedict, *Race: Science and Politics* (New York: Modern Age, 1940); Marvin K. Opler, "Review of *An Anthropologist at Work: Writings of Ruth Benedict*," *American Anthropologist* 62 (1960): 889–91.

105. Anthony K. Webster and Scott Rushforth, "Morris Edward Opler (1907–1996)," *American Anthropologist* 102 (2000): 328–29. The brothers had a falling out over politics that lasted twenty years. While Marvin leaned to the left, Morris leaned right. However, both were assigned to Japanese detainment camps during the war, where they were both were sympathetic toward the Japanese and castigated for it. Oral history interview with Lewis Opler, November 16, 2015.

106. David H. Price, *Threatening Anthropology: McCarthyism and the FBI's Surveillance of Activist Anthropologists* (Durham, NC: Duke University Press, 2004), 196.

107. Opler's mentor Ruth Benedict became a special advisor for the United States Office of War Information in that same year. Her work would result in *The Chrysanthemum and the Sword*. Ruth Benedict, *The Chrysanthemum and the Sword* (Boston: Houghton Mifflin, 1946). Opler would coauthor a book on the Japanese camps. Edward Holland Spicer, Katherine Luomala, Asael T. Hansen, and Marvin K. Opler, *Impounded People: Japanese Americans in the Relocation Centers* (Washington, DC: War Relocation Authority, 1946).

108. Marvin Opler's son Lewis described how his parents continued to fight for the rights of the Japanese detainees after World War II. When he and his parents visited the homes of some of these Japanese Americans in later years his parents were "revered" and treated with great respect. Opler interview.

109. Price, *Threatening Anthropology*, 198.

110. Peter T. Suzuki, "Anthropologists in the Wartime Camps for Japanese Americans: A Documentary Study," *Dialectical Anthropology* 6 (1981): 33. Suzuki argues that both Marvin and Morris Opler were unusual among anthropologists working in the camps for their willingness to condemn the conditions experienced by the detainees.

111. Opler interview.

112. Marvin K. Opler, *Culture, Psychiatry, and Human Values: The Methods and Value of a Social Psychiatry* (Springfield, IL: Charles C. Thomas, 1956).

113. Opler's brother Morris was working at Cornell at this time, but for a different department (Anthropology) at the Ithaca campus. Marvin Opler was hired to work at the Payne Whitney Clinic, which was affiliated to the Department of Psychiatry based in New York City. Since

they were not speaking at the time, it is unlikely that Morris played a role in his younger brother's appointment.

114. Price, *Threatening Anthropology*; Lee Wengraf, "How Women Became Less Than Equal," *International Socialist Review* 63 (2008), https://isre view.org/issue/63/how-women-became-less-equal. Leacock's unpublished autobiography also describes how misogyny also undermined her academic career. Juli McLoone, "Eleanor Leacock, Feminist Anthropologist," *Beyond the Reading Room*, March 30, 2015, https://apps.lib .umich.edu/blogs/beyond-reading-room/eleanor-burke-leacock -feminist-anthropologist.

115. Lewis Opler saw Rennie as a "god-like" figure who figured in his decision to become a psychiatrist. Rennie was a "white coat psychiatrist who my father loved, so unconsciously if I want my father to love me, I'll become Rennie. Um, none of this I can prove, but I believe it has face validity and I think it's true." Opler interview.

116. Srole et al., *Mental Health in the Metropolis*, viii.

117. Opler's contention is echoed by Bloom, who states that Oscar Diethelm, the department chair, was against the research, as it clashed with his "classical European focus on nosology [the classification of disease]." He required Rennie to maintain all his departmental responsibilities as deputy chair, leaving him only two hours per week for research. Samuel L. Bloom, *Word as Scalpel: A History of Medical Sociology* (Oxford: Oxford University Press, 2002), 169–70.

118. Bloom, *Word as Scalpel*, 337; Opler interview.

119. Alexander H. Leighton Papers, Alexander H. Leighton fonds, MS-13-86, Dalhousie University Archives, Halifax, Nova Scotia, Canada, Box 50, Folder 3.

120. Opler interview.

121. Suzuki, "Anthropologists in the Wartime Camps," 49–50.

122. Alexander H. Leighton, "Review of *Culture, Psychiatry, and Human Values*," *Social Problems* 4 (1956): 181. Indeed, a cordial exchange between Opler and Leighton in January 1956 (before Rennie's death) about the former's research on Irish ethnicity further suggests that this review caused tension. "Letters to and from Opler and Leighton, January 12 and January 18, 1956," Box 13, Folder 12, Opler Papers.

123. "Letter from Opler to Leighton, March 20, 1957," Box 13, Folder 12, Opler Papers. *Pace* Opler, the reviews are not all that different. While

Kluckhohn's may have been more effusive in its praise, Leighton's review was largely positive; both described the book as confusing at times and not always clearly written. Clyde Kluckhohn, "Review of *Culture, Psychiatry, and Human Values*," *American Anthropologist* 59 (1957): 192–94.

124. "Opler to Leighton, March 20, 1957," Box 13, Folder 12, Opler Papers.

125. "Srole to Rennie, June 20, 1953," Box 13, Folder 17, Opler Papers. The original wording was "different scientific research competence," but this was toned down, with the last two words scored out and replaced with "approaches and degrees."

126. Oral history interview with Ira Srole, February 17, 2016.

127. Hobart and William Smith Colleges hold Srole's papers, despite his short tenure there. They also host the annual Leo Srole Urban Studies Lecture.

128. Srole's wartime experiences contributed to his interest in community psychiatry. Bloom, *Word as Scalpel*, 121.

129. "Press Release for Srole National Tour," Srole Papers, Box 1, Folder 22a.

130. Srole interview.

131. Srole interview.

132. Opler interview. Ira Srole also confirmed that the two did not get along. Srole interview.

133. "Opler to Leighton, March 20, 1957," Box 13, Folder 12, Opler Papers.

134. "Memo from Leighton to Opler, Srole, and Langner, March 27, 1957," Box 13, Folder 12, Opler Papers.

135. "Opler to Leighton, March 28, 1957," Box 13, Folder 12, Opler Papers.

136. Alexander H. Leighton, foreword to Ira Srole et al., *Mental Health in the Metropolis*, ix.

137. Srole would leave Cornell in 1961, stating in an interview with Samuel Bloom that he had been fired. He finished his career at Columbia. Bloom, *Word as Scalpel*, 170.

138. "Srole to Paul Schneider, Jun 13, 1960," Box 13, Folder 14, Opler Papers.

139. "Opler to Morris Opler, July 9, 1960," Box 13, Folder 14, Opler Papers.

140. Srole et al., *Mental Health in the Metropolis*, 356, 230.

141. The project also found that mental illness was associated with increased age and poor physical health.

142. Srole et al., *Mental Health in the Metropolis*, 340.

143. "Summary of Interview with Srole, 1967," Box 1, Folder 33d, Srole Papers.

144. Leighton, foreword, ix.

145. Srole et al., *Mental Health in the Metropolis*, 327, 328, 335.

146. Srole et al., *Mental Health in the Metropolis*, 342.

147. A number of progressive New York–based psychiatrists, including Max Winsor, Fredric Wertham, and Hilde Mosse, had also argued for better education, fairer juvenile justice, and efforts to combat racism in order to promote better mental health in young people. Dennis Doyle, "'We Didn't Know You Were a Negro': Fredric Wertham and the Ironies of Race, Comic Books, and Juvenile Delinquency in the 1950s," *Journal of Social History* 52 (2018): 153–79.

148. "Summary of Interview with Srole," Srole Papers.

149. Srole et al., *Mental Health in the Metropolis*, 236.

150. Srole and Millman, "Personal History," vii.

151. Srole et al., *Mental Health in the Metropolis*, 6–7.

152. Leo Srole, "Urbanization and Mental Health: Some Reformulations," *American Scientist* 60 (1972): 576–83. Here, and elsewhere, Srole cited *The Intellectuals Versus the City*, which was published in the same year as *Mental Health in the Metropolis* and chronicled the history of anti-city thought in the United States. Morton White and Lucia White, *The Intellectuals Versus the City: From Thomas Jefferson to Frank Lloyd Wright* (Cambridge, MA: Harvard University Press, 1962).

153. Srole, "Urbanization and Mental Health, 579; Bruce P. Dohrenwend and Barbara S. Dohrenwend, "Psychiatric Disorder in Urban Settings," in *American Handbook of Psychiatry*, ed. S. Arieti (New York: Basic Books, 1974), 2:423–47.

154. Srole also observed that the blurring of the boundary between rural and urban caused by suburbanization and the automobile made it more difficult to assess which setting was better for mental health.

155. Srole, "Urbanization and Mental Health," 583. In a footnote, Srole quoted a report from the *New York Times* that claimed that one million Americans were being forced from agricultural communities because of technological innovations that rendered their occupations redundant.

156. "Correspondence, General, 1956–62," Box 13, Folder 3, Opler Papers.

157. Marvin K. Opler, *Culture and Social Psychiatry* (New York: Atherton, 1967), 34.

158. Opler did previously describe how rural areas were found to have high rates of mental illness in his previous book, *Culture, Society, and Human Values.*

159. "Who Cares for the Mentally Ill?" *New York Times* (November 5, 1981), 26.

160. Bryce Nelson, "Mental Illness Cited Among Many Homeless," *New York Times*, October 2, 1983, 25.

161. Ellen Baxter and Kim Hopper, *Private Lives, Public Spaces* (New York: Community Service Society, 1981).

5. FROM COVE TO WOODLOT

1. Alexander H. Leighton, *My Name Is Legion: Foundations for a Theory of Man in Relation to Culture* (New York: Basic Books, 1959).

2. Marc-Adélard Tremblay, "Alexander H. Leighton and Jane M. Murphy's Scientific Contributions in Psychiatric Epidemiology," paper given to the Canadian Anthropology Society, Halifax, May 10, 2003. M. Kingsbury, E. Sucha, N. J. Horton, H. Sampasa-Kanyinga, J. M. Murphy, S. E. Gilman, and I. Colman, "Lifetime Experience of Multiple Common Mental Disorders and 19-Year Mortality: Results from a Canadian Population-Based Cohort," *Epidemiology and Psychiatric Sciences* 29 (2019): e18.

3. Leighton, *My Name Is Legion*, 3.

4. Alexander H. Leighton Papers, Alexander H. Leighton fonds, MS-13-86, Dalhousie University Archives, Halifax, Nova Scotia, Canada, Box 46, Folder 25.

5. Marjorie C. Meehan, "The Stirling County Study of Psychiatric Disorder and Sociocultural Environment," *JAMA* 187 (1964): 785; Oral history interview with Theodore Leighton, June 1, 2021. Alexander Leighton also wanted to involve a historian but lacked the budget for one. "Letter from Alexander Leighton to Pendleton Herring, June 21, 1954," Social Science Research Council Records (FA021), Rockefeller Archive Center, Series 1, Box 422, Folder 5091.

6. These funders provided over $500,000 during the first five years of the project. In later years, however, its investigators struggled to keep it going financially. Leighton Papers, Box 46, Folder 25; Alexander H. Leighton, *Caring for Mentally Ill People: Psychological and Social Barriers in Historical Context* (Cambridge: Cambridge University Press, 1982), x.

7. In this way, it was similar to Eaton and Weil's contemporaneous study of Hutterite communities. Joseph W. Eaton and Robert J. Weil, *Culture and Mental Disorders: A Comparative Study of the Hutterites and Other Populations* (Glencoe, IL: Free Press, 1955).

8. Leighton, *Caring for Mentally Ill People*, 1.

9. Leighton Papers, Box 46, Folder 25.

10. These can be accessed at https://archives.novascotia.ca/collier/results/.

11. Nancy J. Parezo, "Dorothea Cross Leighton: Anthropologist and Activist," in *Their Own Frontier: Women Intellectuals Re-Visioning the American West*, ed. Shirley A. Leckie and Nancy J. Parezo (Lincoln: University of Nebraska Press, 2008), 318.

12. Leighton, *My Name Is Legion*, 46.

13. Leighton, *Caring for Mentally Ill People*, 224–25.

14. Leighton interview.

15. "Atlantic Voice: World Renowned Health Survey, Right Under Our Noses," CBC News, https://www.cbc.ca/news/canada/nova-scotia /atlantic-voice-world-renowned-health-survey-right-under-our -noses-1.3083959. The Leightons' son Ted doubted that many people would be able to identify Stirling County from the map in *People of Cove and Woodlot*, since few would be familiar with that part of Nova Scotia, but the point I am making is that anyone who *wanted* to discover where Stirling County was (such as myself) could do so easily. Leighton interview.

16. Charles C. Hughes, Marc-Adelard Tremblay, Robert N. Rapoport, and Alexander H. Leighton, *People of Cove and Woodlot* (New York: Basic Books, 1960), 18.

17. Naomi Rogers, *Dirt and Disease: Polio Before FDR* (New Brunswick, NJ: Rutgers University Press, 1992), chap. 1. The Leightons' escape from Philadelphia is reminiscent of the yellow fever epidemic that struck the city in 1793, which saw twenty thousand residents flee. The

contemporary accounts of this epidemic, including one from a pair of Black clergymen, are particularly vivid and illustrate the controversies that ensued. Richard Allen and Absalom Jones, *A Narrative of the Proceedings of the Black People, During the Late Awful Calamity in Philadelphia, in the Year 1793: and a Refutation of Some Censures, Thrown Upon Them in Some Late Publications* (Philadelphia: William W. Woodward, 1794).

18. Leighton interview.

19. Leighton interview.

20. Alexander H. Leighton, "A Porcupine Throws Quills," *Journal of Mammalogy* 7 (1926): 61.

21. Hughes et al., *People of Cove and Woodlot*, 8–9. Alexander Leighton described how they also considered situating the study in the Ramah region of New Mexico because of its considerable ethnic diversity, consisting of the Navajo and Zuni, as well as Latinos, Mormons, and newcomers from Texas. The site was rejected, however, both because it was deemed to be too linguistically and culturally diverse and because the region was undergoing rapid change. Barkow, "Interview," 245–46.

22. Barkow, "Interview," 247.

23. Parezo, "Dorothea Cross Leighton," 312–13.

24. Barkow, "Interview," 243–44.

25. Parezo, "Dorothea Cross Leighton," 310.

26. In 1893, Johns Hopkins became the first elite medical school on the East Coast to accept women.

27. Parezo, "Dorothea Cross Leighton," 311.

28. Parezo, "Dorothea Cross Leighton," 313.

29. Barkow, "Leighton Interview," 244.

30. Robert C. Angell, "Review of *Human Relations in a Changing World,*" *AJS* 55 (1949): 305.

31. Parezo, "Dorothea Cross Leighton," 317–19. Neither of the Leightons would practice medicine after they completed their medical training. Leighton interview.

32. Dorothea Cross Leighton, cited in Parezo, "Dorothea Cross Leighton," 320–21.

33. Alexander H. Leighton and Dorothea C. Leighton, *The Navajo Door* (Cambridge, MA: Harvard University Press, 1944).

34. Clyde Kluckhohn and Dorothea Leighton, *The Navajo* (Cambridge, MA: Harvard University Press, 1946); Dorothea Cross Leighton and Clyde Kluckhohn, *Children of the People: The Navajo Individual and His Development* (Cambridge, MA: Harvard University Press, 1948); Dorothea Cross Leighton and John Adair, *People of the Middle Place: A Study of the Zuni Indians* (New Haven, CT: Human Relations Area Files Press, 1966).

35. *The Governing of Men* was effectively a government report written largely for a military audience, so its focus on "governing men," rather than working with them, should be understood in that context. But it also locates a difference between Dorothea Leighton's and Alexander Leighton's views on how to apply anthropological insights. Whereas Parezo has emphasized Dorothea Leighton's empathetic and relativistic approach to understanding the Navajo, Alexander Leighton's writing at times suggests that anthropological study can also inform how best to design administrative structures that can be used as a means of control. This comes across not only in *The Governing of Men* but also *Caring for Mentally Ill People* (1982). Alexander H. Leighton, *The Governing of Men: General Principles and Recommendations Based on Experience at a Japanese Relocation Camp* (Princeton, NJ: Princeton University Press, 1945).

36. Marc-Adélard Tremblay, "Alexander Hamilton Leighton, 17 July 1908–11 August 2007," *Proceedings of the American Philosophical Society* 153 (2009): 479.

37. Barkow, "Leighton Interview," 238–43.

38. Alexander H. Leighton, *Human Relations in a Changing World: Observations on the Use of the Social Sciences* (New York: E. P. Dutton, 1949). As indicated by his book's title, Leighton stressed how the social sciences could be utilized to solve many of the world's problems. In this way, his book shared similarities with William Menninger's *Psychiatry in a Troubled World*, which argued the same for psychiatry.

39. Peter T. Suzuki, "Anthropologists in the Wartime Camps for Japanese Americans: A Documentary Study," *Dialectical Anthropology* 6 (1981): 57.

40. Leighton, *Caring for Mentally Ill People*, 96.

41. This echoes what David Mechanic has said about the political views of social psychiatrists: "They were liberal in the political sense. That is, they believed in helping the poor, they believed in broader distribution

of income. They believed in poverty programs. They believed in providing decent housing to people who are poor. They're liberal in their social instincts but their psychiatric instincts are not driven by politics." Oral history interview with David Mechanic, February 9, 2015.

42. Parezo, "Dorothea Cross Leighton," 326–27.

43. Leighton interview. Dorothea Leighton's role was certainly overlooked in a 1989 interview of Alexander Leighton, a celebration of his and Jane Murphy's accomplishments in 2003, and in a biographical article that followed his death. Barkow, "Leighton Interview"; Tremblay, "Alexander H. Leighton"; Tremblay, "Alexander Hamilton Leighton."

44. Theodore Leighton has explained how his mother was genuinely a "co-investigator" on the study (despite formally being assistant to the director, Alexander Leighton) and that she and his father "steered" it together. In addition to her extensive anthropological insights, her calmness and practicality were vital in helping resolve problems. Leighton interview.

45. Hughes et al., *People of Cove and Woodlot*, 9.

46. Hughes et al., *People of Cove and Woodlot*, 21, 22.

47. Hughes et al., *People of Cove and Woodlot*, 25–26. The introduction of year-round logging resulted in the decline of an iconic Canadian occupation: the log driver, who, during the spring thaw, would propel logs downstream. An animation of the *Log-Driver's Waltz*, written by Wade Hemsworth and sung by Kate and Anna McGarrigle in 1979, continues to be one of the Canadian National Film Board's most popular films. Wade Hemsworth, "Log-Driver's Waltz," Canada Vignettes, Canadian National Film Board, https://www.nfb.ca/film/log_drivers _waltz/.

48. Hughes et al., *People of Cove and Woodlot*, 27.

49. Hughes et al., *People of Cove and Woodlot*, 31, 32, 29.

50. Hughes et al., *People of Cove and Woodlot*, 37.

51. In *People of Cove and Woodlot*, the number of deportees was given as six thousand, but now the figure is thought to be higher. N. E. S. Griffiths, *From Migrant to Acadian: A North American Border People, 1604–1755* (Montreal: McGill-Queen's University Press, 2005).

52. Hughes et al., *People of Cove and Woodlot*, 40.

53. Hughes et al., *People of Cove and Woodlot*, 253.

54. John Collier Jr., quoted in Hughes et al., *People of Cove and Woodlot*, 244–45. None of Collier Jr.'s pictures in *People of Cove and Woodlot* depicted people from these communities. Collier Jr. was the son of John Collier, who headed the Bureau of Indian Affairs during the 1930s.

55. Hughes et al., *People of Cove and Woodlot*, 248.

56. John Collier Jr., quoted in Hughes et al., *People of Cove and Woodlot*, 246.

57. In *The Character of Danger*, however, the authors discussed how their own "background influences," formed by living in Stirling County for extended periods, "colored many of our perceptions and interpretations." Perhaps this is because the lead author of this volume was Dorothea Leighton. Dorothea C. Leighton, John S. Harding, David B. Macklin, Allister M. Macmillan, and Alexander H. Leighton, *The Character of Danger: Psychiatric Symptoms in Selected Communities* (New York: Basic Books, 1963), 9.

58. Hughes et al., *People of Cove and Woodlot*, 58–59, 284–87, 7.

59. Leighton et al., *Character of Danger*, 355, 323.

60. Leighton et al., *Character of Danger*, 365.

61. The collapse of fishing, mining, and other industries elsewhere in Nova Scotia in subsequent decades have been linked to mental disorder, substance abuse, and suicide. See Lachlan MacKinnon, *Closing Sysco: Industrial Decline in Atlantic Canada's Steel City* (Toronto: University of Toronto Press, 2019).

62. Leighton et al., *Character of Danger*, 367–68.

63. Leighton et al., *Character of Danger*, 367, 330, 332, 335–37.

64. Leighton et al., *Character of Danger*, 368–69.

65. Leighton et al., *Character of Danger*, 388.

66. This contrasted with Freud's early theories. Sigmund Freud, *Drei Abhandlungen zur Sexualtheorie* (Leipzig: Franz Deuticke, 1905); Sigmund Freud, *Totem und Tabu* (Leipzig: Hugo Heller, 1913).

67. Clifford Shaw's Chicago School research on juvenile delinquency also separated the roles of social disintegration and poverty, contending that the former was the real culprit. Ernest W. Burgess, "Mental Health in Modern Society," in *Mental Health and Mental Disorder: A Sociological Approach*, ed. Arnold M. Rose (London: Routledge and Kegan Paul, 1956), 9.

68. Alexander H. Leighton, "Poverty and Social Change," *Scientific American* 212 (1965): 21.

69. Mical Raz, *What's Wrong with the Poor? Psychiatry, Race, and the War on Poverty* (Chapel Hill: University of North Carolina Press, 2013).

70. Carl C. Bell, *The Sanity of Survival: Reflections on Community Mental Health and Wellness* (Chicago: Third World, 2004), xi.

71. Marvin Karno and Donald A. Schwartz, *Community Mental Health: Reflections and Explorations* (New York: John Wiley and Sons, 1974), 3–4.

72. Gerald Caplan, *An Approach to Community Mental Health* (London: Tavistock, 1961), vii–viii. Caplan was affiliated with the Harvard School of Public Health, where he taught Bertram S. Brown (1931–2020), NIMH director from 1970–1977. He also influenced Robert Felix's views on community mental health.

73. Pedro Ruiz, "The Fiscal Crisis in New York City: Effects on the Mental Health Care of Minority Populations," *AJP* 136 (1979): 93–96.

74. Caplan, *An Approach to Community Mental Health*, chaps. 2–4.

75. Karno and Schwartz, *Community Mental Health*, 7.

76. Leighton, *Caring for Mentally Ill People*, 52, 65, 67, 68.

77. Leighton, *Caring for Mentally Ill People*, 68, 112

78. "Atlantic Voice."

79. Leighton, *Caring for Mentally Ill People*, 72.

80. Harry R. Brickman, "Foreword," in Marvin Karno and Donald A. Schwartz, *Community Mental Health: Reflections and Explorations* (New York: John Wiley and Sons, 1974), viii.

81. Leighton, *Caring for Mentally Ill People*, 84, 105, 109.

82. See also Matthew P. Dumont and Dora M. Dumont, "Deinstitutionalization in the United States and Italy: A Historical Survey," *International Journal of Mental Health* 37 (2008): 61–70.

83. "Harry Brickman Interview, 1999," California Social Welfare Archives, USC Libraries, https://calisphere.org/item/29e7b15735f61db3db7e87e2 400dfa85/.

84. "J. R. Elpers Interview, February 9, 2010," UCLA/Los Angeles County Department of Mental Health.

85. Hale describes how, in 1954, the annual income of hospital psychiatrists was $9,000, compared to $22,000 for private analysts. University

psychiatrists earned $15,000, while private psychiatrists who employed somatic and directive therapies earned $25,000. As a group, psychiatrists earned less than most physicians, but the income of psychoanalysts was above average. Nathan G. Hale Jr., *The Rise and Crisis of Psychoanalysis in the United States: Freud and the Americans, 1917–1985* (New York: Oxford University Press, 1995), 247–48.

86. Leighton, *Caring for Mentally Ill People*, 99, 97.

87. The Short-Doyle Act was preceded by community mental health legislation drafted by the California Department of Mental Hygiene in 1955 but was then stalled by the "very conservative California Medical Association," which was "alarmed" by its apparently socialist implications. Karno and Schwartz, *Community Mental Health*, 38.

88. Alfred Auerback, "The Short-Doyle Act: California Community Mental Health Services Program: Background and Status After One Year," *California Medicine* 90 (1959): 335–38. The state proportion would increase to 75 percent in 1963 and 90 percent in 1969.

89. Edward Rudin and Robert S. McInnes, "Community Mental Health Services Act: Five Years of Operation Under the California Law," *California Medicine* 99 (1963): 9–11.

90. Karno and Schwartz, *Community Mental Health*, 39.

91. Just before these efforts were underway in California, the sociologist Elaine Cumming and psychiatrist John Cumming undertook an experiment to see if mental health education could reduce stigma in two small towns in Saskatchewan. They found that it could not. Elaine Cumming and John Cumming, *Closed Ranks: An Experiment in Mental Health Education* (Cambridge, MA: Harvard University Press, 1957); Kathleen Kendall, "From Closed Ranks to Open Doors: Elaine and John Cumming's Mental Health Education Experiment in 1950s Saskatchewan," *Histoire Sociale/Social History* 44 (2011): 257–86.

92. Ruth J. Levy, "Community Mental Health Services: Operation in San Jose," *California Medicine* 92 (1960): 346.

93. Levy, "Community Mental Health Services," 346.

94. Rudin and McInnes, "Community Mental Health Services Act," 11.

95. Both Karno and Schwartz left community mental health for academia, but they insisted this was not out of disillusionment. They did note, however, that many people attracted to community mental health were

drawn to it in part because they thought it would allow them to escape the politics that came with working in larger institutions. Unfortunately, this was not to be the case. CMHCs merely had different power dynamics. Karno and Schwartz, *Community Mental Health*, 53, 134.

96. Karno and Schwartz, *Community Mental Health*, 137, 35–36.

97. Donald A. Schwartz, "Community Mental Health: An Underview," *Psychiatric Quarterly* 44 (1970): 348.

98. For more on how mental health care evolved in California, see Howard Padwa, Marcia Meldrum, Jack R. Friedman, and Joel T. Braslow, "A Mental Health System in Recovery: The Era of Deinstitutionalisation in California," in *Deinstitutionalisation and After: Post-War Psychiatry in the Western World*, ed. Despo Kritsotaki, Vicky Long, and Matthew Smith (Basingstoke: Palgrave, 2016), 241–65.

99. Rebecca Miller, Allison N. Ponce, and Kenneth S. Thompson, "Deinstitutionalization and the Community Mental Health Center Movement (1954–1976)," in *Classics of Community Psychiatry: Fifty Years of Public Mental Health Outside the Hospital*, ed. Michael Rowe, Martha Lawless, Kenneth Thompson, and Larry Davidson (Oxford: Oxford University Press, 2011), 11.

100. Malin VanAntwerp, "The Route to Primary Prevention," *Community Mental Health Journal* 7 (1971): 183–88.

101. E. Fuller Torrey, *American Psychosis: How the Federal Government Destroyed the Mental Illness Treatment System* (Oxford: Oxford University Press, 2013), 64–65.

102. John Cody, quoted in Raymond M. Glasscote, James N. Sussex, Elaine Cumming, and Lauren H. Smith, *The Community Mental Health Center: An Interim Appraisal* (Washington, DC: APA, 1969), 97. The report detailed the activities of CMHCs in Denver and Houston. While the preventive activities of the Denver Center focused mainly on consultation, the Houston Center worked closely with the local Neighborhood Centers Association, which focused in part on meeting the basic living needs of families.

103. Andrea M. Vayda and Felice D. Perlmutter, "Primary Prevention in Community Mental Health Centers: A Survey of Current Activities," *Community Mental Health Journal* 13 (1977): 343–51.

104. Vayda and Perlmutter, "Primary Prevention," 343.

105. Gerald N. Grob, *From Asylum to Community, Mental Health Policy in Modern America* (Princeton, NJ: Princeton University Press, 1991), 251.

106. David F. Musto, "Whatever Happened to Community Mental Health?" *Public Interest* 39 (1975): 53–79.

107. Eli M. Bower, "Primary Prevention of Mental and Emotional Disorders: A Conceptual Framework and Action Possibilities," *American Journal of Orthopsychiatry* 33 (1963): 824.

108. VanAntwerp, "Route to Primary Prevention."

109. Oral history interview with Hunter McQuistion, August 9, 2016.

110. Grob, *From Asylum to Community*, 255.

111. Anthony Broskowski and Frank Baker, "Professional, Organizational, and Social Barriers to Primary Prevention," *American Journal of Orthopsychiatry* 44 (1974): 707–19.

112. Grob, *From Asylum to Community*, chap. 10. Some also argued that CMHCs attempted to avoid treating more seriously ill patients. David Mechanic, *Mental Health and Social Policy* (Englewood Cliffs, NJ: Prentice Hall, 1969). An analysis of the use of CMHCs also suggested that the mental health education conducted by CMHCs encouraged individuals to seek their support for a wider array of problems. This may have redirected efforts away from patients with more serious symptoms. Joseph Veroff, Richard A. Kulka, and Elizabeth Douvan, *Mental Health in America: Patterns of Health-Seeking from 1957 to 1976* (New York: Basic Books, 1981), chap. 8.

113. President Richard Nixon also wanted to terminate CMHC funding but was prevented by Congress. Richard Nixon, "Statement About the Community Mental Health Centers Amendments of 1970," March 16, 1970, American Presidency Project, https://www.presidency.ucsb.edu/documents/statement-about-the-community-mental-health-centers-amendments-1970; Steven S. Sharfstein, "Whatever Happened to Community Mental Health?" *Psychiatric Services* 51 (2000): 616–20.

114. A joint NIMH-NAMH conference on primary prevention in 1976 also spurred the President's commission. Although much of the content focused on the sort of top-down consultations that had been already occurring, a few papers, including one on a Harlem CMHC, focused on tackling underlying social problems. Donald C. Klein and

Stephen E. Goldston, *Primary Prevention: An Idea Whose Time Has Come* (Rockville, MD: NIMH, 1976).

115. In an oral history, the former NIMH psychologist Stephen Goldston stated that the prevention panel was largely thanks to the efforts of Beverly Long (1920–2015), then the president of the National Mental Health Association of Georgia and a friend of Rosalynn Carter. It is also notable that there were more psychologists on the prevention panel than psychiatrists and that sociologists and anthropologists were not represented. President's Commission on Mental Health, *Report to the President*, vol. 4: *Appendix* (Washington, DC: U.S. Government Printing Office, 1978), 1823; "Oral History of Stephen Goldston, October 5, 1999," Office of NIH History and Stetten Museum. For more on the work of PCMH, see Gerald N. Grob, "Public Policy and Mental Illnesses: Jimmy Carter's Presidential Commission on Mental Health," *Millbank Memorial Quarterly* 83 (2005): 425–56.

116. President's Commission on Mental Health, *Report to the President*, 1836.

117. President's Commission on Mental Health, *Report to the President*, 1855.

118. Henry A. Foley and Steven S. Sharfstein, *Madness and Government: Who Cares for the Mentally Ill?* (Washington, DC: American Psychiatric Press, 1983), 130, 129–34.

119. Foley and Sharfstein, *Madness and Government*, 135.

120. Stephen E. Goldston, "Primary Prevention: Historical Perspectives and a Blueprint for Action," *American Psychologist* 41 (1986): 453–60.

121. Roy R. Grinker, "Psychiatry Rides Off Madly in All Directions," *Archives of General Psychiatry* 10 (1964): 228–37; Leighton, *Caring for Mentally Ill People*, 15.

122. Grob, "Public Policy and Mental Illnesses," 425, 448.

123. Grob, "Public Policy and Mental Illnesses," 429, 448.

6. THE DECLINE OF SOCIAL PSYCHIATRY

1. John W. Gardner, "No Easy Victories," *American Statistician* 22 (1968): 14–16.

2. Matthew P. Dumont, *The Absurd Healer: A Personal Account of a Community Psychiatrist's Involvement with the City as Patient* (1968; New York: Viking, 1971).

3. Leonard J. Duhl, foreword to Dumont, *Absurd Healer*, 15.

4. Perhaps touching on the calls of social psychiatrists for ever more research, as well as the difficulty in defining mental illness, Dumont argued that "asking for definite proof that poverty 'causes' mental illness is asking for the impossible." There could never "be a single cause of anything so complex as an arbitrarily defined collection of behavior characteristics." Dumont, *Absurd Healer*, 25–26.

5. Dumont, *Absurd Healer*, 80. In the book's front matter there was a disclaimer from NIMH and the Department of Public Health stating that the opinions expressed therein did not represent their official policy. They likely had passages such as this one in mind.

6. Matthew P. Dumont, *Treating the Poor: A Personal Sojourn Through the Rise and Fall of Community Mental Health* (Belmont, MA: Dymphna, 1992), 10–11, 116, 5, 16, 143, 142.

7. Dumont, *Treating the Poor*, 136. Emphasis in original.

8. Bruce Mazlish, *In Search of Richard Nixon: A Psychohistorical Inquiry* (New York: Basic Books, 1972); E. Fuller Torrey, *American Psychosis: How the American Federal Government Destroyed the Mental Illness Treatment System* (Oxford: Oxford University Press, 2014), 75–84.

9. Those still involved in social psychiatry believed that worsening socioeconomic factors were having a detrimental impact on mental health. John J. Schwab and Mary E. Schwab, *Sociocultural Roots of Mental Illness: An Epidemiologic Survey* (New York: Plenum, 1978), viii.

10. Michael B. Katz, *The Undeserving Poor: America's Enduring Confrontation with Poverty* (Oxford: Oxford University Press, 2013), x; Mical Raz, *What's Wrong with the Poor? Psychiatry, Race, and the War on Poverty* (Chapel Hill: University of North Carolina Press, 2013), 37, 40.

11. Oscar Lewis, *Five Families: Mexican Case Studies in the Culture of Poverty* (New York: Basic Books, 1959).

12. Raz, *What's Wrong*, 37.

13. Eleanor Burke Leacock, *The Culture of Poverty: A Critique* (New York: Simon and Schuster, 1991), 11.

14. Raz, *What's Wrong*, 38.

15. Raz, *What's Wrong*, 38–40.

16. Daniel P. Moynihan, *The Negro Family: The Case for National Action* (Washington, DC: United States Department of Labor), 5, 29.

17. Kathleen W. Jones, *Taming the Troublesome Child: American Families, Child Guidance, and the Limits of Psychiatric Authority* (Cambridge, MA: Harvard University Press, 1992); Raz, *What's Wrong*; John Stewart, *Child Guidance in Britain: The Dangerous Age of Childhood, 1918–1955* (London: Routledge, 2014).

18. Alice O'Connor, *Poverty Knowledge: Social Science, Social Policy, and the Poor in Twentieth-Century American History* (Princeton, NJ: Princeton University Press, 2001).

19. Raz, *What's Wrong*, chap. 3.

20. Katz, *Undeserving Poor*, 114–15.

21. Eleanor Leacock, who had participated on MMS, also edited a volume critiquing the notion of the culture of poverty. Leacock, *Culture of Poverty*. Marvin Opler, with whom she had sparred during Midtown, also disliked the term. Marvin K. Opler, "International and Cultural Conflicts Affecting Mental Health: Violence, Suicide, and Withdrawal," *American Journal of Psychotherapy* 23 (1969): 608–20.

22. Also influential in shaping white attitudes about Black Americans, as Elizabeth Hinton has written, was the parallel "war" on crime that Johnson also launched, which targeted Black Americans. This "war" also reinforced Moynihan's notion that Black communities were inherently flawed and required correction. Similarly, the "war" on drugs, a phrase typically traced to Nixon but found in an earlier speech by New York's Governor Nelson Rockefeller, also disproportionately affected Black Americans and deflected from government's focusing on structural problems. "Speech from Nelson A. Rockefeller to New York Association of Community Mental Health Boards," May 26, 1970, Nelson A. Rockefeller gubernatorial records, Speeches, Series 33 (FA372), Box 75, Folder 3036, Rockefeller Archive Center; Elizabeth Hinton, *From the War on Poverty to the War on Crime: The Making of Mass Incarceration in America* (Cambridge, MA: Harvard University Press, 2016).

23. Dumont, *Absurd Healer*, 60. Emphasis in original.

24. Jill Quadagno, *The Color of Welfare: How Racism Undermined the War on Poverty* (Oxford: Oxford University Press, 1996), 145.

25. O'Connor, *Poverty Knowledge*, 134.

26. O'Connor, *Poverty Knowledge*.

27. Dumont, *Treating the Poor*, 38.

28. Oral history interview with John Talbott, March 17, 2015.

29. Aaron Levin, "APA Members Speak Out During Vietnam War," *Psychiatric News* January 12, 2016.

30. Lucas Richert, *Break on Through: Radical Psychiatry and the American Counterculture* (Cambridge, MA: MIT Press, 2019), 23–24.

31. Richert, *Break on Through*, 45.

32. Katz, *Undeserving Poor*, 156.

33. The gradual recognition that mental illness continued to be a problem in communist countries also undermined the idea that socialist systems would eliminate mental illness. Melvin Sabshin, "Melvin Sabshin Reflects on Two Decades at the Helm of the APA," *Psychiatric Services* 48 (1997): 1164–67; Mat Savelli and Sarah Marks, *Psychiatry in Communist Europe* (Basingstoke: Palgrave, 2015).

34. Nathan G. Hale Jr., *The Rise and Crisis of Psychoanalysis in the United States: Freud and the Americans* (New York: Oxford University Press, 1995), 322–44.

35. Martin Halliwell, *Therapeutic Revolutions: Medicine, Psychiatry, and American Culture, 1945–1970* (New Brunswick, NJ: Rutgers University Press, 2013), 267–70.

36. Halliwell, *Therapeutic Revolutions*, chap. 2; Andrew Scull, *Madness in Civilization: A Cultural History of Insanity from the Bible to Freud, from the Madhouse to Modern Medicine* (London: Thames and Hudson, 2015), 351–57; Ben Parker, "The Western Film and Psychoanalysis," *Film Quarterly* 68 (2014): 22–30; Alexander Dunst, *Madness in Cold War America: Mad America* (London: Routledge, 2017).

37. There was also an assumption that psychoanalysis was ineffective with people from lower socioeconomic classes. Dumont argued that this was not because the poor were less verbal or because they were less curious about their emotional lives than others. Rather, they were "forced to deal more with what happened yesterday than with what happened in one's childhood, though much happened then as well." As a result, emotions did not tend to be repressed but were expressed, often violently or destructively. Psychotherapy, he argued, was effective with the poor, but the resources to deliver it were dwindling. Dumont, *Treating the Poor*, 6–10.

38. Dumont, *Treating the Poor*, 17.

39. Talbott interview.

40. Oisín Wall, *The British Anti-Psychiatrists: From Institutional Psychiatry to the Counter-Culture, 1960–1971* (London: Routledge, 2018), 20–21. Many of these "antipsychiatrists" did not associate themselves with the term, and, subsequently, historians have also debated the use of the term. In her recent article on Frantz Fanon, for instance, Camille Robcis uses radical psychiatry as more of a catch-all, limiting antipsychiatry to British and Italian efforts to overturn the asylum system and ideas about the social construction of mental illness. Here, I define antipsychiatry more broadly. Camille Robcis, "Frantz Fanon, Institutional Psychotherapy, and the Decolonization of Psychiatry," *Journal of the History of Ideas* 81 (2020): 303–25.

41. Thomas S. Szasz, *The Myth of Mental Illness: Foundations of a Theory of Personal Conduct* (New York: Harper and Row, 1961); Michel Foucault, *Folie et déraison. Histoire de la folie a l'âge classique* (Paris: Librarie Plon, 1965).

42. I say "most" because the 1960s and 1970s comprised a period when new conditions, such as what would become attention deficit hyperactivity disorder and post-traumatic stress disorder, were being added to the list of psychiatric disorders commonly diagnosed and others, such as homosexuality, were being removed. There was, therefore, considerable debate even among conventional psychiatrists about what constituted a mental illness. Allan Young, *Harmony of Illusions: Inventing Post-Traumatic Stress Disorder* (Princeton, NJ: Princeton University Press, 1997); Matthew Smith, *Hyperactive: The Controversial History of ADHD* (London: Reaktion, 2012).

43. Dariel Telfer, *The Caretakers* (New York: Simon and Schuster, 1959); Richard Condon, *The Manchurian Candidate* (New York: McGraw-Hill, 1959); Ken Kesey, *One Flew Over the Cuckoo's Nest* (New York: Viking, 1962).

44. Michael Staub, *Madness Is Civilization: When the Diagnosis Was Social* (Chicago: University of Chicago Press, 2011), 2.

45. Staub, *Madness Is Civilization*, 3.

46. Norman Dain, "Anti-Psychiatry in the United States," in *Discovering the History of Psychiatry*, ed. Mark S. Micale and Roy Porter (Oxford: Oxford University Press, 1994), 430.

47. Gerald N. Grob, "The Attack of Psychiatric Legitimacy in the 1960s: Rhetoric and Reality," *Journal of the History of the Human Sciences* 47 (2011): 398–416.

48. Richert, *Break on Through*.

49. John A. Talbott, "Radical Psychiatry: An Examination of the Issues," *AJP* 131 (1974): 121–28.

50. Talbott, "Radical Psychiatry," 127.

51. Robert S. Garber, "The Presidential Address: The Proper Business of Psychiatry," *AJP* 128 (1971): 2–3.

52. Walter E. Barton, "Robert Slocum Garber, M.D. Ninety-Ninth President, 1970–1971," *AJP* 128 (1971): 14–18.

53. Grob, "Attack of Psychiatric Legitimacy," 400.

54. Richert, *Break on Through*, 63–64. See also Diana Ralph, *Work and Madness: The Rise of Community Psychiatry* (Montreal: Black Rose, 1983).

55. Talbott, "Radical Psychiatry."

56. Richert, *Break on Through*.

57. The publications of Erika Dyck, Lucas Richert, and Michael Pollan have helped reignite debates about the therapeutic use of psychedelics today. Erika Dyck, *Psychedelic Psychiatry: LSD from Clinic to Campus* (Baltimore, MD: Johns Hopkins University Press, 2008); Lucas Richert, *Strange Trips: Science, Culture, and the Regulation of Drugs* (Montreal: McGill-Queen's University Press, 2019); Michael Pollan, *How to Change Your Mind: The New Science of Psychedelics* (New York: Penguin, 2018).

58. An example of this is the food additive–free Feingold diet, developed during the early 1970s to treat children diagnosed with hyperactivity. Many parents opted for the diet because they found that conventional treatments (for example, the stimulant drug Ritalin) were either ineffective or caused too many side effects. Matthew Smith, *An Alternative History of Hyperactivity: Food Additives and the Feingold Diet* (New Brunswick, NJ: Rutgers University Press, 2011).

59. John Burnham, "Deinstitutionalisation and the Great Sociocultural Shift to Consumer Culture," in *Deinstitutionalisation and After: Post-War Psychiatry in the Western World*, ed. Despo Kritisotaki, Vicky Long, and Matthew Smith (Basingstoke: Palgrave, 2016), 39–56; Dunst, *Madness in Cold War America*, chap. 3.

60. Elizabeth Lunbeck, *The Americanization of Narcissism* (Cambridge, MA: Harvard University Press, 2014).

61. I have chosen to use the term "psychiatric survivors' movement," but many other terms have also been used to refer to mental patient rights groups since the 1960s. These include the ex-patients' movement, mad pride movement, mad people's movement, mental patients' liberation movement, mental health users' movement, and service users' movement. The psychiatric survivors' movement remains active through websites, such as mindfreedom.org and madinamerica.org, and publications, such as the UK-based *Asylum* magazine. It has also influenced the development of the neurodiversity movement, which advocates for more flexibility and accommodation for neurologically atypical individuals, who are often labeled with neurological disorders such as autism and ADHD. The term "Mad Studies" has also been coined to represent academic inquiry into madness (a term that has been co-opted by the movement). Judi Chamberlin, *On Our Own: Patient-Controlled Alternatives to the Mental Health System* (New York: Hawthorn, 1978); Barbara Everett, *A Fragile Revolution: Consumers and Psychiatric Survivors Confront the Power of the Mental Health System* (Waterloo, ON: Wilfred Laurier University Press, 2000); Linda J. Morrison, *Talking Back to Psychiatry: The Psychiatric Consumer/Survivor/Ex-Patient Movement* (New York: Routledge, 2005); Robert Menzies, Brenda A. LeFrançois, and Geoffrey Reaume, "Introducing Mad Studies," in *Mad Matters: A Critical Reader in Canadian Mad Studies*, ed. Brenda A. LeFrançois, Robert Menzies, and Geoffrey Reaume (Toronto: Canadian Scholars' Press, 2013), 1–22.

62. Judi Chamberlin, "The Ex-Patients' Movement: Where We've Been and Where We're Going," *Journal of Mind and Behavior* 11 (1990): 323–36.

63. Erika Dyck, Lesley Baker, Lanny Beckman, Geertje Boschma, Chris Dooley, Kathleen Kendall, Eugène LeBlanc, et al., "After the Asylum in Canada: Surviving Deinstitutionalisation and Revising History," in *Deinstitutionalisation and After: Post-War Psychiatry in the Western World*, ed. Despo Kritisotaki, Vicky Long, and Matthew Smith (Basingstoke: Palgrave, 2016), 75–95.

64. There was also a distinction between the aims of the psychiatric survivors' movement and the service user or consumer movement.

"Psychiatric survivors," as the term suggests, were more critical of psychiatry and the medical model of mental illness. Those who identified themselves as consumers were more reform oriented and less likely to critique biomedical ideas about mental illness. Alexandra L. Adame, "'There Needs to Be a Place in Society for Madness': The Psychiatric Survivor Movement and New Directions in Mental Health Care," *Journal of Humanistic Psychology* 54 (2013): 456–75.

65. Oryx Cohen, "How Do We Recover? An Analysis of Psychiatric Survivor Oral History Histories," *Journal of Humanistic Psychology* 45 (2005): 333–54; Morrison, *Talking Back to Psychiatry*; Menzies, LeFrançois, and Reaume, "Introducing Mad Studies."

66. For alternative, patient-centered approaches, see Bruce M. Z. Cohen, *Mental Health User Narratives: New Perspectives on Illness and Recovery* (Basingstoke: Palgrave, 2008); Mark Rapley, Joanna Moncrieff, and Jacqui Dillon, *De-Medicalizing Misery: Psychiatry, Psychology, and the Human Condition* (Basingstoke: Palgrave, 2011); Ewen Speed, Joanna Moncrieff, and Mark Rapley, *De-Medicalizing Misery II: Society, Politics, and the Mental Health Industry* (Basingstoke: Palgrave, 2017).

67. Herb Kutchins and Stuart A. Kirk, *Making Us Crazy: DSM: The Psychiatric Bible and the Creation of Mental Disorders* (New York: Free Press, 1997); Ethan Waters, *Crazy Like Us: The Globalization of the American Psyche* (New York: Simon and Schuster, 2010); Allan V. Horwitz, *DSM: A History of Psychiatry's Bible* (Baltimore, MD: Johns Hopkins University Press, 2021).

68. Jack D. Pressman, *Last Resort: Psychosurgery and the Limits of Medicine* (Cambridge: Cambridge University Press, 1998); Edward Shorter and David Healy, *Shock Therapy: A History of Electroconvulsive Treatment in Mental Illness* (New Brunswick, NJ: Rutgers University Press, 2013).

69. Melvin Sabshin, "The Anti-Community Mental Health 'Movement,'" *AJP* 125 (1969): 1005–12.

70. Jonathan Michel Metzl, *Prozac on the Couch: Prescribing Gender in the Era of Wonder Drugs* (Durham, NC: Duke University Press, 2003).

71. Anselm Strauss, Leonard Schatzman, Rue Bucher, Danuta Ehlrich, and Melvin Sabshin, *Psychiatric Ideologies and Institutions* (New York: Free Press of Glencoe, 1964).

72. Matthew Smith, "Psychiatry Limited: Hyperactivity and the Evolution of American Psychiatry, 1957–1980," *Social History of Medicine* 21 (2008): 541–59.

73. Oral history interview with Wes Sowers, April 26, 2016.

74. Charles E. Rosenberg, *Explaining Epidemics and Other Studies in the History of Medicine* (Cambridge: Cambridge University Press, 1992), 245–56.

75. David Healy, *The Creation of Psychopharmacology* (Cambridge, MA: Harvard University Press, 2002), chap. 2.

76. Joel Braslow, *Mental Ills and Bodily Cures: Psychiatric Treatment in the First Half of the Twentieth Century* (Berkeley: University of California Press, 1997), 35–37.

77. Healy, *Creation of Psychopharmacology*, chap. 3.

78. There is a rich historiography of psychiatric drugs that can supplement this very brief summary. Although most of these histories showcase the pitfalls of psychopharmacology, the histories written about psychedelics have been more enthusiastic. It is notable that LSD, as with Valium and, to a lesser extent, Ritalin, fell into disfavor in medical circles once it began to be used recreationally. David Healy, *The Antidepressant Era* (Cambridge, MA: Harvard University Press, 1997); Andrea Tone, *The Age of Anxiety: A History of America's Turbulent Affair with Tranquilizers* (New York: Basic Books, 2008); Dyck, *Psychedelic Psychiatry*; David Herzberg, *Happy Pills in America: From Miltown to Prozac* (Baltimore, MD: Johns Hopkins University Press, 2008); Joanna Moncrieff, *The Myth of the Chemical Cure: A Critique of Psychiatric Drug Treatment* (Basingstoke: Palgrave, 2008); Smith, *Hyperactive*, chap. 4; Nicolas Henckes, "Magic Bullet in the Head? Psychiatric Revolutions and Their Aftermath," in *Therapeutic Revolutions: Pharmaceuticals and Social Change in the Twentieth Century*, ed. Jeremy A. Greene, Flurin Condrau, and Elizabeth Siegel Watkins (Chicago: University of Chicago Press, 2016), 65–88; Richert, *Strange Trips*.

79. Siddhartha Mukherjee, *The Emperor of All Maladies: A Biography of Cancer* (New York: Scribner, 2010).

80. Maurice Laufer, quoted in Robert Reinhold, "Drugs That Help Control the Unruly Child," *New York Times*, July 5, 1970.

81. Frank Stahnisch, *A New Field in Mind: A History of Interdisciplinarity in the Early Brain Sciences* (Montreal: McGill-Queen's Press, 2020).

82. Stephen T. Casper, "A Revisionist History of American Neurology," *Brain* 133 (2010): 638–42; David Schuster, *Neurasthenic Nation: America's Search for Health, Happiness, and Comfort, 1869–1920* (New Brunswick, NJ: Rutgers University Press, 2011).

83. Elan D. Louis, "The Neurological Study Unit: 'A Combined Attack on a Single Problem from Many Angles,'" *Canadian Bulletin of Medical History* 38 (2021): 233–52. Yale's Neurological Unit suffered some of the same growing pangs as its mental hygiene center.

84. Penfield's collaborator was the psychiatrist Ewen Cameron (1901–1967), who would later be revealed to have contributed to the CIA's MK-Ultra mind control experiments. Yvan Prkachin, "Two Solitudes: Wilder Penfield, Ewen Cameron, and the Search for a Better Lobotomy," *Canadian Bulletin of Medical History* 38 (2021): 253–84.

85. Stephen T. Casper, *The Neurologists: A History of A Medical Specialty in Modern Britain, c. 1789–2000* (Manchester: Manchester University Press, 2014), 171.

86. John Forrester, "Introduction," in Sigmund Freud, *Interpreting Dreams* (1899; London: Folio, 2015), xxxiv.

87. Peter Falkai, Andrea Schmitt, and Nancy Andreason, "Forty Years of Structural Brain Imaging in Mental Disorder: Is It Clinically Useful or Not?" *Dialogues in Clinical Neuroscience* 20 (2018): 179–86.

88. Fernando Vidal, "Brainhood, Anthropological Figure of Modernity," *History of the Human Sciences* 22 (2009): 5–36.

89. Edmund T. Rolls, *Neuroculture: On the Implications of Brain Science* (Oxford: Oxford University Press, 2012). For critiques of "neuroculture," see Charles T. Wolfe, *Brain Theory: Essays in Critical Neurophilosophy* (Basingstoke: Palgrave, 2014); Fernando Vidal and Francesco Ortega, *Being Brains: Making the Cerebral Subject* (New York: Fordham University Press, 2017).

90. Theodore M. Porter, *Genetics in the Madhouse: The Unknown History of Human Heredity* (Princeton, NJ: Princeton University Press, 2018).

91. A search of terms such as "genetic" and "hereditary" in *AJP* during the twentieth century indicates that psychiatrists remained interested in

such explanations for mental illness throughout the heyday of psychoanalysis and social psychiatry. After the 1970s, however, this interest began to accelerate and continues to remain strong.

92. Daniel B. Borenstein, "Presidential Address: Bridging the Millennia: Mind Meets Brain," *AJP* 158 (2001): 1597.

93. Laura D. Hirshbein, "Stella Chess and the History of American Child Psychiatry," *Social History of Medicine* 34 (2021): 788–807.

94. Ilina Singh, "Doing Their Jobs: Mothering with Ritalin in a Culture of Mother-Blame," *Social Science and Medicine* 59 (2004): 1193–205; Adam Feinstein, *A History of Autism: Conversations with the Pioneers* (Chichester: Wiley, 2010); Smith, *Hyperactive.*

95. Jennifer Singh, *Multiple Autisms: Spectrums of Advocacy and Genomic Science* (Minneapolis: University of Minnesota Press, 2016).

96. Iain McClure and Matthew Smith, "Neurodevelopmental Disorders," in *An Introduction to Mental Health and Illness: Critical Perspectives,* ed. Mat Savelli, James Gillett, and Gavin Andrews (Don Mills, ON: Oxford University Press, 2020), 179–203.

97. Hannah Decker, *The Making of DSM-III: A Diagnostic Manual's Conquest of American Psychiatry* (Oxford: Oxford University Press, 2013); Horwitz, *DSM.*

98. Decker, *Making of DSM-III,* xviii.

99. Kutchins and Kirk, *Making Us Crazy.*

100. Social psychiatrists also used diagnostic categories, but far fewer of them. They would typically divide patients into those suffering from psychoses and neuroses, and then split up certain types, for example schizophrenia (see chapter 2). But they also emphasized that diagnosis was an imprecise art and tended to issue caveats to that effect in their statistical analysis.

101. *DSM-III* helped spur the unhelpful craze in retrospectively diagnosing historical figures with mental disorders.

102. Decker, *Making of DSM-III,* 326.

103. When I worked as a youth counselor in Canada during the late 1990s and early 2000s, this was precisely the process by which ADHD was diagnosed, except there was no need to worry about insurance. Smith, *Hyperactive,* preface.

104. Dumont, *Treating the Poor,* 127.

105. The dichotomy of mental illness being perceived as a disorder that affects only specific individuals versus a phenomenon that can afflict anyone was beautifully illustrated in the lead-up to the first heavyweight bout between Tyson Fury and Deontay Wilder. While Fury argued that depression was an "illness, just like cancer" and affected only specific individuals, Wilder countered that, with respect to mental illness: "We have all been there—I can tell you stories about myself." "Tyson Fury Says It Is His 'Calling' to Help People with Mental Health Problems," BBC Sport, https://www.bbc.com/sport/boxing/46107708.

106. David Herzberg, *White Market Drugs: Big Pharma and the Hidden History of Addiction in America* (Chicago: University of Chicago Press, 2020).

EPILOGUE: SOCIAL PSYCHIATRY AND UNIVERSAL BASIC INCOME

1. Anna Macintyre, Daniel Ferris, Briana Gonçalves, and Neil Quinn, "What Has Economics Got to Do with It? The Impact of Socioeconomic Factors on Mental Health and the Case for Collective Action," *Humanities and Social Sciences Communications* 4 (2018): https://www.nature.com/articles/s41599-018-0063-2.

2. Vincent J. Felitti, Robert F. Anda, Dale Nordenberg, David F. Williamson, Alison M. Spitz, Valerie Edwards, Mary P. Koss, and James S. Marks, "Relationship of Childhood Abuse and Household Dysfunction to Many of the Leading Causes of Death in Adults," *American Journal of Preventive Medicine* 14 (1998): P245–58; Michael Smith, "Capability and Adversity: Reframing the 'Causes of the Causes' for Mental Health," *Humanities and Social Sciences Communications* 4 (2008): https://www.nature.com/articles/s41599-018-0066-z.

3. Richard Wilkinson and Kate Pickett, *The Spirit Level: Why Equal Societies Almost Always Do Better* (London: Allen Lane, 2009); Richard Wilkinson and Kate Pickett, *The Inner Level: How More Equal Societies Reduce Stress, Restore Sanity, and Improve Everyone's Well-Being* (London: Allen Lane, 2018).

4. World Health Organization, *Social Determinants of Mental Health* (Geneva: WHO, 2014), https://apps.who.int/iris/bitstream/handle/10665/112828/9789241506809_eng.pdf.

5. Clancy Blair and C. Cybele Raver, "Poverty, Stress, and Brain Development: New Directions for Prevention and Intervention," *Academic Pediatrics* 16 (2016): S30–36.

6. Louise Haagh, *The Case for Universal Basic Income* (Cambridge: Polity, 2019); Malcolm Torrey, *Basic Income: A History* (Cheltenham: Edward Elgar, 2021).

7. Joint Commission on Mental Health of Children, *Crisis in Child Mental Health: Challenge for the 1970s* (New York: Harper and Row, 1970). The digest of the full report was published by JCMHC in 1969 and distributed widely to politicians and public health officials.

8. Reginald Lourie, "The Joint Commission on Mental Health of Children," *AJP* 122 (1966): 1280–81.

9. Benjamin Pasamanick, "Statement of the American Orthopsychiatric Association on the Joint Commission on Mental Health of Children," *American Journal of Orthopsychiatry* 38 (1968): 402–9.

10. JCMHC, *Digest of Crisis in Child Mental Health: Challenge for the 1970s* (Washington, DC: JCMHC, 1969), 8–20.

11. Daniel P. Moynihan, *The Politics of a Guaranteed Income: The Nixon Administration and the Family Assistance Plan* (New York: Vintage, 1973); Alice O'Connor, "The False Dawn of Poor-Law Reform: Nixon, Carter, and the Quest for a Guaranteed Income," *Journal of Policy History* 10 (1998): 99–129. The Greens have been one of the few parties to support UBI consistently. Peter Sloman, "Universal Basic Income in British Politics, 1918–2018: From a 'Vagabond's Wage' to a Global Debate," *Journal of Social Policy* 47 (2018): 625–42.

12. One exception is this statement from Psychologists for Social Change: http://www.psychchange.org/basic-income-psychological-impact-assessment.html.

13. John Henley, "Finnish Basic Income Pilot Improved Wellbeing, Study Finds," *Guardian*, May 7, 2020, https://www.theguardian.com/society/2020/may/07/finnish-basic-income-pilot-improved-wellbeing-study-finds-coronavirus. Naomi Wilson and Shari McDaid, "The Mental Health Effects of a Universal Basic Income: A Synthesis of the Evidence from Previous Pilots," *Social Science and Medicine* 287 (2021): https://doi.org/10.1016/j.socscimed.2021.114374.

14. Evelyn J. Forget, "New Questions, New Data, Old Interventions: The Health Effect of a Guaranteed Annual Income," *Preventive Medicine* 57 (2013): 925–28.

15. E. Jane Costello, Alaattin Erkanli, William Copeland, and Adrian Angold, "Association of Family Income Supplements in Adolescence with Developments of Psychiatric and Substance Use Disorders in Adulthood Among an American Indian Population," *JAMA* 303 (2010): 1954–60.

16. Natalie Paddon, "'I may end up homeless again': Six Ontarians Talk About Their Life Before, After, and Once Again, Without Basic Income," *Toronto Star*, August 2, 2018.

17. Wilson and McDaid, "Mental Health Effects."

18. Ken Loach, *I, Daniel Blake* (2016), https://www.imdb.com/title /tt5168192/; Sarah Gavron, *Rocks* (2019), https://www.imdb.com/title /tt9067182/; Chloe Zhao, *Nomadland* (2020), https://www.imdb.com /title/tt9770150/.

19. Carl C. Bell has persuasively discussed many of these factors in his writing and interviews, many of which are rooted in racism and poverty. *The Sanity of Survival: Reflections on Community Mental Health and Wellness* (Chicago: Third World, 2004); Oral history interview with Carl C. Bell, April 22, 2016.

20. Megan Sutter and Paul B. Perrin, "Discrimination, Mental Health, and Suicidal Ideation in LGBTQ People of Color," *Journal of Counselling Psychology* 63 (2016): 98–105; David R. Williams, Jourdyn Lawrence, and Brigette Davis, "Racism and Health: Evidence and Needed Research," *Annual Review of Public Health* 40 (2019): 105–25; Zheng Wu and Christoph M. Schimmele, "Perceived Religious Discrimination and Mental Health," *Ethnicity and Health* 22 (2019): 1–18.

21. Emily Brignone, Daniel R. George, Lawrence Sinoway, Curren Katz, Charity Sauder, Andrea Murray, Robert Gladden, and Jennifer Kraschnewski, "Trends in the Diagnosis of Diseases of Despair in the United States, 2009–2018: A Retrospective Study," *BMJ Open* 10 (2020): e037679, doi:10.1136/bmjopen-2020-037679.

22. Donna Lu, "Universal Basic Income Seems to Improve Employment and Well-Being," *New Scientist*, May 6, 2020, https://www.newscientist .com/article/2242937-universal-basic-income-seems-to-improve -employment-and-well-being/.

23. Herbert J. Gans, *The Urban Villagers: Group and Class in the Life of Italian-Americans* (New York: Free Press of Glencoe, 1962).

24. The Independent Sector values each hour of volunteer time at $28.54, suggesting that significant economic benefit could accrue if UBI freed more people up to volunteer in ways that they enjoyed, rather than to work at low-paid, unmeaningful jobs.

25. Deborah K. Padgett, "There's No Place Like (a) Home: Ontological Security Among Persons with Serious Mental Illness in the United States," *Social Science and Medicine* 64 (1982): 1925–36; Jack Tsai, Thomas O'Toole, and Lisa K. Kearney, "Homelessness as a Public Mental Health and Social Problem: New Knowledge and Solutions," *Psychological Services* 14 (2017): 113–17.

BIBLIOGRAPHY

Adame, Alexandra L. "'There Needs to Be a Place in Society for Madness': The Psychiatric Survivor Movement and New Directions in Mental Health Care." *Journal of Humanistic Psychology* 54 (2013): 456–75.

Adams, Jon, and Edmund Ramsden. "Rat Cities and Beehive Worlds: Density and Design in the Modern City." *Comparative Studies in Society and History* 53 (2011): 722–56.

Adams, Julia, and David L. Weakliem. "August B. Hollingshead's 'Four Factor Index of Social Status': From Unpublished Paper to Citation Classic." *Yale Journal of Sociology* 8 (2011): 11–19.

Adams, Walter A. "Review of *Mental Disorders in Urban Areas*." *Social Service Review* 13 (1939): 545–46.

Adams, Zoe M., and Naomi Rogers. "'Services Not Mausoleums': Race, Politics, and the Concept of Community in American Medicine (1963–1970)." *Journal of Medical Humanities* 41 (2020): 515–29.

Addams, Jane. *Twenty Years at Hull House*. New York: Macmillan, 1911.

Adler, Herman M. "The Relation Between Psychiatry and the Social Sciences." *AJP* 83 (1927): 661–69.

Allen, Richard, and Absalom Jones. *A Narrative of the Proceedings of the Black People, During the Late Awful Calamity in Philadelphia, in the Year 1793: and a Refutation of Some Censures, Thrown Upon Them in Some Late Publications*. Philadelphia: William W. Woodward, 1794.

American Journal of Sociology. "Notes and Abstracts." *AJS* 6 (1901): 575–76.

——. "Recent Literature." *AJS* 25 (1931): 123–44.

American Psychiatric Association. *Proceedings of the First Colloquium on Personality Investigation*. New York: APA, 1928.

——. *Diagnostic and Statistical Manual of Mental Disorders*. 2nd ed. Washington, DC: American Psychiatric Association, 1968.

——. *Diagnostic and Statistical Manual of Mental Disorders*. 3rd ed. Washington, DC: American Psychiatric Association, 1980.

American Sociological Association. "Manhattan Study: A Classic." *Footnotes* 16 (1988): 10.

Anderson, Nels. *The Hobo: The Sociology of the Homeless Man*. 1923; Chicago: University of Chicago Press, 1965.

Angell, Robert C. "Review of *Human Relations in a Changing World*." *AJS* 55 (1949): 305.

Apple, Rima. *Perfect Motherhood: Science and Childrearing in America*. New Brunswick, NJ: Rutgers University Press, 2006.

Aragona, Massimiliano. "The Influence of Max Weber on the Concept of Empathetic Understanding (*Verstehen*) in the Psychopathology of Karl Jaspers." *History of Psychiatry* 30 (2019): 293–99.

"Atlantic Voice: World Renowned Health Survey, Right Under Our Noses." CBC News. https://www.cbc.ca/news/canada/nova-scotia/atlantic-voice -world-renowned-health-survey-right-under-our-noses-1.3083959.

Auerback, Alfred. "The Short-Doyle Act: California Community Mental Health Services Program: Background and Status After One Year." *California Medicine* 90 (1959): 335–38.

Bailey, Martha J., and Nicholas J. Duquette. "How Johnson Fought the War on Poverty: The Economics and Politics of Funding at the Office of Economic Opportunity." *Journal of Economic History* 74 (2014): 351–88.

Baker, Mike, Jennifer Valentio-DeVries, Manny Fernandez, and Michael LaForgia. "Three Words. 70 Cases. The Tragic History of 'I Can't Breathe.'" *New York Times*, June 29, 2020.

Bakker, Nelleke. "Child Guidance, Dynamic Psychology and Psychopathologisation of Child Rearing (c. 1920–1940): A Transnational Perspective." *History of Education* 49 (2020): 617–35.

Barkow, Jerome. "Interview with Alec Leighton." *Anthropologica* 31 (1989): 237–61.

Barton, Walter E. "Robert Slocum Garber, M.D. Ninety-Ninth President, 1970–1971." *AJP* 128 (1971): 14–18.

Bauer, Nicole. "'This weather always gets me down': A Psychological Perspective on Mental Illness." *Health* 23 (2019): 180–96.

Baxter, Ellen, and Kim Hopper. *Private Lives, Public Spaces*. New York: Community Service Society, 1981.

Beard, George M. *American Nervousness, Its Causes and Consequences: A Supplement to Neurasthenia (Nervous Exhaustion)*. New York: G. P. Putnam's Sons, 1881.

Beers, Clifford Whittingham. *A Mind That Found Itself: An Autobiography*. New York: Longmans, Green, 1908.

Bell, Carl C. *The Sanity of Survival: Reflections on Community Mental Health and Wellness*. Chicago: Third World, 2004.

Bell, Norman W., and John P. Spiegel. "Social Psychiatry: Vagaries of a Term." *Archives of General Psychiatry* 14 (1966): 337–45.

Bellack, Leopold. *Handbook of Community Psychiatry and Community Mental Health*. New York: Grune & Stratton, 1964.

Benedict, Ruth. *The Chrysanthemum and the Sword*. Boston: Houghton Mifflin, 1946.

——. *Patterns of Culture*. Boston: Houghton Mifflin, 1934.

——. *Race: Science and Politics*. New York: Modern Age, 1940.

Bernard, Viola W. "Psychoanalysis and Members of Minority Groups." *Journal of the American Psychoanalytic Association* 1 (1953): 256–67.

Beyer, Christof. "'Islands of Reform': Early Transformation of the Mental Health Service in Lower Saxony, Germany in the 1960s." In *Deinstitutionalisation and After: Post-War Psychiatry in the Western World*, ed. Despo Kritsotaki, Vicky Long, and Matthew Smith, 99–114. Basingstoke: Palgrave, 2016.

Blain, Daniel. "Twenty-Five Years of Hospital and Community Psychiatry." *Hospital and Community Psychiatry* 26 (1975): 605–9.

Blair, Clancy, and C. Cybele Raver. "Poverty, Stress, and Brain Development: New Directions for Prevention and Intervention." *Academic Pediatrics* 16 (2016): S30–36.

Blanchard, Sessi Kuwabara. "How the Young Lords Took Lincoln Hospital, Left a Health Activism Legacy." *Filter*, October 30, 2018. https://filtermag.org/how-the-young-lords-took-lincoln-hospital-and-left-a-health-activism-legacy/.

Blazer, Dan. *Age of Melancholy: Major Depression and Its Social Origins*. New York: Routledge, 2005.

Bloom, Samuel L. *Word as Scalpel: A History of Medical Sociology*. Oxford: Oxford University Press, 2002.

Borenstein, Daniel B. "Presidential Address: Bridging the Millennia: Mind Meets Brain." *AJP* 158 (2001): 1597–1600.

Bower, Eli M. "Primary Prevention of Mental and Emotional Disorders: A Conceptual Framework and Action Possibilities." *American Journal of Orthopsychiatry* 33 (1963): 832–48.

Braslow, Joel. *Mental Ills, Bodily Cures: Psychiatric Treatment in the First Half of the Twentieth Century*. Berkeley: University of California Press, 1997.

Brickman, Harry R. "Foreword." In *Community Mental Health: Reflections and Explorations*, by Marvin Karno and Donald A. Schwartz. New York: John Wiley and Sons, 1974.

Brignone, Emily, Daniel R. George, Lawrence Sinoway, Curren Katz, Charity Sauder, Andrea Murray, Robert Gladden, and Jennifer Kraschnewski. "Trends in the Diagnosis of Diseases of Despair in the United States, 2009–2018: A Retrospective Study." *BMJ Open* 10 (2020): e037679. doi:10.1136/bmjopen-2020-037679.

Brody, Eugene B., and Frederick C. Redlich. *Psychotherapy with Schizophrenics*. New York: International Universities Press, 1952.

Broskowski, Anthony, and Frank Baker. "Professional, Organizational, and Social Barriers to Primary Prevention." *American Journal of Orthopsychiatry* 44 (1974): 707–19.

Brown, Bertram S., and Harold Goldstein. "The Lightning Rod of Human Service Delivery." In *Controversy in Psychiatry*, ed. John Paul Brady and H. Keith H. Brodie, 1041–54. Philadelphia: W. B. Saunders, 1978.

Brown, L. Guy. "The Field and Problems of Social Psychiatry." In *Fields and Methods of Sociology*, ed. L. L. Bernard, 129–45. New York: Ray Long and Richard R. Smith Publishers, 1934.

Bulmer, Martin. *The Chicago School of Sociology*. Chicago: University of Chicago Press, 1984.

Burgess, Ernest W. "The Influence of Sigmund Freud Upon Sociology in the United States." *AJS* 45 (1939): 356–74.

——. "Introduction." In *Mental Disorder in Urban Areas: An Ecological Study of Schizophrenia and Other Psychoses*, by Robert E. L. Faris and H. Warren Dunham. Chicago: University of Chicago Press, 1939.

——. "Problems of Social Psychiatry and Theoretical Overview." In *Mental Health and Mental Disorder: A Sociological Approach*, ed. Arnold M. Rose, 3–17. London: Routledge and Kegan Paul, 1956.

Burgess, Ernest W., and Donald J. Bogue, eds. *Contributions to Urban Sociology*. Chicago: University of Chicago Press, 1964.

Burnham, John. "Deinstitutionalisation and the Great Sociocultural Shift to Consumer Culture." In *Deinstitutionalisation and After: Post-War Psychiatry in the Western World*, ed. Despo Kritisotaki, Vicky Long, and Matthew Smith, 39–56. Basingstoke: Palgrave, 2016.

Calhoun, John B. "Population Density and Social Pathology." *Scientific American* 206 (1962): 139–48.

——. "Space and the Strategy of Life." In *Behavior and Environment*, ed. A. H. Esser, 329–86. New York: Plenum, 1971.

Caplan, Gerald. *An Approach to Community Mental Health*. London: Tavistock, 1961.

Carey, James T. *Sociology and Public Affairs: The Chicago School*. London: Sage, 1975.

Casper, Stephen T. *The Neurologists: A History of a Medical Specialty in Modern Britain, c. 1789–2000*. Manchester: Manchester University Press, 2014.

——. "A Revisionist History of American Neurology." *Brain* 133 (2010): 638–42.

Caudill, William, and Bertram H. Roberts. "Pitfalls in the Organization of Interdisciplinary Research." *Human Organization* 10 (1951): 12–15.

Cavan, Ruth Shonle. "The Chicago School of Sociology, 1918–1933." *Urban Life* 11 (1983): 407–20.

——. *Suicide*. Chicago: University of Chicago Press, 1928.

Chamberlin, Judi. "The Ex-Patients' Movement: Where We've Been and Where We're Going." *Journal of Mind and Behavior* 11 (1990): 323–36.

——. *On Our Own: Patient-Controlled Alternatives to the Mental Health System*. New York: Hawthorn, 1978.

Clark, Jr., Gordon H. *Community Psychiatry: Problems and Possibilities*. Spring House, PA: McNeil Pharmaceutical, 1987.

Cobb, Stanley, and Erich Lindemann. "Symposium on the Management of the Cocoanut Grove Burns at the Massachusetts General Hospital: Neuropsychiatric Observations." *Annals of Surgery* 117 (1943): 814–24.

Cohen, Bruce M. Z. *Mental Health User Narratives: New Perspectives on Illness and Recovery.* Basingstoke: Palgrave, 2008.

Cohen, Oryx. "How Do We Recover? An Analysis of Psychiatric Survivor Oral Histories." *Journal of Humanistic Psychology* 45 (2005): 333–54.

Comez-Días, Lillian, Gordon Nagayama Hall, and Helen A. Neville. "Racial Trauma: Theory, Research, and Healing: Introduction to the Special Issue." *American Psychologist* 74 (2019): 1–5.

Condon, Richard. *The Manchurian Candidate.* New York: McGraw-Hill, 1959.

Cortese, Anthony J. "The Rise, Hegemony, and Decline of the Chicago School of Sociology, 1892–1945." *Social Science Journal* 32 (1995): 235–54.

Costello, E. Jane, Alaattin Erkanli, William Copeland, and Adrian Angold. "Association of Family Income Supplements in Adolescence with Developments of Psychiatric and Substance Use Disorders in Adulthood Among an American Indian Population." *JAMA* 303 (2010): 1954–60.

Crabb, Mary Katherine. "An Epidemic of Pride: Pellagra and the Culture of the American South." *Anthropologica* 34 (1992): 89–103.

Cumming, Elaine, and John Cumming. *Closed Ranks: An Experiment in Mental Health Education.* Cambridge, MA: Harvard University Press, 1957.

Dain, Norman. "Anti-Psychiatry in the United States." In *Discovering the History of Psychiatry,* ed. Mark S. Micale and Roy Porter, 415–44. Oxford: Oxford University Press, 1994.

——. *Clifford W. Beers: Advocate for the Insane.* Pittsburgh, PA: University of Pittsburgh Press, 1980.

Danto, Elizabeth Ann. *Freud's Free Clinics: Psychoanalysis and Social Justice, 1918–1938.* New York: Columbia University Press, 2005.

Decker, Hannah. *The Making of DSM-III: A Diagnostic Manual's Conquest of American Psychiatry.* Oxford: Oxford University Press, 2013.

Deutsch, Albert. *The Mentally Ill in America: A History of their Care and Treatment from Colonial Times.* Garden City, NY: Doubleday, Doran and Company, 1937.

——. *The Shame of the States.* 1948; New York: Arno, 1973.

Devereux, Georges. "Review of *Mental Disorders in Urban Areas.*" *Psychoanalytic Review* 27 (1940): 251–52.

Diamond, Andrew J. *Chicago on the Make: Power and Inequality in a Modern City.* Berkeley: University of California Press, 2017.

Dohrenwend, Bruce P., and Barbara S. Dohrenwend. "Psychiatric Disorder in Urban Settings." In *American Handbook of Psychiatry*, ed. S. Arieti, 2:423–47. New York: Basic Books, 1974.

Dollard, John. *Caste and Class in a Southern Town*. New Haven, CT: Yale University Press, 1937.

——. "Scratch a New Yorker, and What Do You Find?" *New York Times*, April 22, 1962.

Dowbiggin, Ian. *Keeping America Sane: Psychiatry and Eugenics in the United States and Canada, 1880–1940*. Ithaca, NY: Cornell University Press, 1997.

Doyle, Dennis. *Psychiatry and Racial Liberalism in Harlem, 1936–1968*. Rochester, NY: University of Rochester Press, 2016.

——. "'We Didn't Know You Were a Negro': Fredric Wertham and the Ironies of Race, Comic Books, and Juvenile Delinquency in the 1950s." *Journal of Social History* 52 (2018): 153–79.

Drescher, Jack. "Out of *DSM*: Depathologizing Homosexuality." *Behavioral Sciences* 5 (2015): 565–75.

Duff, Raymond S., and August B. Hollingshead. *Sickness and Society*. New York: Harper and Row, 1968.

Dumont, Matthew P. *The Absurd Healer: A Personal Account of a Community Psychiatrist's Involvement with the City as Patient*. Foreword by Leonard J. Duhl. 1968; New York: Viking, 1971.

——. *Treating the Poor: A Personal Sojourn Through the Rise and Fall of Community Mental Health*. Belmont, MA: Dymphna, 1992.

Dumont, Matthew P., and Dora M. Dumont. "Deinstitutionalization in the United States and Italy: A Historical Survey." *International Journal of Mental Health* 37 (2008): 61–70.

Dunham, H. Warren. "Community Psychiatry: The Newest Therapeutic Bandwagon." *Archives of General Psychiatry* 12 (1965): 303–13.

——. "The Ecology of Functional Psychoses in Chicago." *American Sociological Review* 2 (1937): 467–79.

——. "The Field of Social Psychiatry." In *Mental Health and Mental Disorder: A Sociological Approach*, ed. Arnold M. Rose, 61–86. London: Routledge and Kegan Paul, 1956.

——. "Mental Disorders in Urban Areas: A Retrospective View." In *Community Surveys of Psychiatric Disorders*, ed. Myrna M. Weissman,

Jerome K. Myers, and Catherine E. Ross, 65–76. New Brunswick, NJ: Rutgers University Press, 1986.

——. "Social Psychiatry." *American Sociological Review* 13 (1948): 183–97.

——. "Social Structures and Mental Disorders: Competing Hypotheses of Explanation." *Milbank Memorial Fund Quarterly* 39 (1961): 259–311.

——. *Sociological Theory and Mental Disorder.* Detroit, MI: Wayne State University Press, 1959.

——. "Some Persistent Problems in the Epidemiology of Mental Orders." *AJP* 109 (1953): 567–75.

Dunst, Alexander. *Madness in Cold War America: Mad America.* London: Routledge, 2017.

Durkheim, Émile. *Le suicide. Étude de sociologie.* Paris: Ancienne Librairie Germer Bailière et Cte., 1897.

Dwyer, Ellen. "Psychiatry and Race During World War II." *Journal of the History of Medicine and Allied Sciences* 61 (2006): 117–43.

Dyck, Erika. *Facing Eugenics: Reproduction, Sterilization, and the Politics of Choice.* Toronto: University of Toronto Press, 2013.

——. *Psychedelic Psychiatry: LSD from Clinic to Campus.* Baltimore, MD: Johns Hopkins University Press, 2008.

Dyck, Erika, Lesley Baker, Lanny Beckman, Geertje Boschma, Chris Dooley, Kathleen Kendall, et al. "After the Asylum in Canada: Surviving Deinstitutionalisation and Revising History." In *Deinstitutionalisation and After: Post-War Psychiatry in the Western World*, ed. Despo Kritisotaki, Vicky Long, and Matthew Smith, 75–95. Basingstoke: Palgrave, 2016.

Eaton, J. S., and L. S. Goldstein. "Psychiatry in Crisis." *AJP* 134 (1977): 642–45.

Eaton, Joseph W., and Robert J. Weil. *Culture and Mental Disorders: A Comparative Study of the Hutterites and Other Populations.* Glencoe, IL: Free Press, 1955.

Eldridge, Seba. *Problems of Community Life: An Outline of Applied Sociology.* New York: Thomas Y. Crowell, 1915.

Eliot, Thomas D. "Interactions of Psychiatric and Social Theory Prior to 1940." In *Mental Health and Mental Disorder: A Sociological Approach*, ed. Arnold M. Rose, 18–41. London: Routledge and Kegan Paul, 1956.

Engel, Jonathan W. "Early Psychiatry at Yale: Milton C. Winternitz and the Founding of the Department of Psychiatry and Mental Hygiene." *Yale Journal of Biology and Medicine* 67 (1994): 33–47.

Etheridge, Elizabeth W. *The Butterfly Caste: A Social History of Pellagra in the South.* Westport, CT: Greenwood, 1972.

Everett, Barbara. *A Fragile Revolution: Consumers and Psychiatric Survivors Confront the Power of the Mental Health System.* Waterloo, ON: Wilfred Laurier University Press, 2000.

Falkai, Peter, Andrea Schmitt, and Nancy Andreason. "Forty Years of Structural Brain Imaging in Mental Disorder: Is It Clinically Useful or Not?" *Dialogues in Clinical Neuroscience* 20 (2018): 179–86.

Faris, Jack. "Robert E. Lee Faris, ASA Past President, 1907–1998." *Footnotes* 26 (1998): 8.

Faris, Robert E. L. *Chicago Sociology: 1920–1932.* Chicago: University of Chicago Press, 1967.

——. "Cultural Isolation and the Schizophrenic Personality." *AJS* 40 (1934): 155–64.

——. "Insanity Distribution by Local Areas." *Journal of the American Statistical Association* 27 (1932): 53–57.

——. "Reflections of Social Disorganization in the Behavior of a Schizophrenic Patient." *AJS* 50 (1944): 134–41.

——. "Reflections on the Ability Dimension in Human Society." *American Sociological Review* 26 (1961): 835–43.

——. "Sociological Factors in the Development of Talent and Genius." *Journal of Educational Sociology* 9 (1936): 538–44.

Faris, Robert E. L., and H. Warren Dunham. *Mental Disorders in Urban Areas: An Ecological Study of Schizophrenia and Other Psychoses.* Chicago: University of Chicago Press, 1939.

Feinstein, Adam. *A History of Autism: Conversations with the Pioneers.* Chichester: Wiley, 2010.

Felitti, Vincent J., Robert F. Anda, Dale Nordenberg, David F. Williamson, Alison M. Spitz, Valerie Edwards, Mary P. Koss, and James S. Marks. "Relationship of Childhood Abuse and Household Dysfunction to Many of the Leading Causes of Death in Adults." *American Journal of Preventive Medicine* 14 (1998): P245–58.

Felix, Robert H., and R. V. Bowers. "Mental Hygiene and Socio-Environmental Factors." *Milbank Memorial Fund Quarterly* 26 (1948): 125–47.

Fink, Paul J., and Stephen P. Weinstein. "Whatever Happened to Psychiatry? The Deprofessionalization of Community Mental Health Centers." *AJP* 136 (1979): 406–9.

Foley, Henry A., and Steven S. Sharfstein. *Madness and Government: Who Cares for the Mentally Ill?* Washington, DC: American Psychiatric Press, 1983.

Föllmer, Moritz. "The Sociology of Individuality and the History of Urban Society." *Urban History* 47 (2020): 311–26.

For the People's Health. "Untitled Article by Health Revolutionary Unity Movement from *For the People's Health.*" Reprinted in *Berkeley Tribe*, February 18–March 2, 1972.

Forget, Evelyn J. "New Questions, New Data, Old Interventions: The Health Effect of a Guaranteed Annual Income." *Preventive Medicine* 57 (2013): 925–28.

Forrester, John. "Introduction." In *Interpreting Dreams*, by Sigmund Freud, ii–l. 1899; London: Folio, 2015.

Foucault, Michel. *Folie et déraison. Histoire de la folie a l'âge classique.* Paris: Librarie Plon, 1965.

Frank, Lawrence K. "Society as Patient." *AJS* 42 (1936): 335–44.

Fraser, C. Gerald. "Community Takes Over Control of Bronx Mental Health Service." *New York Times*, March 6, 1969.

Frasquilho, Diana, Margarida Gaspar Matos, Ferdinand Salonna, Diogo Guerreiro, Cláudia C. Storti, Tânia Gaspar, and José M. Caldas-de-Almeida. "Mental Health Outcomes in Times of Economic Recession: A Systematic Literature Review." *BMC Public Health* 16 (2016): doi:10.1186/s12889-016-2720-y.

Frazier, E. Franklin. *The Negro Family in Chicago.* Chicago: University of Chicago Press, 1931.

Frederick, Calvin J., Peter Loewenberg, and Robert O. Pasnau. "In Memoriam: Frederick C. Redlich." University of California. https://senate.universityofcalifornia.edu/_files/inmemoriam/html/FrederickC.Redlich.htm.

Freedman, Daniel X. "Community Mental Health: Slogan and a History of the Mission." In *Controversy in Psychiatry*, ed. John Paul Brady and H. Keith H. Brodie, 1060–70. Philadelphia: W. B. Saunders, 1978.

Freud, Sigmund. *Drei Abhandlungen zur Sexualtheorie.* Leipzig: Franz Deuticke, 1905.

——. *Totem und Tabu.* Leipzig: Hugo Heller, 1913.

Fried, Marc. "Grieving for a Lost Home: The Psychological Costs of Relocation." In *Urban Renewal: The Record and the Controversy*, ed. James Q. Wilson, 359–79. Cambridge, MA: MIT Press, 1966.

Fritz, Jan M. "The History of Clinical Sociology." *Sociological Practice* 7 (1989): 72–95.

Frumkin, Robert M. "Occupation and Major Mental Disorder." In *Mental Health and Mental Disorder: A Sociological Approach*, ed. Arnold M. Rose, 136–60. London: Kegan Paul, 1956.

Gabriel, Joseph M. "Mass Producing the Individual: Mary C. Jarret, Elmer E. Southard, and the Industrial Origin of Psychiatric Social Work." *Bulletin of the History of Medicine* 79 (2005): 430–58.

Gans, Herbert J. *The Levittowners: Ways of Life and Politics in a New Suburban Community*. 1966; New York: Columbia University Press, 2017.

——. *The Urban Villagers: Group and Class in the Life of Italian-Americans*. New York: Free Press of Glencoe, 1962.

Garber, Robert S. "The Presidential Address: The Proper Business of Psychiatry." *AJP* 128 (1971): 1–11.

Gardner, John W. "No Easy Victories." *American Statistician* 22 (1968): 14–16.

Gavron, Sarah. *Rocks*. 2019. https://www.imdb.com/title/tt9067182/.

Gerard, D. L., and L. G. Houston. "Family Setting and the Social Ecology of Schizophrenia." *Psychiatric Quarterly* 27 (1953): 90–101.

Gill, Merton Max, Frederick C. Redlich, and Richard Newman. *The Initial Interview in Psychiatric Practice*. New York: International Universities Press, 1954.

Glasscote, Raymond M., James N. Sussex, Elaine Cumming, and Lauren H. Smith. *The Community Mental Health Center: An Interim Appraisal*. Washington, DC: APA, 1969.

Goffman, Erving. *Asylums: Essays on the Social Situation of Mental Patients and Other Patients*. New York: Anchor, 1961.

Goldberg, E. M., and S. L. Morrison. "Schizophrenia and Social Class." *British Journal of Psychiatry* 109 (1963): 785–802.

Goldston, Stephen E. "Primary Prevention: Historical Perspectives and a Blueprint for Action." *American Psychologist* 41 (1986): 453–60.

Gonzalez, Evelyn. *The Bronx*. New York: Columbia University Press, 2004.

Graham, Stephen. *The Gentle Art of Tramping*. New York: Appleton, 1926.

Grant, Julia. *Raising Baby by the Book: The Education of American Mothers*. New Haven, CT: Yale University Press, 1998.

de Greef, Guillaume. "Introduction to Sociology: IV." Trans. Eben Mumford. *AJS* 9 (1903): 69–104.

Griffin, J. D. M., S. R. Laycock, and W. Line. *Mental Hygiene: A Manual for Teachers.* New York: American Book Company, 1940.

Griffiths, N. E. S. *From Migrant to Acadian: A North American Border People, 1604–1755.* Montreal: McGill-Queen's University Press, 2005.

Grinker, Roy R. "Psychiatry Rides Off Madly in All Directions." *Archives of General Psychiatry* 10 (1964): 228–37.

Grinker, Roy R., and John P. Spiegel. *Men Under Stress.* Philadelphia: Blakiston, 1945.

——. *War Neuroses in North Africa: The Tunisian Campaign, January–May 1943.* New York: Josiah Macy Jr. Foundation, 1943.

Grob, Gerald N. "The Attack of Psychiatric Legitimacy in the 1960s: Rhetoric and Reality." *Journal of the History of the Human Sciences* 47 (2011): 398–416.

——. *From Asylum to Community: Mental Health Policy in Modern America.* Princeton, NJ: Princeton University Press, 1991.

——. *The Mad Among Us: A History of the Care of America's Mentally Ill.* New York: Free Press, 1994.

——. *Mental Illness in American Society, 1875–1940.* Princeton, NJ: Princeton University Press, 1983.

——. "Presidential Address: Psychiatry's Holy Grail: The Search for the Mechanisms of Mental Diseases." *Bulletin of the History of Medicine* 72 (1998): 189–219.

——. "Public Policy and Mental Illnesses: Jimmy Carter's Presidential Commission on Mental Health." *Millbank Memorial Quarterly* 83 (2005): 425–56.

——. *The State and the Mentally Ill: A History of the Worcester State Hospital in Massachusetts, 1830–1920.* Chapel Hill: University of North Carolina Press, 1966.

Group for the Advancement of Psychiatry. *The Social Responsibility of Psychiatry: A Statement of Orientation.* New York: GAP, 1950.

Groves, Ernest R. "Sociology and Psycho-Analytic Psychology: An Interpretation of the Freudian Hypothesis." *AJS* 23 (1917): 107–16.

Gruenberg, Ernest. "Review of *Mental Health in the Metropolis.*" *Millbank Memorial Fund Quarterly* 41 (1963): 79.

Haagh, Louise. *The Case for Universal Basic Income.* Cambridge: Polity, 2019.

Hale Jr., Nathan G. *The Rise and Crisis of Psychoanalysis in the United States: Freud and the Americans, 1917–1985.* Vol. 2. Oxford: Oxford University Press, 1995.

Halliwell, Martin. *Therapeutic Revolutions: Medicine, Psychiatry, and American Culture, 1945–1970.* New Brunswick, NJ: Rutgers University Press, 2013.

Hallowitz, Emanuel. "The Role of a Neighborhood Service Center in Community Mental Health." *American Journal of Orthopsychiatry* 28 (1968): 705–14.

Hallowitz, Emanuel, and Frank Riessman. "The Role of the Indigenous Nonprofessional in a Community Mental Health Neighborhood Service Center Program." *American Journal of Orthopsychiatry* 37 (1967): 766–78.

Halpern, Werner I. "The Community Mental Health Aide." *Mental Hygiene* 53 (1969): 78–83.

Harrington, Michael. *The Other America: Poverty in the United States.* New York: Simon and Schuster, 1962.

Harvey, Lee. *Myths of the Chicago School of Sociology.* Aldershot: Avebury, 1986.

Healey, Michael N. "Assembling Adjustment: Parergasia, Paper Technologies, and the Revision of Recovery." *Culture, Medicine, and Psychiatry* 45 (2021): 405–28.

Healy, David. *The Antidepressant Era.* Cambridge, MA: Harvard University Press, 1997.

——. *The Creation of Psychopharmacology.* Cambridge, MA: Harvard University Press, 2002.

Hedegaard, Holly, Sally C. Curtin, and Margaret Warner. "Suicide Rates in the United States Continue to Increase." *NCHS Data Brief* 309 (2018). https://www.cdc.gov/nchs/data/databriefs/db309.pdf.

Henckes, Nicolas. "Magic Bullet in the Head? Psychiatric Revolutions and Their Aftermath." In *Therapeutic Revolutions: Pharmaceuticals and Social Change in the Twentieth Century,* ed. Jeremy A. Greene, Flurin Condrau, and Elizabeth Siegel Watkins. Chicago: University of Chicago Press, 2016.

Henley, John. "Finnish Basic Income Pilot Improved Wellbeing, Study Finds." *Guardian,* May 7, 2020. https://www.theguardian.com/society

/2020/may/07/finnish-basic-income-pilot-improved-wellbeing-study
-finds-coronavirus.

Herman, Ellen. *Romance of American Psychology: Political Culture in the Age of Experts*. Berkeley: University of California Press, 1995.

Herzberg, David. *Happy Pills in America: From Miltown to Prozac*. Baltimore, MD: Johns Hopkins University Press, 2010.

———. *White Market Drugs: Big Pharma and the Hidden History of Addiction in America*. Chicago: University of Chicago Press, 2020.

Hinton, Elizabeth. *From the War on Poverty to the War on Crime: The Making of Mass Incarceration in America*. Cambridge, MA: Harvard University Press, 2016.

Hirshbein, Laura D. "Stella Chess and the History of American Child Psychiatry." *Social History of Medicine* 34 (2021): 788–807.

Hollingshead, August B. *Elmtown's Youth: The Impact of Social Class on Adolescents*. New York: John Wiley and Sons, 1949.

———. "Commentary on 'The Indiscriminate State of Social Class Measurement.'" *Social Forces* 49 (1971): 563–67.

———. "Four Factor Index of Social Status." *Yale Journal of Sociology* 8 (2011): 21–52.

Hollingshead, August B., and Frederick C. Redlich. *Social Class and Mental Illness*. New York: John Wiley and Sons, 1958.

Hollman, Suzanne. "White's Restraint and Progressive American Psychiatry at St. Elizabeth's Hospital: 1903–1937." PhD diss., University College London, 2020.

Horwitz, Allan V. *DSM: A History of Psychiatry's Bible*. Baltimore, MD: Johns Hopkins University Press, 2021.

Hughes, Charles C., Marc-Adelard Tremblay, Robert N. Rapoport, and Alexander H. Leighton. *People of Cove and Woodlot*. New York: Basic Books, 1960.

Hutchins, Robert M. "An Institute of Human Relations." *AJS* 35 (1929): 187–93.

Iverson, Noel. "Nels Anderson: A Profile." *Labour/Le Travail* 63 (2009): 181–205.

Jackson, Kenneth T. *Crabgrass Frontier: The Suburbanization of the United States*. New York: Oxford University Press, 1985.

Jackson, Mark. *The Age of Stress: Science and the Search for Stability*. Oxford: Oxford University Press, 2013.

———. *The Borderland of Imbecility: Medicine, Society, and the Fabrication of the Feeble Mind in Victorian and Edwardian Britain*. Manchester: Manchester University Press, 2000.

———. "Men and Women Under Stress: Neuropsychiatric Models of Resilience During and After the Second World War." In *Stress in Post-War Britain, 1945–1980*, ed. Mark Jackson, 111–29. London: Routledge, 2015.

Jacobs, Jane. *The Death and Life of Great American Cities*. New York: Random House, 1961.

Jaffe, A. J., and Ethel Shanas. "Economic Differentials in the Probability of Insanity." *AJS* 39 (1944): 534–39.

Jahoda, Marie. "Toward a Social Psychology of Mental Health." In *Symposium on the Healthy Personality*, ed. Milton J. E. Senn, 211–30. New York: Josiah Macy Jr. Foundation, 1950.

Jaye, Lola. "Why Race Matters When It Comes to Mental Health." BBC, August 12, 2020. https://www.bbc.com/future/article/20200804-black-lives-matter-protests-race-mental-health-therapy.

Jazbinsek, Dietmar. "The Metropolis and the Mental Life of Georg Simmel: On the History of an Antipathy." *Journal of Urban History* 30 (2003): 102–25.

Joint Commission on Mental Health of Children. *Crisis in Child Mental Health: Challenge for the 1970s*. New York: Harper and Row, 1970.

———. *Digest of Crisis in Child Mental Health: Challenge for the 1970s*. Washington, DC: JCMHC, 1969.

Joint Committee on Mental Illness and Health. *Action for Mental Health: Final Report of the Joint Commission on Mental Illness and Health*. New York: Basic Books, 1961.

Jones, Kathleen W. *Taming the Troublesome Child: American Families, Child Guidance, and the Limits of Psychiatric Authority*. Cambridge, MA: Harvard University Press, 1999.

Jones, Maxwell. *Social Psychiatry: In the Community, in Hospitals, and in Prisons*. Springfield, IL: Charles C. Thomas, 1962.

Junod, Henri A. *The Life of a South African Tribe*. Vol. 2: *The Psychic Life*. Neuchatel: Attinger-Frêres, 1913.

Kaplan, Seymour R., and Melv Roman. *The Organization and Delivery of Mental Health Services in the Ghetto*. New York: Praeger, 1973.

Kapp, Steven, K., ed. *Autistic Community and the Neurodiversity Movement: Stories from the Frontline*. Basingstoke: Palgrave, 2020.

Karno, Marvin, and Donald A. Schwartz. *Community Mental Health: Reflections and Explorations.* New York: John Wiley and Sons, 1974.

Kasanin, Jacob S. "Review of *Analysis of Parergasia.*" *American Journal of Orthopsychiatry* 9 (1939): 817–18.

Katz, Michael B. *The Undeserving Poor: America's Enduring Confrontation with Poverty.* 2nd ed. Oxford: Oxford University Press, 2013.

Kayipmaz, Selvi, Ishak San, Eren Usul, and Semih Korkut. "The Effect of Meteorological Variables on Suicide." *International Journal of Biometeorology* 64 (2020): 1593–98.

Kendall, Kathleen. "From Closed Ranks to Open Doors: Elaine and John Cumming's Mental Health Education Experiment in 1950s Saskatchewan." *Histoire Sociale/Social History* 44 (2011): 257–86.

Kennedy, John F. "Special Message to the Congress on Mental Illness and Mental Retardation." February 5, 1963. https://www.presidency.ucsb.edu /documents/special-message-the-congress-mental-illness-and-mental -retardation.

Kesey, Ken. *One Flew Over the Cuckoo's Nest.* New York: Viking, 1962.

Kingsbury, M., E. Sucha, N. J. Horton, H. Sampasa-Kanyinga, J. M. Murphy, S. E. Gilman, and I. Colman. "Lifetime Experience of Multiple Common Mental Disorders and 19-Year Mortality: Results from a Canadian Population-Based Cohort." *Epidemiology and Psychiatric Sciences* 29 (2019): e18.

Klein, Donald C., and Stephen E. Goldston. *Primary Prevention: An Idea Whose Time Has Come.* Rockville, MD: NIMH, 1976.

Kluckhohn, Clyde. "Review of *Culture, Psychiatry, and Human Values.*" *American Anthropologist* 59 (1957): 192–94.

Kluckhohn, Clyde, and Dorothea Leighton. *The Navajo.* Cambridge, MA: Harvard University Press, 1946.

Kohn, Melvin L. "Social Class and Schizophrenia: A Critical Review." In *Social Psychology and Mental Illness,* ed. Henry Weschler, Leonard Solomon, and Bernard M. Kramer, 113–28. New York: Holt, Rinehart, and Winston, 1970.

Kraut, Maurice H. "The Province of Social Psychiatry." *Journal of Abnormal and Social Psychology* 28 (1933): 155–59.

Kritsotaki, Despo. "From 'Social Aid' to "Social Psychiatry': Mental Health and Social Welfare in Post-War Greece (1950s–1960s)." *Humanities and*

Social Sciences Communications 4 (2018), https://www.nature.com/articles /s41599-018-0064-1.

Kritsotaki, Despo, Vicky Long, and Matthew Smith. *Deinstitutionalisation and After: Post-War Psychiatry in the Western World.* Basingstoke: Palgrave Macmillan, 2016.

——. *Preventing Mental Illness: Past, Present, and Future.* Basingstoke: Palgrave, 2018.

Kroeber, A. L. "Anthropology of Hawaii." *American Anthropologist* 23 (1921): 129–37.

——. "Totem and Taboo: An Ethnic Psychoanalysis." *American Anthropologist* 22 (1920): 48–55.

Krumer-Nevo, Michal, and Orly Benjamin. "Critical Poverty Knowledge: Contesting Othering and Social Distancing." *Current Sociology* 58 (2010): 693–714.

Kutchins, Herb, and Stuart A. Kirk. *Making Us Crazy: DSM: The Psychiatric Bible and the Creation of Mental Disorders.* New York: Free Press, 1997.

Kusmer, Kenneth L. *Down and Out, On the Road: The Homeless in American History.* Oxford: Oxford University Press, 2002.

Kutz, Lester R. *Evaluating Chicago Sociology.* Chicago: University of Chicago Press, 1984.

Lamb, S. D. *Pathologist of the Mind: Adolf Meyer and the Origins of American Psychiatry.* Baltimore, MD: Johns Hopkins University Press, 2014.

——. "Social Skills: Adolf Meyer's Revision of Clinical Skill for the New Psychiatry of the Twentieth Century." *Medical History* 59 (2015): 443–64.

Langner, Thomas S., and Stanley T. Michael. *Life Stress and Mental Health: The Midtown Manhattan Study.* New York: Free Press of Glencoe, 1963.

Lapouse, Rema, Mary A. Monk, and Milton Terrace. "The Drift Hypothesis and Socioeconomic Differentials in Schizophrenia." *American Journal of Public Health* 46 (1956): 978–86.

Leacock, Eleanor Burke. *The Culture of Poverty: A Critique.* New York: Simon and Schuster, 1991.

LeFrançois, Brenda A., Robert Menzies, and Geoffrey Reaume. *Mad Matters: A Critical Reader in Canadian Mad Studies.* Toronto: Canadian Scholars' Press, 2013.

Leighton, Alexander H. *Caring for Mentally Ill People: Psychological and Social Barriers in Historical Context*. Cambridge: Cambridge University Press, 1982.

——. *The Governing of Men: General Principles and Recommendations Based on Experience at a Japanese Relocation Camp*. Princeton, NJ: Princeton University Press, 1945.

——. *Human Relations in a Changing World: Observations on the Use of the Social Sciences*. New York: E. P. Dutton, 1949.

——. *My Name is Legion: Foundations for a Theory of Man in Relation to Culture*. New York: Basic Books, 1959.

——. "A Porcupine Throws Quills." *Journal of Mammalogy* 7 (1926): 61.

——. "Poverty and Social Change." *Scientific American* 212 (1965): 21–27.

——. "Review of *Culture, Psychiatry, and Human Values*." *Social Problems* 4 (1956): 181.

Leighton, Alexander H., and Dorothea C. Leighton. *The Navajo Door*. Cambridge, MA: Harvard University Press, 1944.

Leighton, Dorothea Cross, and Clyde Kluckhohn. *Children of the People: The Navajo Individual and His Development*. Cambridge, MA: Harvard University Press, 1948.

Leighton, Dorothea Cross, and John Adair. *People of the Middle Place: A Study of the Zuni Indians*. New Haven, CT: Human Relations Area Files Press, 1966.

Leighton, Dorothea C., John S. Harding, David B. Macklin, Allister M. Macmillan, and Alexander H. Leighton. *The Character of Danger: Psychiatric Symptoms in Selected Communities*. New York: Basic Books, 1963.

Levin, Aaron. "APA Members Speak Out During Vietnam War." *Psychiatric News*, January 12, 2016.

Levy, Ruth J. "Community Mental Health Services: Operation in San Jose." *California Medicine* 92 (1960): 345–47.

Lewis, Oscar. *Five Families: Mexican Case Studies in the Culture of Poverty*. New York: Basic Books, 1959.

Loach, Ken. *I, Daniel Blake*. 2016. https://www.imdb.com/title/tt5168192/.

Louis, Elan D. "The Neurological Study Unit: 'A Combined Attack on a Single Problem from Many Angles.'" *Canadian Bulletin of Medical History* 38 (2021): 233–52.

Lourie, Reginald. "The Joint Commission on Mental Health of Children." *AJP* 122 (1966): 1280–81.

Lu, Donna. "Universal Basic Income Seems to Improve Employment and Well-Being." *New Scientist*, May 6, 2020. https://www.newscientist.com /article/2242937-universal-basic-income-seems-to-improve-employ- ment-and-well-being/.

Lunbeck, Elizabeth. *The Americanization of Narcissism*. Cambridge, MA: Harvard University Press, 2014.

Macintyre, Anna, Daniel Ferris, Briana Gonçalves, and Neil Quinn. "What Has Economics Got to Do with It? The Impact of Socioeconomic Fac- tors on Mental Health and the Case for Collective Action." *Humanities and Social Sciences Communications* 4 (2018). https://www.nature.com /articles/s41599-018-0063-2.

MacKinnon, Lachlan. *Closing Sysco: Industrial Decline in Atlantic Canada's Steel City*. Toronto: University of Toronto Press, 2019.

Malzberg, Benjamin. "Migration and Mental Disease Among Negroes in New York State." *American Journal of Physical Anthropology* 21 (1936): 107–13.

March, Dana, and Gerald M. Oppenheimer. "Social Disorder and Diagnostic Order: The U.S. Mental Hygiene Movement, the Midtown Manhattan Study, and the Study of Psychiatric Epidemiology in the 20th Century." *International Journal of Epidemiology* 43 Supplement (2014): 129–142.

Markowitz, Gerald, and Daniel Rosner. *Children, Race, and Power: Kenneth and Mamie Clark's Northside Center*. Charlottesville: University of Vir- ginia Press, 1996.

May, Mark A. "A Retrospective View of the Institute of Human Relations at Yale." *Behavior Science Notes* 6 (1971): 141–72.

Mazlish, Bruce. *In Search of Richard Nixon: A Psychohistorical Inquiry*. New York: Basic Books, 1972.

McBee, Marian. "A Mental Hygiene Clinic in a High School: An Evalua- tion of Problems, Methods, and Results in the Cases of 328 Students." *Mental Hygiene* 19 (1935): 238–80.

McLoone, Juli. "Eleanor Leacock, Feminist Anthropologist." *Beyond the Reading Room*, March 30, 2015. https://apps.lib.umich.edu/blogs/beyond -reading-room/eleanor-burke-leacock-feminist-anthropologist.

McClure, Iain, and Matthew Smith. "Neurodevelopmental Disorders." In *An Introduction to Mental Health and Illness: Critical Perspectives*, ed. Mat Savelli, James Gillett, and Gavin Andrews, 179–203. Don Mills, ON: Oxford University Press, 2020.

McConnell, John W. *The Evolution of Social Classes*. Washington, DC: American Council on Public Affairs, 1942.

McCord, Clinton P. "Social Psychiatry—Its Significance as a Specialty." *AJP* 82 (1925): 233–40.

McGonigal, Kathryn, and John F. Galliher. *Mabel Agnes Elliott: Pioneering Feminist, Pacifist Sociologist*. Lanham, MD: Lexington, 2009.

McNally, Kiernan. *A Critical History of Schizophrenia*. Basingstoke: Palgrave, 2016.

Mead, Margaret. *Coming of Age in Samoa*. New York: William Morrow, 1928.

Mechanic, David. *Mental Health and Social Policy*. Englewood Cliffs, NJ: Prentice Hall, 1969.

Meehan, Marjorie C. "The Stirling County Study of Psychiatric Disorder and Sociocultural Environment." *JAMA* 187 (1964): 785.

Mendes, Gabriel N. *Under the Strain of Color: Harlem's Lafargue Clinic and the Promise of an Antiracist Psychiatry*. Ithaca, NY: Cornell University Press, 2015.

Menninger, William C. "Presidential Address." *AJP* 106 (1949): 2–12.

——. *Psychiatry in a Troubled World: Yesterday's War and Today's Challenge*. New York: Macmillan, 1948.

Menzies, Robert, Brenda A. LeFrançois, and Geoffrey Reaume. "Introducing Mad Studies." In *Mad Matters: A Critical Reader in Canadian Mad Studies*, ed. Brenda A. LeFrançois, Robert Menzies, and Geoffrey Reaume, 1–22. Toronto: Canadian Scholars' Press, 2013.

Metzl, Jonathan Michel. *The Protest Psychosis: How Schizophrenia Became a Black Disease*. Boston: Beacon, 2009.

——. *Prozac on the Couch: Prescribing Gender in the Era of Wonder Drugs*. Durham, NC: Duke University Press, 2003.

Meyer, Adolf. "Presidential Address." *AJP* 85 (1928): 1–31.

Miller, Rebecca, Allison N. Ponce, and Kenneth S. Thompson. "Deinstitutionalization and the Community Mental Health Center Movement (1954–1976)." In *Classics of Community Psychiatry: Fifty Years of Public Mental Health Outside the Hospital*, ed. Michael Rowe, Martha Lawless, Kenneth Thompson, and Larry Davidson, 9–20. Oxford: Oxford University Press, 2011.

Miller, S. M., and Elliott G. Mishler. "Social Class, Mental Illness, and American Society: An Expository Review." *Millbank Memorial Fund Quarterly* 37 (1959): 174–99.

Moncrieff, Joanna. *The Myth of the Chemical Cure: A Critique of Psychiatric Drug Treatment*. Basingstoke: Palgrave, 2008.

Morawski, J. G. "Organizing Knowledge and Behavior at Yale's Institute of Human Relations." *Isis* 77 (1986): 219–42.

Morel, Jules. "Prevention of Mental Diseases." Trans. C. R. Henderson. *AJS* 5 (1899): 72–97.

Morrison, Linda J. *Talking Back to Psychiatry: The Psychiatric Consumer/Survivor/Ex-Patient Movement*. New York: Routledge, 2005.

Moyer, Imogene L. "Ruth Shonle Cavan (1896–1993): A Tribute." *Women and Criminal Justice* 7 (1996): 3–22.

Moynihan, Daniel P. *The Negro Family: The Case for National Action*. Washington, DC: United States Department of Labor, 1965.

——. *The Politics of a Guaranteed Income: The Nixon Administration and the Family Assistance Plan*. New York: Vintage, 1973.

Mueller, John H. "Review of *Mental Disorders in Urban Areas*." *Journal of Abnormal and Social Psychology* 35 (1940): 593.

Mukherjee, Siddhartha. *The Emperor of All Maladies: A Biography of Cancer*. New York: Scribner, 2010.

Mullan, Fitzhugh. *White Coat, Clenched Fist: The Political Education of an American Physician*. 1976; Ann Arbor: University of Michigan Press, 2006.

Musto, David F. "Whatever Happened to Community Mental Health?" *Public Interest* 39 (1975): 53–79.

Myers, Jerome K., and Bertram H. Roberts. *Family and Class Dynamics in Mental Illness*. New York: John Riley and Sons, 1959.

Myers, Jerome K., and L. L. Bean. *A Decade Later: A Follow-up of Social Class and Mental Illness*. New York: John Wiley and Sons, 1968.

Myers, Jerome K., and Robert Straus. "A Sociological Profile of August B. Hollingshead." *Sociological Inquiry* 59 (1989): 1–6.

Myerson, Abraham. "Review of *Mental Disorders in Urban Areas*." *AJP* 96 (1940): 996–97.

Nelson, Alondra. "'Genuine Struggle and Care: An Interview with Cleo Silvers." *American Journal of Public Health* 106 (2016): 1744–48.

Nelson, Bryce. "Mental Illness Cited Among Many Homeless." *New York Times*, October 2, 1983.

Neugebauer, R., B. P. Dohrenwend, and B. S. Dohrenwend. "Formulation of Hypotheses About the True Prevalence of Functional Psychiatric

Disorders Among Adults in the United States." In *Mental Illness in the United States*, ed. B. P. Dohrenwend, 45–94. New York: Praeger, 1980.

Neve, Michael. "Commentary on the History of Social Psychiatry and Psychotherapy in Twentieth-Century Germany, Holland, and Great Britain." *Medical History* 48 (2004): 407–12.

Nixon, Richard. "Statement About the Community Mental Health Centers Amendments of 1970." March 16, 1970. American Presidency Project. https://www.presidency.ucsb.edu/documents/statement-about-the-community-mental-health-centers-amendments-1970.

Noll, Richard. *American Madness: The Rise and Fall of Dementia Praecox*. Cambridge, MA: Harvard University Press, 2011.

O'Brien, Robert C. *Mrs. Frisby and the Rats of NIMH*. New York: Athenaeum, 1971.

O'Connor, Alice. "The False Dawn of Poor-Law Reform: Nixon, Carter, and the Quest for a Guaranteed Income." *Journal of Policy History* 10 (1998): 99–129.

——. *Poverty Knowledge: Social Science, Social Policy, and the Poor in Twentieth-Century American History*. Princeton, NJ: Princeton University Press, 2001.

Office of the Surgeon General. *Mental Health: Culture, Race, and Ethnicity: A Supplement to Mental Health: A Report of the Surgeon General*. Rockville, MD: Substance Abuse and Mental Health Services Administration, 2001. https://www.ncbi.nlm.nih.gov/books/NBK44246/.

Oosterhuis, Harry. "Between Institutional Psychiatry and Mental Health Care: Social Psychiatry in the Netherlands, 1916–2000." *Medical History* 48 (2004): 413–28.

Opler, Marvin K. *Culture, Psychiatry, and Human Values: The Methods and Value of a Social Psychiatry*. Springfield, IL: Charles C. Thomas, 1956.

——. "International and Cultural Conflicts Affecting Mental Health: Violence, Suicide, and Withdrawal." *American Journal of Psychotherapy* 23 (1969): 608–20.

——. "Review of *An Anthropologist at Work: Writings of Ruth Benedict*." *American Anthropologist* 62 (1960): 889–91.

Osterweis, Rollin G. *Three Centuries of New Haven*. New Haven, CT: Yale University Press, 1953.

Ozarin, Lucy D. "Daniel Blain: Founder of This Journal." *Psychiatric Services* 50 (1999): 1563.

——. "Recent Community Mental Health Legislation: A Brief Review." *American Journal of Public Health* 52 (1962): 436–42.

Paddon, Natalie "'I may end up homeless again': Six Ontarians Talk About Their Life Before, After, and Once Again, Without Basic Income." *Toronto Star*, August 2, 2018.

Padgett, Deborah K. "There's No Place Like (a) Home: Ontological Security Among Persons with Serious Mental Illness in the United States." *Social Science and Medicine* 64 (1982): 1925–36.

Padwa, Howard, Marcia Meldrum, Jack R. Friedman, and Joel T. Braslow. "A Mental Health System in Recovery: The Era of Deinstitutionalisation in California." In *Deinstitutionalisation and After: Post-War Psychiatry in the Western World*, ed. Despo Kritsotaki, Vicky Long, and Matthew Smith, 241–65. Basingstoke: Palgrave, 2016.

Page, James D. "Review of *Mental Disorder in Urban Areas.*" *Journal of Educational Psychology* 30 (1939): 707.

Parezo, Nancy J. "Dorothea Cross Leighton: Anthropologist and Activist." In *Their Own Frontier: Women Intellectuals Re-Visioning the American West*, ed. Shirley A. Leckie and Nancy J. Parezo, 303–33. Lincoln: University of Nebraska Press, 2008.

Paris, Joel. *Overdiagnosis in Psychiatry: How Modern Psychiatry Lost Its Way While Creating a Diagnosis for Almost All of Life's Misfortunes.* 2nd ed. Oxford: Oxford University Press, 2020.

Park, Robert E. *The Principles of Human Behavior.* Chicago: Zalaz Corporation, 1915.

——. "Review of *Problems of Community Life: An Outline of Applied Sociology.*" *AJS* 21 (1915): 121.

Park, Robert E., and Ernest W. Burgess. *Introduction to the Science of Sociology.* Chicago: University of Chicago Press, 1921.

Park, Robert E., Ernest W. Burgess, Roderick Duncan Mackenzie, and Louis Wirth. *The City.* Chicago: University of Chicago Press, 1925.

Parker, Ben. "The Western Film and Psychoanalysis." *Film Quarterly* 68 (2014): 22–30.

Pasamanick, Benjamin. "Statement of the American Orthopsychiatric Association on the Joint Commission on Mental Health of Children." *American Journal of Orthopsychiatry* 38 (1968): 402–9.

Perry, Melissa J. "The Relationship Between Social Class and Mental Disorder." *Journal of Primary Prevention* 17 (1996): 18–30.

Plant, James S. "Review of *Mental Disorders in Urban Areas*." *AJS* 44 (1939): 1000–1001.

Pleck, Elizabeth. *Domestic Tyranny: The Making of Social Policy Against Family Violence from Colonial Times to the Present.* New York: Oxford University Press, 1987.

Pollan, Michael. *How to Change Your Mind: The New Science of Psychedelics.* New York: Penguin, 2018.

Pols, Hans. "Anomie in the Metropolis: The City in American Sociology and Psychiatry." *Osiris* 18 (2003): 194–211.

Pols, Hans, and Stephanie Oak. "War and Mental Health: The U.S. Psychiatric Response in the 20th Century." *American Journal of Public Health* 97 (2007): 2132–42.

Porter, Theodore M. *Genetics in the Madhouse: The Unknown History of Human Heredity.* Princeton, NJ: Princeton University Press, 2018.

Prescott, Heather Munro. *A Doctor of Their Own: The History of Adolescent Medicine.* Cambridge, MA: Harvard University Press, 1998.

President's Commission on Mental Health. *Report to the President.* Vol. 4: *Appendix.* Washington, DC: U.S. Government Printing Office, 1978.

Pressman, Jack D. *Last Resort: Psychosurgery and the Limits of Medicine.* Cambridge: Cambridge University Press, 1998.

Price, David H. *Threatening Anthropology: McCarthyism and the FBI's Surveillance of Activist Anthropologists.* Durham, NC: Duke University Press, 2004.

Prkachin, Yvan. "Two Solitudes: Wilder Penfield, Ewen Cameron, and the Search for a Better Lobotomy." *Canadian Bulletin of Medical History* 38 (2021): 253–84.

Quadagno, Jill. *The Color of Welfare: How Racism Undermined the War on Poverty.* Oxford: Oxford University Press, 1996.

Queen, Stuart A. "The Ecological Study of Mental Disorders." *American Sociological Review* 5 (1940): 201–9.

Ralph, Diana. *Work and Madness: The Rise of Community Psychiatry.* Montreal: Black Rose, 1983.

Ramsden, Edmund. "Rats, Stress, and the Built Environment." *History of the Human Sciences* 25 (2012): 123–47.

——. "The Urban Animal: Population Density and Social Pathology in Rodents and Humans." *Bulletin of the World Health Organization* 87 (2009): 82.

Ramsden, Edmund, and Matthew Smith. "Remembering the West End: Social Science, Mental Health, and the American Urban Environment, 1939–1968." *Urban History* 45 (2018): 128–49.

Rapley, Mark, Joanna Moncrieff, and Jacqui Dillon. *De-Medicalizing Misery: Psychiatry, Psychology, and the Human Condition.* Basingstoke: Palgrave, 2011.

Raushenbush, Winifred. *Robert E. Park: Biography of a Sociologist.* Durham, NC: Duke University Press, 1979.

Ray, Isaac. *Mental Hygiene.* Boston: Ticknor and Fields, 1863.

Raz, Mical. *What's Wrong with the Poor? Psychiatry, Race, and the War on Poverty.* Chapel Hill: University of North Carolina Press, 2013.

Reckless, Walter. *Vice in Chicago.* Chicago: University of Chicago Press, 1933.

Reckless, Walter, and Mapheus Smith. *Juvenile Delinquency.* New York: McGraw-Hill, 1932.

Redlich, Frederick C. *Hitler: Diagnosis of a Destructive Prophet.* New York: Oxford University Press, 1999.

Reinhold, Robert. "Drugs That Help Control the Unruly Child." *New York Times,* July 5, 1970.

Rennie, Thomas A. C. "Adolf Meyer (1866–1950)." *Psychosomatic Medicine* 12 (1950): 71–72.

——. "National Planning for Psychiatric Education." *Mental Hygiene* 30 (1946): 186–98.

——. "Psychiatric Social Work." *AJP* 102 (1946): 542–44.

——. "Social Psychiatry: A Definition." *International Journal of Social Psychiatry* 1 (1955): 5–13.

Rennie, Thomas A. C., and Luther E. Woodward. *Mental Health in Modern Society.* New York: Commonwealth Fund, 1948.

Richardson, Theresa R. *The Century of the Child: The Mental Hygiene Movement and Social Policy in the United States and Canada.* Albany: State University of New York Press, 1989.

Riessman, Frank. "Strategies and Suggestions for Training Nonprofessionals." *Community Mental Health Journal* 3 (1967): 103–10.

Riessman, Frank, Jerome Cohen, and Arthur Pearl. *Mental Health of the Poor.* New York: Free Press of Glencoe, 1964.

Richert, Lucas. *Break on Through: Radical Psychiatry and the American Counterculture.* Cambridge, MA: MIT Press, 2019.

——. *Strange Trips: Science, Culture, and the Regulation of Drugs.* Montreal: McGill-Queen's University Press, 2019.

Robcis, Camille. "Frantz Fanon, Institutional Psychotherapy, and the Decolonization of Psychiatry." *Journal of the History of Ideas* 81 (2020): 303–25.

Robertson, Stephen. *Crimes Against Children: Sexual Violence and Legal Culture in New York City, 1880–1960.* Chapel Hill: University of North Carolina Press, 2005.

Rogers, Naomi. *Dirt and Disease: Polio Before FDR.* New Brunswick, NJ: Rutgers University Press, 1992.

Rogler, Lloyd H., and August B. Hollingshead. *Trapped: Families and Schizophrenia.* New York: John Wiley and Sons, 1965.

Rolls, Edmund T. *Neuroculture: On the Implications of Brain Science.* Oxford: Oxford University Press, 2012.

Romano, Serena. *Moralising Poverty: The "Undeserving" Poor in the Public Gaze.* London: Routledge, 2017.

Rose, Nikolas, and Des Fitzgerald. *The Urban Brain: Mental Health in the Vital City.* Princeton, NJ: Princeton University Press, 2022.

Rosenau, Milton J. *Preventive Medicine and Hygiene.* New York: D. Appleton and Co., 1913.

Rosenberg, Charles E. *Explaining Epidemics and Other Studies in the History of Medicine.* Cambridge: Cambridge University Press, 1992.

——. "Pathologies of Progress: The Idea of Civilization at Risk." *Bulletin of the History of Medicine* 72 (1998): 714–30.

Rose, Nikolas, and Des Fitzgerald. *The Urban Brain: Mental Health in the Vital City.* Princeton, NJ: Princeton University Press, 2022.

Rothman, David J. *The Discovery of the Asylum: Social Order and Disorder in the New Republic.* Boston: Little, Brown, 1971.

Rudin, Edward, and Robert S. McInnes. "Community Mental Health Services Act: Five Years of Operation Under the California Law." *California Medicine* 99 (1963): 9–11.

Ruiz, Pedro. "The Fiscal Crisis in New York City: Effects on the Mental Health Care of Minority Populations." *AJP* 136 (1979): 93–96.

——. "A Seven-Year Evaluation of a Career-Escalation Training Program for Indigenous Nonprofessionals." *Hospital and Community Psychiatry* 27 (1976): 253–57.

Ryan, Joanna. *Class and Psychoanalysis: Landscapes of Inequality.* London: Routledge, 2017.

Sabshin, Melvin. "The Anti-Community Mental Health 'Movement.'" *AJP* 125 (1969): 1005–12.

——. "Melvin Sabshin Reflects on Two Decades at the Helm of the APA." *Psychiatric Services* 48 (1997): 1164–67.

Sacco, Lynn. *Unspeakable: Father-Daughter Incest in American History.* Baltimore, MD: Johns Hopkins University Press 2009.

Said, Edward. *Orientalism.* New York: Pantheon, 1978.

Salmon, Thomas W. "Mental Hygiene." In *Preventive Medicine and Hygiene*, ed. Milton Joseph Rosenau, 298–303. New York: D. Appleton and Co., 1913.

——. "Mental Hygiene." In *Preventive Medicine and Hygiene*, ed. Milton Joseph Rosenau, 298–303. New York: D. Appleton and Co., 1916.

Sapir, Edward. "The Contribution of Psychiatry to an Understanding of Behavior in Society." *AJS* 42 (1937): 862–70.

Satin, David G. *Community Mental Health, Erich Lindemann, and Social Conscience in American Psychiatry.* 3 vols. New York: Routledge, 2020.

——. "Erich Lindemann as Humanist, Scientist, and Change Agent." *American Journal of Community Psychology* 12 (1984): 519–27.

Savelli, Mat, and Sarah Marks. *Psychiatry in Communist Europe.* Basingstoke: Palgrave, 2015.

Schermerhorn, R. A. "Review of *Sociological Theory and Mental Disorder*." *Social Forces* 39 (1961): 364–65.

Schmiedebach, Heinz-Peter, and Stefan Priebe. "Social Psychiatry in Germany in the Twentieth Century: Ideas and Models." *Medical History* 48 (2004): 449–72.

Schroeder, Clarence W. "Mental Disorder in Cities." *AJS* 48 (1942): 40–47.

Schumacher, Henry C. "The Depression and Its Effect on the Mental Health of the Child." *American Journal of Public Health* 24 (1934): 367–71.

Schuster, David. *Neurasthenic Nation: America's Search for Health, Happiness, and Comfort, 1869–1920.* New Brunswick, NJ: Rutgers University Press, 2011.

Schwab, John J., and Mary E. Schwab. *Sociocultural Roots of Mental Illness: An Epidemiological Survey.* New York: Plenum, 1978.

Schwartz, Donald A. "Community Mental Health: An Underview." *Psychiatric Quarterly* 44 (1970): 333–58.

Schweinfurth, Georg. *The Heart of Africa.* Vol. 2. Trans. Ellen E. Frewer. New York: Harper and Brothers, 1874.

Scoville, Mildred C. "An Inquiry Into the Status of Psychiatric Social Work." *American Journal of Orthopsychiatry* 1 (1931): 145–51.

Scull, Andrew. *Decarceration: Community and the Deviant—a Radical View.* Englewood Cliffs, NJ: Prentice Hall, 1977.

——. *Madness in Civilization: A Cultural History of Insanity from the Bible to Freud, from the Madhouse to Modern Medicine.* London: Thames and Hudson, 2015.

——. "The Mental Health Sector and the Social Sciences in Post–World War II USA. Part 1: Total War and Its Aftermath." *History of Psychiatry* 22 (2010): 3–19.

——. "The Mental Health Sector and the Social Sciences in Post–World War II USA. Part 2: The Impact of Federal Research Funding and the Drugs Revolution." *History of Psychiatry* 22 (2011): 268–84.

Searcy, J. T. "An Epidemic of Acute Pellagra." *Transactions of the Medical Association of the State of Alabama*, April 1907, 387–97.

——. "The Sociology of Insanity." *Southern Bench and Bar Review* 1 (1913): 286–89.

Seger, Shane. "Memorial Fund Continues to Support Training in Social Psychiatry." Yale School of Medicine, February 14, 2013. https://medicine.yale.edu/news-article/4783/.

Segrest, Mab. *Administrations of Lunacy: Racism and the Haunting of American Psychiatry at the Milledgeville Asylum.* New York: New Press, 2020.

Selye, Hans. "The General Adaptation Syndrome and the Diseases of Adaptation." *Journal of Clinical Endocrinology* 6 (1946): 117–230.

Sharfstein, Steven S. "Whatever Happened to Community Mental Health?" *Psychiatric Services* 51 (2000): 616–20.

Shaw, Clifford R. *Brothers in Crime.* Chicago: University of Chicago Press, 1938.

——. *The Jack-Roller.* Chicago: University of Chicago Press, 1930.

——. *The Natural History of a Delinquent Career.* Chicago: University of Chicago Press, 1931.

Shaw, Robert, and Carol J. Eagle. "Programmed Failure: The Lincoln Hospital Story." *Community Mental Health Journal* 7 (1971): 255–63.

Shaw, Clifford, and Frederick Zorbaugh. *Delinquency Areas: A Study of the Geographic Distribution of School Truants, Juvenile Delinquents, and Adult Offenders in Chicago.* Chicago: University of Chicago Press, 1929.

Shorter, Edward. *A Historical Dictionary of Psychiatry*. Oxford: Oxford University Press, 2005.

——. *A History of Psychiatry: From the Era of the Asylum to the Age of Prozac*. New York: Wiley, 1997.

——. "History of Urban Mental Illness." In *Mental Health and Illness in the City*, ed. N. Okkels, C. Kristiansen, and P. Munk-Jorgensen, 17–24. Singapore: Springer, 2017.

——. *The Kennedy Family and the Story of Mental Retardation*. Philadelphia: Temple University Press, 2000.

Shorter, Edward, and David Healy. *Shock Therapy: A History of Electroconvulsive Therapy in Mental Illness*. New Brunswick, NJ: Rutgers University Press, 2007.

Silvers, Cleo, Leon Fink, and Brian Greenberg. *Upheaval in the Quiet Zone: A History of Hospital Workers' Union 1199*. Urbana: University of Illinois Press, 1989.

Simmel, Georg. "The Metropolis and Mental Life." In *The Urban Sociology Reader*, ed. Jan Lin and Christopher Mele, 23–31. London: Routledge, 2012.

Singh, Ilina. "Doing Their Jobs: Mothering with Ritalin in a Culture of Mother-Blame." *Social Science and Medicine* 59 (2004): 1193–205.

Singh, Jennifer. *Multiple Autisms: Spectrums of Advocacy and Genomic Science*. Minneapolis: University of Minnesota Press, 2016.

Sletcher, Michael. *New Haven: From Puritanism to the Age of Terrorism*. Charleston, SC: Arcadia, 2004.

Sloman, Peter. "Universal Basic Income in British Politics, 1918–2018: From a 'Vagabond's Wage' to a Global Debate." *Journal of Social Policy* 47 (2018): 625–42.

Smith, Matthew. *An Alternative History of Hyperactivity: Food Additives and the Feingold Diet*. New Brunswick, NJ: Rutgers University Press, 2011.

——. "A Fine Balance: Individualism, Society, and the Prevention of Mental Illness in the United States, 1945–1968." *Humanities and Social Sciences Communications* 2 (2016): 1–11.

——. *Hyperactive: The Controversial History of ADHD*. London: Reaktion, 2012.

——. "Mixing with Medics," *Social History of Medicine* 24 (2011): 142–50.

——. "Psychiatry Limited: Hyperactivity and the Evolution of American Psychiatry, 1957–1980." *Social History of Medicine* 21 (2008): 541–59.

Smith, Michael. "Capability and Adversity: Reframing the 'Causes of the Causes' for Mental Health." *Humanities and Social Sciences Communications* 4 (2008): https://www.nature.com/articles/s41599-018-0066-z.

Smuts, Alice. *Science in the Service of Children, 1893–1935.* New Haven, CT: Yale University Press, 2006.

Solenberger, Alice. *One Thousand Homeless Men: A Study of Original Records.* Philadelphia: Wm. F. Fell Co., 1911.

Southard, E. E. "Alienists and Psychiatrists: Notes on Divisions and Nomenclature of Mental Hygiene." *Mental Hygiene* 1 (1917): 567–71.

Speed, Ewen, Joanna Moncrieff, and Mark Rapley. *De-Medicalizing Misery II: Society, Politics, and the Mental Health Industry.* Basingstoke: Palgrave, 2017.

Spicer, Edward Holland, Katherine Luomala, Asael T. Hansen, and Marvin K. Opler. *Impounded People: Japanese Americans in the Relocation Centers.* Washington, DC: War Relocation Authority, 1946.

Spinney, Robert G. *City of Big Shoulders: A History of Chicago.* Dekalb: Northern Illinois Press, 2000.

Srole, Leo. "Urbanization and Mental Health: Some Reformulations." *American Scientist* 60 (1972): 576–83.

Srole, Leo, and Anita K. Fischer. *Mental Health in the Metropolis: The Midtown Manhattan Study.* Rev. and enlarged ed. New York: New York University Press, 1978.

Srole, Leo, and Ernest Joel Millman. *Personal History and Health: The Midtown Longitudinal Study, 1954–1974.* New Brunswick, NJ: Transaction, 1997.

Srole, Leo, Thomas S. Langner, Stanley T. Michael, Marvin K. Opler, and Thomas A. C. Rennie. *Mental Health in the Metropolis: The Midtown Manhattan Study.* New York: McGraw Hill, 1962.

Stahnisch, Frank. *A New Field in Mind: A History of Interdisciplinarity in the Early Brain Sciences.* Montreal: McGill-Queen's Press, 2020.

Staub, Michael. *Madness Is Civilization: When the Diagnosis Was Social, 1948–1980.* Chicago: University of Chicago Press, 2011.

"Staying Healthy to Age 85." *US News and World Report*, June 22, 1964.

Stead, William T. *If Christ Came to Chicago!* Chicago: Laird and Lee, 1894.

Stearns, A. W. "Review of *Mental Disorders in Urban Areas*." *Annals of the American Academy of Political and Social Science* 204 (1939): 223–24.

Stevens, H. C. "Review of *The Mental Health of the Schoolchild*." *AJS* 21 (1915): 272–74.

Stewart, John. *Child Guidance in Britain: The Dangerous Age of Childhood, 1918–1955*. London: Routledge, 2014.

Strauss, Anselm, Leonard Schatzman, Rue Bucher, Danuta Ehlrich, and Melvin Sabshin. *Psychiatric Ideologies and Institutions*. New York: Free Press of Glencoe, 1964.

Substance Abuse and Mental Health Services Administration. *Behavioral Health Spending and Use Accounts, 1986–2014*. Rockville, MD: Department of Health and Human Services, 2016. https://store.samhsa.gov/product/Behavioral-Health-Spending-and-Use-Accounts-1986-2014/SMA16-4975.

Summers, Martin. "Inner City Blues: African Americans, Psychiatry, and the Post-War 'Urban Crisis.'" Seminar paper given to the University of Strathclyde, March 16, 2021.

——. *Madness in the City of Magnificent Intentions: A History of Race and Mental Illness in the Nation's Capital*. Oxford: Oxford University Press, 2019.

Sutherland, E. H. "Review of *Delinquency Areas: A Study of the Geographic Distribution of School Truants, Juvenile Delinquents, and Adult Offenders in Chicago*." *AJS* 36 (1930): 139–40.

Sutherland, J. F. "Geographical Distribution of Lunacy in Scotland." *British Association for Advancement of Science* (1901): 742–43.

Sutter, Megan, and Paul B. Perrin. "Discrimination, Mental Health, and Suicidal Ideation in LGBTQ People of Color." *Journal of Counselling Psychology* 63 (2016): 98–105.

Suzuki, Peter T. "Anthropologists in the Wartime Camps for Japanese Americans: A Documentary Study." *Dialectical Anthropology* 6 (1981): 23–60.

Sweetser, William. *Mental Hygiene or an Examination of the Intellect and Passions Designed to Illustrate their Influence on Health and the Duration of Life*. New York: J & H. G. Langley, 1843.

Szasz, Thomas. *The Myth of Mental Illness: Foundations of a Theory of Personal Conduct*. New York: Hoeber-Harper, 1961.

Talbott, John A. *The Death of the Asylum: A Critical Study of State Hospital Management, Services, and Care.* New York: Grune and Stratton, 1978.

——. "Radical Psychiatry: An Examination of the Issues." *AJP* 131 (1974): 121–28.

Talbott, John, Anita M. Ross, Alan F. Skerrett, Marion D. Curry, Stuart I. Marcus, Helen Theodorou, and Barbara J. Smith. "The Paraprofessional Teaches the Professional." *AJP* 130 (1973): 805–8.

Telfer, Dariel. *The Caretakers.* New York: Simon and Schuster, 1959.

Terry, Gladys C., and Thomas A. C. Rennie. *Analysis of Parergasia.* New York: Nervous and Mental Disease Monographs, 1938.

Third World Newsreel. *Lincoln Hospital.* New York: Third World Newsreel, 1970, https://www.twn.org/catalog/pages/responsive/cpage.aspx?rec=905 &card=price.

Thomas, William I., and Florian Znaiecki. *The Polish Peasant in Europe and America.* New York: Knopf, 1927.

Thomson, Elnora E. "Case Work in the Field of Mental Hygiene." *Annals of the American Academy of Political and Social Science* 77 (1918): 71–78.

Thrasher, Frederick. *The Gang: A Study of 1,313 Gangs in Chicago.* Chicago: University of Chicago Press, 1927.

Tone, Andrea. *Age of Anxiety: A History of America's Turbulent Affair with Tranquilizers.* New York: Basic Books, 2009.

Tönnies, Ferdinand. "Community and Society." In *The Urban Sociology Reader,* ed. Jan Lin and Christophe Mele, 16–22. London: Routledge, 2012.

Torrey, E. Fuller. *American Psychosis: How the Federal Government Destroyed the Mental Illness Treatment System.* Oxford: Oxford University Press, 2013.

Torrey, Malcolm. *Basic Income: A History.* Cheltenham: Edward Elgar, 2021.

Tosti, Gustavo. "Suicide in the Light of Recent Studies." *AJS* 3 (1898): 464–78.

Tremblay, Marc-Adélard. "Alexander H. Leighton and Jane M. Murphy's Scientific Contributions in Psychiatric Epidemiology." Paper given to the Canadian Anthropology Society, Halifax, May 10, 2003.

——. "Alexander Hamilton Leighton, 17 July 1908–11 August 2007." *Proceedings of the American Philosophical Society* 153 (2009): 478–88.

Tsai, Jack, Thomas O'Toole, and Lisa K. Kearney. "Homelessness as a Public Mental Health and Social Problem: New Knowledge and Solutions." *Psychological Services* 14 (2017): 113–17.

Turner, Jonathan H. "The Mixed Legacy of the Chicago School of Sociology." *Sociological Perspectives* 31 (1988): 325–38.

United States Army Medical Department. *Neuropsychiatry in World War II*. Vol. 1. Washington, DC: Office of the Surgeon General, 1966.

United States Department of Housing and Urban Development. *The Applicability of Housing First Models to Homeless Persons with Serious Mental Illness*. Rockville, MD: U.S. Department of Housing and Urban Development, 2007. https://www.huduser.gov/portal/publications/hsgfirst.pdf.

VanAntwerp, Malin. "The Route to Primary Prevention." *Community Mental Health Journal* 7 (1971): 183–88.

Vayda, Andrea M., and Felice D. Perlmutter. "Primary Prevention in Community Mental Health Centers: A Survey of Current Activities." *Community Mental Health Journal* 13 (1977): 343–51.

Veroff, Joseph, Richard A. Kulka, and Elizabeth Douvan. *Mental Health in America: Patterns of Health-Seeking from 1957 to 1976*. New York: Basic Books, 1981.

Vidal, Fernando. "Brainhood, Anthropological Figure of Modernity." *History of the Human Sciences* 22 (2009): 5–36.

Vidal, Fernando, and Francesco Ortega. *Being Brains: Making the Cerebral Subject*. New York: Fordham University Press, 2017.

Wake, Naoko. "The Military, Psychiatry, and 'Unfit' Soldiers, 1939–1942." *Journal of the History of Medicine and Allied Sciences* 62 (2007): 461–94.

——. *Private Practices: Harry Stack Sullivan, the Science of Homosexuality, and American Liberalism*. New Brunswick, NJ: Rutgers University Press, 2011.

Wall, Oisín. *The British Anti-Psychiatrists: From Institutional Psychiatry to the Counter-Culture, 1960–1971*. London: Routledge, 2018.

Wang, Wen-Ji. "Neurasthenia, Psy Sciences and the 'Great Leap Forward' in Maoist China." *History of Psychiatry* 30 (2019): 443–56.

Washington, Robert. "Robert E. Park Reconsidered." *International Journal of Politics, Culture, and Society* 7 (1993): 97–107.

Waters, Ethan. *Crazy Like Us: The Globalization of the American Psyche*. New York: Simon and Schuster, 2010.

Webster, Anthony K., and Scott Rushforth. "Morris Edward Opler (1907–1996)." *American Anthropologist* 102 (2000): 328–29.

Weeks, John H. *Among the Primitive Bakongo*. London: Seeley, Service and Co., 1914.

Wengraf, Lee. "How Women Became Less Than Equal." *International Socialist Review* 63 (2008). https://isreview.org/issue/63/how-women-became-less-equal.

White, Morton, and Lucia White. *The Intellectuals Versus the City: From Thomas Jefferson to Frank Lloyd Wright*. Cambridge, MA: Harvard University Press, 1962.

White, William A. "Geographical Distribution of Insanity in the United States." *Journal of Nervous and Mental Disease* 30 (1903): 257–79.

Wilkinson, Richard, and Kate Pickett. *The Inner Level: How More Equal Societies Reduce Stress, Restore Sanity, and Improve Everyone's Well-Being*. London: Allen Lane, 2018.

——. *The Spirit Level: Why Equal Societies Almost Always Do Better*. London: Allen Lane, 2009.

Williams, David R., Jourdyn Lawrence, and Brigette Davis. "Racism and Health: Evidence and Needed Research." *Annual Review of Public Health* 40 (2019): 105–25.

Wilner, Daniel M., Roseabelle Price Walkley, Thomas C. Pinkerton, and Matthew Tayback. *The Housing Environment and Family Life: A Longitudinal Study of the Effects of Housing on Morbidity and Mental Health*. Baltimore, MD: Johns Hopkins University Press, 1962.

Wilson, Naomi, and Shari McDaid. "The Mental Health Effects of a Universal Basic Income: A Synthesis of the Evidence from Previous Pilots." *Social Science and Medicine* 287 (2021). https://doi.org/10.1016/j.socscimed.2021.114374.

Winston, Ellen. "The Alleged Lack of Mental Diseases Among Primitive Groups." *American Anthropologist* 36 (1934): 234–38.

——. "The Assumed Increase in Mental Disease." *AJS* 40 (1935): 427–39.

Wirth, Louis. "Clinical Sociology." *AJS* 37 (1931): 49–66.

——. *The Ghetto*. Chicago: University of Chicago Press, 1925.

——. "The Ghetto." *AJS* 33 (1927): 68–71.

——. "Urbanism as a Way of Life." *AJS* 44 (1938): 1–24.

Wolfe, Charles T. *Brain Theory: Essays in Critical Neurophilosophy*. Basingstoke: Palgrave, 2014.

Woodward, Luther E., and Thomas A. C. Rennie. *Jobs and the Man*. Springfield, IL: Charles C. Thomas, 1945.

Woolston, Howard B. "The Urban Habit of Mind." *AJS* 17 (1912): 602–14.

World Health Organization. *Mental Disorders*. Geneva: WHO, 2019. https://www.who.int/news-room/fact-sheets/detail/mental-disorders.

——. *Mental Health in the Workplace*. Geneva: WHO, 2019. https://www.who.int/mental_health/in_the_workplace/en/.

——. *Social Determinants of Mental Health*. Geneva: WHO, 2014.

Wu, Harry Yi-Jiu. *Mad by the Millions: Mental Disorders and the Early Years of the World Health Organization*. Cambridge, MA: MIT Press, 2021.

——. "World Citizenship and the Emergence of the Social Psychiatry Project of the World Health Organization, 1948–c.1965." *History of Psychiatry* 26 (2015): 166–81.

Wu, Yu-Chuan. "A Disorder of Qi: Breathing Exercise as a Cure for Neurasthenia in Japan, 1900–1945." *Journal of the History of Medicine and the Allied Sciences* 71 (2016): 322–44.

Wu, Zheng, and Christoph M. Schimmele. "Perceived Religious Discrimination and Mental Health." *Ethnicity and Health* 22 (2019): 1–18.

Young, Allan. *Harmony of Illusions: Inventing Post-Traumatic Stress Disorder*. Princeton, NJ: Princeton University Press, 1997.

Zhao, Chloe. *Nomadland*. 2020. https://www.imdb.com/title/tt9770150/.

Zorbaugh, Harvey W. *The Gold Coast and the Slum*. Chicago: University of Chicago Press, 1927.

ARCHIVES

Adolf Meyer Collection, Alan Mason Chesney Medical Archives of the Johns Hopkins Medical Institutions.

Alexander H. Leighton Papers, Alexander H. Leighton fonds, MS-13-86, Dalhousie University Archives, Halifax, Nova Scotia, Canada.

Commonwealth Fund Records, Rockefeller Archive Center.

Ernest W. Burgess Papers, Special Collections Research Center, University of Chicago Library.

Hanna Holborn Gray Special Collections Research Center, University of Chicago Library.

John B. Calhoun Papers, 1909–1996, National Library of Medicine.

Marvin Kaufmann Opler Papers, 1915–1979, Archives and Special Collections, Columbia University Health Sciences Library.

Melvin Sabshin Library and Archives, American Psychiatric Association: Daniel Blain (1898–1982).

Nelson A. Rockefeller Gubernatorial Records (FA372), Rockefeller Archive Center.

Social Science Research Council Records (FA021), Rockefeller Archive Center.

Leo Srole Papers, 1933–1993, SC-54, Hobart and William Smith Colleges Archives and Special Collections.

ORAL HISTORY INTERVIEWS

Barton, Michael. July 22, 2015. Interview with Matthew Smith. https:// pureportal.strath.ac.uk/en/datasets/social-psychiatry-oral-history -interviews.

Bell, Carl C. April 22, 2016. Interview with Matthew Smith. https:// pureportal.strath.ac.uk/en/datasets/social-psychiatry-oral-history -interviews.

Brickman, Harry. 1999. California Social Welfare Archives, USC Libraries.

Clark Jr., Gordon H. May 20, 2015. Interview with Linsey Robb. https:// pureportal.strath.ac.uk/en/datasets/social-psychiatry-oral-history -interviews.

Elpers, J. R. February 9, 2010. UCLA/Los Angeles County Department of Mental Health.

Faris, Jack. March 9, 2021. Interview with Matthew Smith. https://pureportal .strath.ac.uk/en/datasets/social-psychiatry-oral-history-interviews.

Goldston, Stephen. October 5, 1999. Office of NIH History and Stetten Museum.

Hicks, Beverly. March 10, 2015. Interview with Linsey Robb. https:// pureportal.strath.ac.uk/en/datasets/social-psychiatry-oral-history -interviews.

Leighton, Theodore. June 1, 2021. Interview with Matthew Smith. https:// pureportal.strath.ac.uk/en/datasets/social-psychiatry-oral-history -interviews.

Marin, Robert. August 8, 2016. Interview with Matthew Smith. https:// pureportal.strath.ac.uk/en/datasets/social-psychiatry-oral-history -interviews.

McQuistion, Hunter. August 9, 2016. Interview with Matthew Smith. https://pureportal.strath.ac.uk/en/datasets/social-psychiatry-oral -history-interviews.

Mechanic, David. February 9, 2015. Interview with Linsey Robb. https:// pureportal.strath.ac.uk/en/datasets/social-psychiatry-oral-history -interviews.

Opler, Lewis. November 16, 2015. Interview with Matthew Smith. https:// pureportal.strath.ac.uk/en/datasets/social-psychiatry-oral-history -interviews.

Primm, Annelle. June 5, 2015. Interview with Linsey Robb. https://pureportal .strath.ac.uk/en/datasets/social-psychiatry-oral-history-interviews.

Ralph, Diana. July 12, 2016. Interview with Matthew Smith. https:// pureportal.strath.ac.uk/en/datasets/social-psychiatry-oral-history -interviews.

Ranz, Jules. September 9, 2016. Interview with Matthew Smith. https:// pureportal.strath.ac.uk/en/datasets/social-psychiatry-oral-history -interviews.

Silvers, Cleo. Interview 2. March 12, 2007. Bronx African American History Project, BAAHP Digital Archive at Fordham, https://research .library.fordham.edu/baahp_oralhist/232/.

Sowers, Wes. April 26, 2016. Interview with Matthew Smith. https:// pureportal.strath.ac.uk/en/datasets/social-psychiatry-oral-history -interviews.

Srole, Ira. February 17, 2016. Interview with Matthew Smith. https:// pureportal.strath.ac.uk/en/datasets/social-psychiatry-oral-history -interviews.

Talbott, John. March 17, 2015. Interview with Linsey Robb. https://pureportal .strath.ac.uk/en/datasets/social-psychiatry-oral-history-interviews.

INDEX

Chicago Study, 13, 65–67, 71, 76,
79–104, 303n55
child guidance, 3, 13, 20, 22–37, 39,
50–51, 60–61, 76, 102, 292n49,
297n110. *See also* children; Joint
Commission on the Mental
Health of Children (JCMHC)
children, 173–74, 223, 264–65, 269,
295n89, 326–27n68, 327n88,
348n58; and psychoanalytic
theory, 28–31, 222, 292n49; and
socioeconomic conditions, 31–37
126, 149, 192, 232, 241, 243,
274–75. *See also* child guidance;
Joint Commission on the
Mental Health of Children
(JCMHC)
cities, 45, 66–68, 73–75, 173–74,
191–93, 300n10, 324n35, 325n46;
and mental health, 45, 84–92, 100,
151–60, 191–93, 322n14, 323n28
civilization, impact of, 51–52, 63,
83–84, 97
Clark, Gordon H., Jr., 147–48
class, 14, 73–76, 84, 173, 215–16,
313n43, 314n48; and mental
health, 84, 111–32, 166, 257,
314–15n57, 315n62, 315n65,
316n68. *See also* inequality
climate, 83–84, 304–5n70
clinical sociology, 50–51, 93,
297n109
Cody, John, 230
Collier, John, Jr., 207, 211–13,
215–16, 334n10, 338n54
Columbia University, 116–17, 175,
180, 205

combat shock, 21–22, 54–57, 245.
See also trauma
Commonwealth Fund, 25, 38–44,
58, 290n27, 291n35
community disintegration, 9,
153–54, 188, 193, 278, 314n48.
See also social disintegration
community mental health centers
(CMHCs), 2, 108, 132–50, 197–98,
221–36, 310n6, 341n102, 342n113;
financing of, 4–5, 108, 147–49,
233–34; preventive strategies of,
149, 198–201, 221–223, 227–36,
252–53, 320n131, 342–43n114;
problems facing, 6, 37, 127, 132,
145, 223–27, 230–31, 234–36,
342n112; staffing of, 108, 133–34,
146–49, 226, 247, 318n101,
340–41n95. *See also* Bristol
Mental Health Centre;
Community Mental Health
Center Act; indigenous
paraprofessionals; Lincoln
Hospital Mental Health
Services
Community Mental Health Act
(1963), 2, 15, 108–10, 192, 200,
233, 272
concentric zone theory, 50, 66,
73–76, 88
Cornell University, 18, 162–63, 165,
181–83, 186–87, 196, 208,
329–30n113, 331n137
COVID-19, 9–11, 16, 193, 268–69,
274
crime, 67–68, 79, 85, 134, 157, 159,
216–17, 239, 345n22

Printed and bound by CPI Group (UK) Ltd, Croydon, CR0 4YY

19/02/2024

08239082-0001